FREE Study Skills DVD Offer

Dear Customer,

Thank you for your purchase from Mometrix! We consider it an honor and privilege that you have purchased our product and want to ensure your satisfaction.

As a way of showing our appreciation and to help us better serve you, we have developed a Study Skills DVD that we would like to give you for <u>FREE</u>. **This DVD covers our "best practices" for studying for your exam, from using our study materials to preparing for the day of the test.**

All that we ask is that you email us your feedback that would describe your experience so far with our product. Good, bad or indifferent, we want to know what you think!

To get your **FREE Study Skills DVD**, email <u>freedvd@mometrix.com</u> with "FREE STUDY SKILLS DVD" in the subject line and the following information in the body of the email:

    a. The name of the product you purchased.

    b. Your product rating on a scale of 1-5, with 5 being the highest rating.

    c. Your feedback. It can be long, short, or anything in-between, just your impressions and experience so far with our product. Good feedback might include how our study material met your needs and will highlight features of the product that you found helpful.

    d. Your full name and shipping address where you would like us to send your free DVD.

If you have any questions or concerns, please don't hesitate to contact me directly.

Thanks again!

Sincerely,

Jay Willis
Vice President
<u>jay.willis@mometrix.com</u>
1-800-673-8175

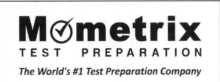

The World's #1 Test Preparation Company

NCLEX-RN SECRETS

Study Guide
Your Key to Exam Success

NCLEX Test Review for the
National Council Licensure Examination for Registered Nurses

Mometrix Test Preparation
NCLEX Exam Secrets Test Prep Team

Written and edited by the NCLEX Exam Secrets Test Prep Team

Printed in the United States of America

This paper meets the requirements of ANSI/NISO Z39.48-1992 (Permanence of Paper).

Mometrix offers volume discount pricing to institutions. For more information or a price quote, please contact our sales department at sales@mometrix.com or 888-248-1219.

NCLEX-RN was developed by the National Council of State Boards of Nursing (NCSBN), which was not involved in the production of, and does not endorse, this product.

ISBN 13: 978-1-5167-0576-4
ISBN 10: 1-5167-0576-9

Dear Future Exam Success Story:

Congratulations on your purchase of our study guide. Our goal in writing our study guide was to cover the content on the test, as well as provide insight into typical test taking mistakes and how to overcome them.

Standardized tests are a key component of being successful, which only increases the importance of doing well in the high-pressure high-stakes environment of test day. How well you do on this test will have a significant impact on your future, and we have the research and practical advice to help you execute on test day.

The product you're reading now is designed to exploit weaknesses in the test itself, and help you avoid the most common errors test takers frequently make.

How to use this study guide

We don't want to waste your time. Our study guide is fast-paced and fluff-free. We suggest going through it a number of times, as repetition is an important part of learning new information and concepts.

First, read through the study guide completely to get a feel for the content and organization. Read the general success strategies first, and then proceed to the content sections. Each tip has been carefully selected for its effectiveness.

Second, read through the study guide again, and take notes in the margins and highlight those sections where you may have a particular weakness.

Finally, bring the manual with you on test day and study it before the exam begins.

Your success is our success

We would be delighted to hear about your success. Send us an email and tell us your story. Thanks for your business and we wish you continued success.

Sincerely,

Mometrix Test Preparation Team

Need more help? Check out our flashcards at: http://MometrixFlashcards.com/NCLEX

TABLE OF CONTENTS

Top 20 Test Taking Tips

1. Carefully follow all the test registration procedures
2. Know the test directions, duration, topics, question types, how many questions
3. Setup a flexible study schedule at least 3-4 weeks before test day
4. Study during the time of day you are most alert, relaxed, and stress free
5. Maximize your learning style; visual learner use visual study aids, auditory learner use auditory study aids
6. Focus on your weakest knowledge base
7. Find a study partner to review with and help clarify questions
8. Practice, practice, practice
9. Get a good night's sleep; don't try to cram the night before the test
10. Eat a well balanced meal
11. Know the exact physical location of the testing site; drive the route to the site prior to test day
12. Bring a set of ear plugs; the testing center could be noisy
13. Wear comfortable, loose fitting, layered clothing to the testing center; prepare for it to be either cold or hot during the test
14. Bring at least 2 current forms of ID to the testing center
15. Arrive to the test early; be prepared to wait and be patient
16. Eliminate the obviously wrong answer choices, then guess the first remaining choice
17. Pace yourself; don't rush, but keep working and move on if you get stuck
18. Maintain a positive attitude even if the test is going poorly
19. Keep your first answer unless you are positive it is wrong
20. Check your work, don't make a careless mistake

Common Nursing Abbreviations

Before we start, here are some common nursing abbreviations that you may see used throughout this guide:

- ADL: activities of daily living.
- BMP: basic metabolic panel
- CBC: complete blood count
- CNS: central nervous system
- DOE: dyspnea on exertion
- ESRD: End-stage Renal Disease
- GI: gastrointestinal
- h: hours
- HA: headache
- MI: myocardial infarction (heart attack)
- MOA: mechanism of action
- N/V/D: nausea, vomiting, and diarrhea.
- ORIF: open reduction internal fixation
- RBC: red blood cell
- ROM: Range of Motion
- S&S: signs and symptoms
- SOB: shortness of breath
- URI: upper respiratory infection
- US: ultrasound
- UTI: urinary tract infection
- WBC: white blood cell

Safe and Effective Care Environment

Management of Care

This domain is defined by the NCSBN as "providing and directing nursing care that enhances the care delivery setting to protect clients and health care personnel." In simpler terms, management of care is the section of the NCLEX exam that will deal with the legal, ethical, and research/quality improvement aspects of nursing care.

Maslow's Hierarchy of Needs

Maslow's Hierarchy of Needs was created by Abraham Maslow as a way to discuss the prioritization of human needs. It is generally represented as a pyramid, with the most basic human needs at the bottom. The principle is that the needs must be met in order, working from bottom to top. Maslow is also used extensively in nursing as a way to prioritize patient needs. It is also a tenant that is basic to the NCLEX exam.
1. Physiological Needs: Basic needs such as air, water, food, sleep, and sex. When these are not satisfied, we may feel sickness, irritation, pain, discomfort, or lack of motivation.
2. Safety/Security Needs: Need for stability and consistency in a chaotic world. These needs are mostly psychological in nature.
3. Love/Belonging: Desire to belong to groups/be accepted: clubs, work groups, religious groups, family, gangs, etc.
4. Esteem Needs: Self-esteem from competence or mastery of a task, as well as recognition from others. Produces satisfaction.
5. Self-Actualization: Defined as "the desire to become more and more what one is, to become everything that one is capable of becoming" - maximize potential.

Theories of Bioethics

Bioethics is a type of philosophy used to guide ethical decisions in health care and nursing. There are several different theories followed by different practices that are used to establish their ethics. The more popular theories of bioethics include:
1. Utilitarianism: Utilitarianism believes that ethical conflicts can be resolved by considering the individuals affected by the decision being made. Utilitarianism works under the premise of doing the most good for the greatest number of people. The theory of utilitarianism believes that maximization of good consequences automatically minimizes bad consequences.
2. Deontology: Deontology functions on the premise of duty or obligation. The deontological theory states that nurses are bound to always do what is right for their patients.
3. Virtue: Virtue is a theory that involves making ethical decisions or taking ethical stands related to health care. The intent is the driving force behind virtue. With virtue, functioning under good intentions makes actions ethical.
4. Egoist: The egoist theory cites objectivism as the main focus. Egoist thought is centered on self-interest of the individual.

Standards of care and ANA's Code of Ethics

While there may be many different ethical belief systems, *standards of care* are the current practice standards used to ensure capable and skillful health care delivery by registered nurses. They are used as a measurement tool for providing quality care; an established norm as a mechanism of providing safe and appropriate care to the public. Nursing standards discuss what would be done in and under the same circumstance by any other nurse with the same level of expertise and knowledge. By following the established standards of care or practice standards, the nurse reduces his/her chances of being found negligent in a court of law. Additionally, nurses must abide by the Nurses' Code of Ethics. Since nursing involves providing for the care and well-being of the sick, injured, and those at risk, nurses must have a code of ethics to govern their behavior and practices. The ANA has developed a Code of Ethics to serve several purposes. First, the code discusses the essential obligations to be upheld by every person who works as a nurse. These obligations set standards of care that are universal to those throughout the nursing profession and include such concepts as patient autonomy and respect for human dignity. The ethics involved in the code are obligatory and are not optional practice. Finally, the code of ethics reflects the nurse's understanding of his/her role as a professional and the requirements of respect and compassion that he/she must give to patients.

In order to decide the most ethical decision, the nurse must use the following steps:
1. Identify the health problem.
2. Define the ethical issue.
3. Gather additional information.
4. Delineate the decision maker.
5. Examine ethical and moral principles.
6. Explore alternative options.
7. Implement decisions.
8. Evaluate and modify actions.

Ethical principles as they relate to Nurses

The nurse should know the ten ethical principles that are used to govern court decisions regarding nursing and medical malpractice:
1. Nurses have a legal duty to always act in the best interest of the individuals they care for.
2. Informed consent is required for testing, procedures, and treatment.
3. All patients should be informed of the consequences of refusing treatment. This should be documented in the permanent patient record.
4. All mentally sound adult patients have the right to refuse treatment, including life-saving treatment.
5. Patients have the right of advance directives to direct care when they are incapacitated.
6. The state may require documented evidence related to refusal of care.
7. Decisions that involve children should be made with the child's best interest in mind.
8. Adolescents are capable of making health care decisions.
9. Health care providers are legally bound to abide by privacy laws.
10. Privacy laws are only breached when the patient is endangering others with his or her decisions.

If the nurse adheres to these guidelines, he/she can avoid charges of negligence and malpractice:

- Negligence: an unintentional tort involving a breach of duty or failure (through an act or an omission) to meet a standard of care, causing patient harm.
- Malpractice: a type of professional liability based on negligence in which the health care professional is held accountable for breach of a duty of care involving special knowledge and skill.

The American Nurses Association also lists six additional ethical principles that a nurse must maintain to be excellent in his/her practice. These include:

1. Autonomy: Autonomy is the individual's self-determination. Autonomy involves personal respect for others. Nurses have an obligation to respect the rights of patients to make unforced, voluntary decisions.
2. Beneficence: Beneficence involves doing well and acting in the patient's best interest.
3. Nonmaleficence: Nonmaleficence is the principle of doing no harm.
4. Justice: The principle of justice involves fair treatment and equal care for all.
5. Veracity: Veracity involves telling the truth. Health care providers are required and responsible to be truthful when providing care to patients.
6. Fidelity: Fidelity is the health care provider's obligation to keep the promises they make to their patients, maintain patient confidentiality, and keep patient information private

Advocacy

Advocacy is an ethical concept that means the act or incidence of beseeching for, supporting, urging public argument, recommending publicity, and espousing actively things that promote the health and well-being of individuals and communities. In simpler terms, advocacy is speaking for those who cannot speak for themselves. Nurses are responsible for recognizing situations that might compromise patients' rights, and advocating for their patients. Nurse advocates accept responsibility to safeguard patient rights, and ensure quality of care for the patients they care for. The role of nurse advocate involves informing the patient of their own rights, providing information needed to make informed decisions, and supporting patient decisions and autonomy.

Nurses' Rights

The primary responsibility of the nurse is to provide safety in health care for all individuals. Nurses are responsible for knowing their scope of practice, the patient's rights, hospital policies and procedures, and standards of care and community norms. Because their primary objective is safety, nurses have the right to refuse assignments that jeopardize the client or the nurse, or place the client in immediate or serious danger. Nurses have the right to refuse to treat patients who are beyond their scope of practice. Nurses have the right to not be abused by clients, coworkers, or employers. Nurses have the right to ask for clarity with assignments, assess his or her personal abilities as they relate to clients and client situations, and assist in identifying options that will fulfill the assignment.

Patient rights

Patients have certain rights when it comes to their medical treatment. A patient's bill of rights is a document that clearly states what rights a patient should be entitled to. Typical rights include:

1. Right to health services provided with dignity and respect for personal and medical needs; this includes effective pain management and cultural consideration.
2. Right to privacy: HIPAA, protection of PHI
3. Right to self-determination: Patients have the right to make health care decisions, and to receive information regarding their care; this includes informed consent and education on procedures, prognosis, and course of treatment.
4. Right to information: Patients should know the cost of health care services being provided and receive notification of discharge or if services are to be terminated.
5. Right to refuse treatment: refuse certain medications, withdraw from a case management program, file a grievance if they feel they have been treated unfairly, and choose a community service agency of their choice.
6. Right to non-discrimination: All patients should receive appropriate care regardless of race, religion, ethnicity, or economic status. Patients cannot be denied care based on age, sexual orientation, marital status, disability, or ability to pay.

Informed consent

Informed consent is the patient's voluntary, autonomous authorization to undergo a medical or surgical procedure. Informed consent is intended to facilitate appropriate, knowledgeable decision making among clients who are hospitalized, receiving specialty services, and/or making any type of decision regarding health care. Informed consent must contain the following elements:

*   Detailed information on the prognosis
*   Potential benefits and risks of the treatment
*   Information related to alternative treatments
*   Risks of refusing treatment
*   Must be directed toward the education and cognitive level of the client; it is the physician's duty to ensure proper understanding of procedure (may require interpreter for language barrier)
*   Signed and acknowledged by both the physician and patient; also includes signature of witness

* Nursing role in informed consent is NOT to obtain informed consent. The physician is responsible for obtaining consent. The nurses' duty is to validate the patient's understanding/ that the patient did indeed give informed consent. The nurse usually witnesses informed consent and may educate the client on informed consent.

There are several prominent situations when obtaining informed consent may not be required. These include:

*   Emergent situations to save life or limb: often occurs in trauma patients, when the client is unconscious, and there is no legal representative of the client available to give consent.
*   Disclosures of therapeutic privilege: where these privileges would have adverse effects on the client/patient (seen in psychiatric patients mostly)

- Lack of decision-making capacity: patient does not have the capacity to make decisions; this includes patients with dementia, delirium, or other cognitive impairments. Informed consent should be obtained from HCPOA/closest family member.
- Waived Right: Patient may waive his/her right to informed consent.
- Court Order: Physician does not believe the decisions being made are in the best interest of the individual; this will involve a court order to treat against patient/client will.

Restraints

Restraints must be used in the following manner:
- Must have a physician's order to apply restraints in acute care and long-term care; renewed every 24 hours.
- Assess patient frequently (every hour with violent/every 2 hours with nonviolent restraints) – circulation, ROM, pain, nutrition and toileting needs.
- Can be delegated to non-licensed personnel; however, nurse is responsible for monitoring.
- More restrictive guidelines with youth/adolescents; the nurse must refer to the institution's individual policy regarding restraints.
  KEY: Use least restrictive device for least amount of time

Advance directives

An advance directive is a legal list of the wishes a patient may have regarding the level and type of health care they want provided in a specific situation. Typical advance directives include code status, (limited treatment measures and Do-Not-Resuscitate [DNR] orders), most often stating the client's wishes regarding end-of-life issues, including feeding decisions and life support. In order to be legally binding, the document is witnessed, and clearly states the wishes of the client regarding health care–related situations. The directive must be drawn up when the patient is of sound mind and mentally and emotionally capable of making these types of decisions. It is encouraged for every patient to have some sort of advance directive, reguardless of age or health. On admission to an acute care facility, every patient should be asked and offered the opportunity to exectute advance directives, and a copy placed on the patient's record. The nurse has some responsibilities when it comes to helping patients with advance directives. First, the nurse helps the patient obtain copies of advance directives, ensuring the forms are filled out correctly. The nurse educates the patient and their family about keeping papers in a safe place and submitting copies to the physician, attorney, and others who may need them. The nurse ensures that copies of all documents are in the chart, and that they are copied and sent if the patient is transferred.

Managed care verses Case management

Managed care is a broad term referring to an organized delivery of care or services. It involves a select panel of care providers who give out their services based on a prepayment arrangement between the provider and the managed care organization. For instance, a hospital may be the managed care organization, and the physicians who are part of the hospital staff are prepaid for the services they render to patients who seek care from that institution. HMOs and PPOs are examples of those types of managed care services. Case management is an individual patient care delivery system specific to the patient, their diagnosis, and their individual needs. The main difference is that managed care is the function of the health care reimbursement system, while case management is the structure used to provide individual patient care to affect expected treatments and outcomes.

Because it guides patient care, a good case management plan must include all of the disciplines that are relevant to the patient's care, and it must be clinically specific to the patient and their condition. The plan must be outcome based, with the best possible outcome for the patient as the goal. The plan must be flexible so that it can be adapted to each individual patient. It must also, however, be standardized for each disease process so that a health care team from any institution could easily implement the plan for a patient with the same condition. An example of this would be a case management plan with community-acquired pneumonia as the disease process. The standard treatments and expected outcomes would be listed in the plan, but the entire plan would be individualized for each patient with pneumonia based on factors such as age, response, health history, and compliance. The plan must also have a financial component emphasizing the most cost-effective way to care for the individual patient.

When developing a plan of care, the nurse should keep the patient's individual needs in mind. By specializing the care to the particular patient, the nurse will increase compliance and involvement by the patient. Ways to involve the patient with the plan of care include:
- Interviewing the patient personally, along with the family, allows the patient to have input and to verbalize what issues they feel are priority
- Asking the patient what goals they have and what they expect the outcomes of their care to be can help the nurse to be realistic about the plan of care.
- Including the family and all members of the health care team to ensure that information is complete and accurate
- Setting goals that the patient feels are achievable will help avoid discouragement
- Ensuring that all education provided within the plan of care is easily understood/appropriate to the educational level and cultural needs of the patient.

Referrals

Referrals occur when a physician consults another physician or specialty group to help care for the patient. Referrals are made in both the inpatient and outpatient settings, and may be from physician to physician (such as the attending physician consulting a pulmonologist for a COPD patient) or physician to a group (social services, dietary, etc.). Physicians should call their own referrals, but it is part of the nurses' responsibilities to ensure all referrals are properly called and charted, and that the patient is aware of them. It is the physician's responsibility to ensure all critical referrals are made, especially if the patient's problem is outside the area of their own expertise. However, the nurse should advocate for the patient if a problem arises, and respect the patient's wishes if the patient requests for a certain referral to be made. It is important that when referrals are made, that the entire care team is aware and communicates together to ensure optimal care for the patient.

Management & Delegation

Management is the process by which a person leads and directs the employees under them in order to achieve institutional and financial goals to improve patient care and outcomes. The nurse manager is usually the first level of authority after the charge nurse, and often has to balance clinical skills and expertise with the business aspects of management, such as creation of a budget and conflict resolution between employees. A good manager will set clear expectations for their employees and create attainable long and short-term goals for their floor. They will also focus on building an environment and culture of teamwork with their employees; often this may be accomplished using shared governance (when employees have a say in the policies and procedures of the floor/unit) or creating committees to help identify and improve different areas. One concept of management is types of power. They include

- Authority: power granted by position
- Reward: power inspired by the promise of retribution (bonuses, time-off, food, etc.).
- Expertise: power granted to an individual based on the belief that they are the expert in an area/ more skilled than most.
- Coercion: power gained by threatening physical/physiological/financial pain if expectations are not met.

While certainly not all nurses will become managers, all Registered Nurses (RNs) have the right to delegate certain tasks to appropriate personnel. Delegation involves handing over the responsibility to complete a task, while maintaining the responsibility for how the task is completed, including the final outcome. It is crucial for the nurse to follow the Five Rights of Delegation to prevent liability if the delegate does not perform the task in an acceptable manner. The Five Rights of Delegation are:

1. Right task – "Is this a task that can be delegated to another person/does it require a higher level of skill?"
2. Right circumstances*- "Is there a circumstance that makes this task require more critical thinking/assessment than normal?"
3. Right person – "Is this person trained and liscenced to complete this task and do I have confidence in them personally to complete it correctly?"
4. Right directions/communication – "Did I thoroughly explain what was expected and how to perform this task?"
5. Right supervision/evaluation – "Did I adequately supervise this task/ did I personally follow up to ensure the task was done correctly?"

The RN should never delegate a task that requires assessment or critical thinking. Example: Feeding a new stroke patient—normally fine to delegate feeding, but stroke patient requires assessment for dysphagia.

Confidentiality

Confidentiality is the principle of maintaining the privacy of client information by not giving out any information about the client without the express permission of the client or his/her health care power of attorney (HCPOA). This includes the client's medical status, location, treatments, and condition. Confidentiality respects the patient's autonomy and privacy, supports a trusting relationship between the nurse and the client, and assists in preventing harm to the client. It is also of legal concern, as the Health Insurance Portability and Accountability Act (HIPAA)* has made the sharing of private health information (PHI) a prosecutable offense.

However, there are some notable exceptions to patient confidentiality. These include:
- Information essential to patient's care to other health care providers (Principle of "Need-to-Know")
- Testifying in court
- Reporting communicable diseases
- Reporting child abuse, spouse abuse, and/or elder abuse
- Reporting suspicious or gunshot wounds
- Information relating to workers' compensation issues

HIPAA protects a patient's privacy and prevents that patient from being denied insurance because of a preexisting condition. It creates a standard for privacy protection among health care providers and institutions, and protects the patient's health record. It is based on the principle of "Need to Know," stating that those not directly involved in the patient's care do not have the right to access his/her health records or other PHI (private health information). It also allows the patient to know how and with whom their information will be shared. Employers are required by law to train employees to practice confidentiality and ensure they understand the consequences of a HIPAA breach.

> **Review Video:** Confidentiality
Visit mometrix.com/academy and enter Code: **765064**

Continuity of care

Continuity of care refers to the idea that every patient should receive the same quality of care throughout their healthcare experience, and that care should be congruous within itself. The nurse plays an integral part of maintaining continuity of care in several areas:
- Report: Nurses should use SBAR or some other standardized method for giving/receiving report. This prevents errors/omissions in the report, and ensures that the patient gets the same care throughout the different changes of shift.
- Terminology: The use of abbreviations should be limited, and only used if they are nationally-approved. Medical jargon should be avoided when speaking with patients to avoid miscommunication.
- Safe Procedures: There should ALWAYS be a "time-out" before surgical or invasive procedures to ensure consent is signed, and that it is the right patient/procedure/body-part, etc. It should also be determined before major or life-altering procedures that the patient will have the resources at home needed for a safe and full recovery; this may mean that the nurse will assist in setting up home-healthcare services or a short-term stay in a rehabilitation center.
- Follow-up: Continuity of care continues after hospitalization as the patient transfers into the community. Every patient should have a follow-up visit scheduled before leaving the facility, and the nurse should ensure they have the time and transport necessary to get there. The patient should also have access to the contact information of the physicians on their care team, and leave with written post-discharge instructions.

Discharge planning

Discharge planning begins as soon as a patient is admitted to hospital. With hospital stays becoming increasingly shorter, the nurse needs to help the patient prepare for discharge as soon as possible to ensure a safe transition into the community. This could include medication management, home safety evaluations, and scheduling/transport to follow-up appointments. It is critical for the nurse to work closely with the case management team, as many different disciplines often need to be consulted, such as physical therapy, social services, etc. The nurse will need to act as a liaison between the patient and different members of the health care team, to ensure a safe and timely discharge.

Correct Nursing Documentation & Error Prevention

Documentation is an essential component of nursing to support communication between caregivers, prevent errors and adverse outcomes, and maintain a record of work should nursing care or judgment come into question. The following are components of correct nursing documentation:
- Detailed and Factual: avoiding opinion or blame; only observations, not diagnosis. Example "Patient speaking with raised voice, asking to speak to manager," not "Patient is angry at staff, being belligerent; probably due to negligence by night shift staff."
- Thorough: Should include all actions that were performed for the patient's plan of care, communication/instructions from physicians, educational information given to the patient and family: "If it's not documented, it's not done!"
- Mistakes: correct mistakes with a single line through the error and mark with initials; NEVER use Wite-Out or scribble out the mistake.
- Timely: Chart in real time whenever possible. Charting that is performed late should be noted within documentation that it is a late entry, to avoid questions about time lapses.

Telephone and direct verbal orders both pose a risk of misinterpretation and error because they rely on the nurse correctly understanding and remembering the orders, especially if there are multiple orders. According to the National Patient Safety Goals, telephone and verbal orders should be written in their entirety and read back and confirmed before the orders are carried out. If the ordering physician is present, the physician should write the orders rather than giving verbal orders. The SBAR technique is used to hand-off a patient from one caregiver to another to provide a systematic method so that important information is conveyed:
- (S) Situation: Overview of current situation and important issues.
- (B) Background: Important history and issues leading to current situation.
- (A) Assessment: Summary of important facts and condition.
- (R) Recommendation: Actions needed.

Data Management & Evidence-Based Practice (EBP)

Data management is a crucial tool to help improve patient outcomes. To effectively use this tool, the interdisciplinary team would meet on a regular basis and utilize the following steps:
1. Discuss the goals/expectations for new plan of care
2. Determine method and criteria for data collection
3. Collect the data
4. Analyze the data and begin evaluating the information
5. Report all of the data, the analysis, and the evaluation

6. Begin documenting the care plan for any patient with the disease
7. Develop expected outcomes and needed interventions
8. Develop the treatment plan
9. Implement the new treatment plan
10. Evaluate effectiveness of new treatment plan; revise as needed.

Two common areas where data management and evidence-based practice are seen in the acute care settings are reducing CLABSI's (central-line-associated blood stream infections) and CAUTI's (catheter-associated urinary tract infections). The following are strategies developed using EBP to reduce the risk of these infections:

Strategies for reducing CLABSI's:
- Site selection away from the internal jugular or femoral veins, using PICC if possible.
- Tunneled catheter or ports used if possible because of lower infection rates than non-tunneled catheters.
- TPN catheters used only for TPN and not other procedures.
- Experienced trained staff to insert intravascular devices.
- Dressings should be transparent, and the site examined frequently by palpation. Change dressings at least weekly.
- Using maximum aseptic technique for insertion.
- Rotation of catheter sites every 72-96 hours (for adults) for short peripheral venous catheters but only as needed for others.
- Avoid antibiotic ointments at insertion site because of danger of fungal infections or resistance.

Strategies for reducing CAUTI's include:
- Using aseptic technique for both straight and indwelling catheter insertion.
- Limiting catheter use by establishing protocols for use, duration, and removal, training staff, issuing reminders to physicians, using straight catheterizations rather than indwelling, using ultrasound to scan the bladder, and using condom catheters.
- Utilizing closed-drainage systems for indwelling catheters.
- Avoiding irrigation unless required for diagnosis or treatment.
- Using sampling port for specimens rather than disconnecting catheter and tubing.
- Maintaining proper urinary flow by proper positioning, securing of tubing and drainage bag, and keeping drainage bag below the level of the bladder.
- Changing catheters only when medically needed.
- Cleansing external meatal area gently each day, manipulating the catheter as little as possible.
- Avoid placing catheterized patients adjacent to those infected or colonized with antibiotic-resistant bacteria to reduce cross-contamination.

When discussing healthcare associated infections (HAI's), it is important to mention *Pseudomonas aeruginosa*. *Pseudomonas aeruginosa* is an opportunistic pathogen, exploiting breaks in host defenses to initiate urinary tract infections, respiratory system infections, dermatitis, soft tissue infections, bacteremia, bone and joint infections, gastrointestinal infections, and a wide variety of nosocomial infections. Particularly active in patients with cancer, cystic fibrosis, severe burns, or immunosuppressed AIDS, this disease has a fatality rate of 50% in these patients. Accounting for 10% of all hospital-acquired infections, *Pseudomonas aeruginosa* is the fourth most commonly isolated nosocomial pathogen. Only the antibiotic drug classes of fluoroquinolones, gentamicin, and imipenem are effective against it, and even these drugs are not effective against all strains. In wounds, it is infamous for the blue-green colored discharge it creates. The futility of treating *Pseudomonas* infections with antibiotics is most dramatically illustrated in cystic fibrosis patients, virtually all of whom eventually become infected with a strain so resistant that it cannot be treated, and death is the general outcome. Treatment includes:

- Intense antibiotic therapy
- Supportive treatment.

Prevention includes:

- Clean mop water and other solutions
- Wash hands, disinfect common areas.

Safety and Infection Control

This domain is defined by the NCSBN as "protecting clients and health care personnel from health and environmental hazards." This section contains information regarding safety measures and standards set in place by healthcare institutions that keep patients and clients safe, as well as prevent the spread of disease.

Nosocomial Infections

Types of nosocomial infections are as follows:

- Exogenous infections: Caused by microorganisms that are not found in normal flora (e.g., Aspergillus, Salmonella).
- Endogenous infections: Microorganism overgrowth causes a different area of the body to become infected (e.g., enterococci (GI) to wound site or E. coli (GI) to urinary tract via Foley catheter).
- Iatrogenic infections: Infections that are caused by procedures (e.g., UTI after Foley insertion or bacteremia after IV insertion).

Infection Control Strategies

The following are some common infection control strategies used by health care workers:

- Transmission-based precautions are appropriate for some patients, especially those who are immunocompromised.
- Handwashing and aseptic techniques are especially important for person-to-person transmission.
- Central venous line precautions include using antimicrobial/antiseptic-coated catheters, using clear dressings that do not obscure site; assess for signs of infection.
- Cleaning equipment used for multiple patients in between uses.
- Temperature monitoring, full body assessments, and questionnaires as appropriate will help identify infections early.
- Post-discharge questionnaires or telephone surveys of patients and physicians can identify potential problems after discharge.
- Preoperative shaving should be replaced with clipping and depilatories, or done immediately prior to procedures.
- Glucose/blood sugar control increases resistance to infection.

- Teach medication compliance: must take all antibiotics exactly as prescribed to decrease antibiotic resistance.
- Protect immunocompromised patients: no fresh flowers/fruit, wear mask, no sick visitors, dedicated equipment.

Surgical terms

The following are terms related to surgery:
- Emergency: Must be done immediately to save the patient's life (e.g., appendectomy, repair of traumatic amputation, internal bleeding).
- Elective: Patient's choice, not always necessary, and palliative in nature (e.g., bunionectomy, hernia repair, plastic surgery).
- Diagnostic: surgical exploration (e.g., laparoscopic, biopsy).
- Ablative: excision or removal of diseased body part (e.g., amputation, appendectomy, debridement of necrotic tissue, cholecystectomy, and colostomy).
- Palliative: relieves or reduces symptoms, pain, will not cure (e.g., colostomy, debridement).
- Reconstructive: restores function or appearance of tissue (e.g., scar revision, ORIF).
- Transplant: replaces failing organs (e.g., kidney, heart, lung, liver, and cornea).
- Constructive: restores function lost or reduced from congenital deformities (e.g., cleft palate and lip, atrial septal defect repair).
- Cosmetic/plastic: improves appearance of client (e.g., facelift, rhinoplasty, and blepharoplasty).

Surgical Wound Infections

Surgical wound infections typically occur on approximately the fifth postoperative day. There may be initial symptoms present during the first 36 to 48 hours following a surgical procedure. Causative agents of surgical wound infections include, but are not limited to, *Staphylococcus aureus*, *Escherichia coli*, *Pseudomonas aeruginosa*, *Proteus vulgaris*, and *Enterobacter aerogenes*. Signs and symptoms include increased temperature, pulse, respirations, and blood pressure; reddened wound; purulent/foul-smelling discharge; swelling; and dehiscence (opening of the wound). Diagnosis is based on culture of wound, physical exam, and blood work (WBCs). Treatment includes:
- Medications: antibiotics (based on culture results), Tylenol
- Monitor for systemic effects.
- Apply and change dressings as ordered
- Wound Assessment: **OREEDA**: **O**dor, **R**edness, **E**dema, **E**cchymosis, **D**rainage, **A**pproximation.
- Drainage Amount: **C-COAL**: **C**olor, **C**onsistency, **O**dor, **A**mount, **L**ocation.

Surgical Asepsis

The principles of surgical asepsis are similar to those used for basic infection control, but stricter as open surgical wounds are at a high risk for infections. The principles are as follows:
1. A sterile object remains sterile only when touched by another sterile object.
2. Only sterile objects may be placed on a sterile field.

3. A sterile object or field out of the range of vision or an object held below a person's waist is contaminated.
4. A sterile object or field becomes contaminated by prolonged exposure to air.
5. When a sterile surface comes in contact with a wet, contaminated surface, the sterile object or field becomes contaminated by capillary action.
6. Fluid flows in the direction of gravity – clean from clean-to-dirty, top-to-bottom.
7. The edges of a sterile field or container are considered to be contaminated about 1 inch from the outer edge.
8. When opening sterile supplies, avoid crossing over the sterile object or sterile field.

Strategies for preventing and controlling transmission of infection in operating rooms include:
- Preoperative surgical hand scrubs for 3-5 minutes and aseptic techniques at all times
- Positive-pressure ventilation with respect to corridors and adjacent areas
- ≥ 15 air exchanges per hour (ACH) with at least 3 fresh air
- Filtering of all recirculated and fresh air though filters with 90% efficiency.
- Horizontal laminar airflow or introduction of air at ceiling and exhaust near the floor level
- Operating room closed except to allow passage of essential equipment and staff
- Clean visible soiling with approved disinfectants between patients
- Wet vacuum operating room at end of each day
- Sterilize surgical equipment and avoid use of flash sterilization.
- Perform environmental sampling of surfaces or air as part of epidemiological investigation.
- Establish protocols for patients with airborne precautions, such as tuberculosis.

Handwashing Procedure

Handwashing is the number one way to prevent disease, if done properly. The proper technique for both is as follows:
- Soap and water:
  - Performed when hands are visibly soiled, beginning/end of shift, after using the restroom, or any other time as needed.
  - Handwashing is done under running water with soap.
  - Hands must be lathered thoroughly and scrubbed for a full 30 seconds, covering all areas of the hands and wrists with soap, and then rinsed.
  - The faucet should be turned off by using the elbow or upper forearm or holding a piece of paper towel as a barrier.
  - Hands should be dried using disposable, clean towels. Keep hands above elbows so water runs in one direction (clean to dirty).
- Alcohol-based scrub:
  - Performed when entering/exiting rooms, taking off gloves, patient contact, etc.
  - All hand surfaces should be thoroughly coated with the alcohol rub, including between the fingers, the wrists, and under the nails
  - Hands rubbed together until the solution evaporates. Hands should not be rinsed.

Surgical handwashing aims to remove and kill transient flora and decrease resident flora to reduce the risk of wound contamination should surgical gloves undergo damage. Agents are the same as those used for hygienic hand washes, the primary difference being that more time is spent in scrubbing, an extra 2-3 minutes, and it includes both wrists and forearms. Sterile disposable or nailbrushes sterilized in an autoclave may be used to clean the fingernails only, but not to scrub the hands. A brush should only be used for the first scrub of the day.   After handwashing with soap and water, a hand rub with an alcohol base formulation (70%) should be used if possible. This enhances the destruction or inhibition of resident skin flora. If an alcohol preparation is used, two applications of 5 mL each is suggested, both rubbed to dryness. Sterile towels should be used to dry the hands thoroughly after washing and before alcohol is applied.

PPE

Personal Protective Equipment (PPE) are devices and wearable items such as surgical gowns, gloves, masks and respirators that act as barriers between the infectious material and the health care provider. The use of PPE alone does not fully protect against acquiring an infection. Handwashing, isolation of patients, and care in coughing or sneezing are also important to minimize risk of infection, and protective clothing should be changed whenever torn or ripped.
- Gloves: worn before touching mucous membranes/nonintact skin, or other potentially infectious substances. Must be removed promptly after use without touching outside; donned last after all other PPE; removed first.
- Goggles/Faceshield: non-vented, worn when there is a risk of splashing/risk to face or eyes.
- Gowns: moisture resistant, worn when there is risk of contamination on clothes from blood/body fluids. Put on first.
- Mask: protect patient from droplets during sterile procedure, but also protect nurse as well. For airborne precautions, a special mask called a N95 respirator should be specially fitted to the nurse and used. Put on after gown.

PPE is listed above in the order in which it should be removed.

Standard/Universal precautions

Standard/ universal precautions are used with all patients to prevent the spread of pathogens. They apply to blood; all body fluids, secretions, and excretions (except sweat), regardless of whether or not they contain visible blood; non-intact skin; and mucous membranes.
- Proper handwashing should be utilized at all times.
- Wear gloves when contact is possible with any body fluids/blood.
- Never recap needles, and immediately place used needles in the closest puncture-resistant container, which should be removed for disposal when about 3/4 full. Never point a needle toward any part of the body or manipulate it using both hands.
- Should mouth-to-mouth resuscitation become necessary, it must be performed only with the use of mouthpieces, resuscitation bags, or other ventilation devices.
- A patient who contaminates the environment and will not (or cannot) follow rules of proper hygiene and environmental control must be placed in a private room.

Contact precautions

Contact precautions reduce the risk of transmitting microorganisms by skin-to-skin contact, whether direct, as occurs when health care personnel perform activities requiring physical contact with a patient, or indirect via contaminated intermediate objects in the patient's environment.

- Patient placement -- a private room when possible
- Gloves and handwashing -- wear gloves, dispose of them and wash hands before leaving a patient's room
- Gowns -- wear when there is any chance of clothing touching a contaminated person or surface
- Patient transport -- limit movement and use barriers to prevent spread of infection
- Patient care equipment – avoid, if possible, using a piece of durable equipment with more than one patient

Droplet precautions

Droplet precautions are used for diseases transmitted through large droplets (larger than 5 µm in size). They infect by making contact with the mucous membranes of the nose or mouth of a target. They are contained in droplets generated from a carrier's cough or sneeze, or even talking.

- Gown/gloves worn when contact with fluids is likely, and a mask should be worn when working within 3 ft of the patient. May also need to wear a mask during suctioning.
- Have patient wear a mask during transport
- Can have door open; private room, or room with cohort
- Used for the following pathogens: **SPIDERMAN**
  - S – sepsis, scarlet fever, streptococcal pharyngitis
  - P - parovirus B19, pneumonia, pertussis
  - I - influenza
  - D - diptheria (pharyngeal)
  - E - epiglottitis
  - R - rubella
  - M - mumps/meningitis/mycoplasma/meningeal pneumonia
  - An - adenovirus

Airborne precautions

Airborne precautions are to be taken with infected patients to prevent transmitting disease through airborne droplets containing suspended microorganisms that can be dispersed by air currents. Place infected patients in a private, closed-off room equipped with a monitored, high-efficiency air filtration system and negative air pressure system, minimum of 6 exchanges per hour. If no private room is available, the patient may be cohorted – placed in a room with another patient with the same infection. All personnel must wear gown, gloves, and respiratory protection when entering the room, using special N95 respirator mask or PAPR machine. Limit movement and transport of patients outside the room to essential purposes only, at which time the patient must wear a surgical mask to minimize dispersal of droplet nuclei.

Organizational plan to address mass influx of patients with communicable diseases

The ICP and the infection control team should develop specific plans for dealing with different bioterrorism agents, and training should be provided to staff. An organized approach should include the following:

- Be on the alert for possible bioterrorism-related infections, based on clusters of patients or symptoms.
- Use personal protection equipment, including respirators when indicated.
- Complete thorough assessment of patient, including medical history, physical examination, immunization record, and travel history.
- Provide a probable diagnosis based on symptoms and lab findings, including cultures.
- Provide treatment, including prophylaxis, while waiting for laboratory findings.
- Use transmission precautions as well as isolation for suspected biologic agents.
- Notify local, state, and federal authorities per established protocol.
- Conduct surveillance and epidemiological studies to identify at-risk populations.
- Develop plans to accommodate large numbers of patients:
  - Restricting elective admissions
  - Transferring patients to other facilities.

Biological weapons

A number of different infections could be part of a bioterrorism attack. The type of barrier/isolation needed is dependent upon the symptoms and the mode of transmission. Knowledge of typical presenting symptoms and prompt precautions are essential to prevent spread of disease.

Anthrax
Anthrax (*Bacillus anthracis*) usually occurs from contact with animals, but as a bioterrorism weapon, anthrax would most likely be aerosolized and inhaled. It is not transferred from person to person. There are 3 types:
- Inhalation: fever, cough, shortness of breath, and general debility
- Cutaneous: small non-painful sores that blister and ulcerate with necrosis at the center
- Gastrointestinal: nausea, vomiting, diarrhea, and abdominal pain

The inhaled form of anthrax is the most severe with about a 50% mortality rate. The vaccine for anthrax is not yet available to the public.

Precautions include:
- Prophylaxis with antibiotics after exposure.
- Standard precautions
- Contact precautions for wounds if there are cutaneous lesions.

Viral hemorrhagic fevers
Viral hemorrhagic fevers are zoonoses (spread from animals to humans) and comprise a number of different diseases: Ebola, Lassa, Marburg, yellow, Argentine and Crimean-Congo. Some hemorrhagic fevers can spread person to person, notably Ebola, Marburg, and Lassa, through close contact with body fluids or contaminated items. Hemorrhagic fevers are

extremely contagious multi-system diseases, and those in contact with infected patients are at risk of infection. Symptoms vary somewhat according to the disease but present with flu-like symptoms that progress to bleeding under the skin and internally, and some people develop kidney failure and central nervous system symptoms, such as coma and seizures. Treatment is supportive and mortality rates are high. Only yellow fever and Argentine have vaccines.

Precautions are as follows:
- Maximum precautions must be used with full barrier precautions, with care used in any handling of blood and body fluids or wastes.
- Screening: ask patient if they have been out of the country in the last 3-6 months.

Pandemic influenza

Pandemic influenza is a worldwide epidemic of influenza that causes serious respiratory illness and/or death in large populations of people. Pandemics can occur when a virus mutates, creating a new subtype that infects humans and spreads easily from person to person. Should a global outbreak and a pandemic occur, the implications for health care are profound because the potential number of infected patients will be overwhelming to the medical system.

Precautions are as follows:
- Standard precautions with careful hand hygiene
- Contact precautions with gloves and gown for all patient contact and goggles when within 3 feet
- Dedicated equipment
- Airborne precautions in isolated negative pressure rooms and use of N-95 filter respirator

Pneumonic plague

Yersinia pestis causes pneumonic plague, which is normally carried by fleas from infected rats but can be aerosolized to use as a biologic weapon. There are 3 forms of plague, but they sometimes occur together and bubonic and septicemic plague can develop into pneumonic, which is the primary concern related to bioterrorism:
- Bubonic occurs when a person is bitten by an infected flea.
- Pneumonic occurs with inhalation and results in pneumonia with fever, headache, cough, and progressive respiratory failure.
- Septicemic occurs when *Y. pestis* invades the bloodstream, often after initial bubonic or pneumonic plague.

Pneumonic plague can spread easily from person to person. There is no vaccine available.

Precautions:
- Immediate antibiotics within first 24 hours are necessary, so early diagnosis is critical.
- Prophylaxis with antibiotics may protect those exposed.
- Droplet precautions should be used with appropriate barriers, such as surgical mask.

Botulism

Clostridium botulinum produces an extremely poisonous toxin that causes botulism. The organism can be aerosolized or used to infect food. There are 3 primary forms of botulisms:

- Foodborne botulism results from contamination of food. This type poses the greatest threat from bioterrorism. Symptoms usually appear 12-36 hours after ingestion but may be delayed for 2 weeks, and include nausea, vomiting, dyspnea, dysphagia, slurred speech, progressive weakness, and paralysis
- Infant botulism results from C. botulinum ingested into the intestinal tract. Constipation, poor feeding, and progressive weakness are presenting symptoms.
- Wound botulism results from contamination of open skin, but symptoms are similar to foodborne botulism.

Botulism is not transmitted from person to person, but contaminated food has the potential to infect many people, especially if the contaminated food is manufactured and widely distributed.

Precautions include:

- Antitoxin after exposure and as early in disease as possible.
- Standard precautions
- Do not feed honey to infants, as there is a risk of spore ingestion.

Tularemia

Francisella tularensis causes tularemia, which is usually transmitted from small mammals to humans through insect bites, ingestion of contaminated food or water, inhalation, or handling of infected animals. Although there is no evidence of person-to-person transmission, *F. tularensis* has the potential to be aerosolized for use in bioterrorism because it is highly infective and requires only about 10 organisms to infect. Flu-like symptoms appear in 3-5 days after exposure and progress to severe respiratory infection and pneumonia. A vaccine for laboratory workers was available until recently, but the FDA is currently reviewing it, and it is unavailable in the United States.

- Prophylaxis with antibiotics within 24 hours may prevent disease.
- Standard precautions are sufficient.
- Biologic safety measures should be used for laboratory specimens.
- Autopsy procedures that may cause tissue to be aerosolized should be avoided.

SARS

Severe Acute Respiratory Syndrome (SARS) is caused by a coronavirus (CoV) and presents as a respiratory illness with fever, cough, dyspnea, and general malaise. It is extremely virulent, spreading easily from person to person through close contact by way of contaminated droplets produced by coughing or sneezing. SARS has a high mortality rate. Some possibility exists that SARS may also have airborne transmission, in some cases with aerosol-producing procedures. High rates of infection have occurred in health care workers and others in contact with infected patients, so prompt diagnosis and proper isolation are essential. Precautions are as follows:

- Contact and droplet precautions, including eye protection and appropriate personal protection equipment
- Airborne precautions (recommended by the CDC), especially with aerosol-producing procedures (ventilators, nebulizers, intubation)

- Immediate notification of public health authorities and institution of contact tracing
- Activity restrictions of exposed health care workers planned in coordination with public health officials

Smallpox

The variola virus causes smallpox, which has been eradicated worldwide since 1980, but has the potential for use as a biological weapon because people are no longer vaccinated. Smallpox is extremely contagious and has a high mortality rate (about 30%). Flu-like symptoms appear about 7-17 days after exposure with fever, weakness, vomiting, and rash that begins on the face and arms and spreads. The rash becomes pustular, crusts, scabs over, and then sloughs off, leaving scars. People remain infective from the first rash until all scabs are gone. The disease can spread through contact with infective fluid from lesions or from contact with clothes or bedding. Aerosol spread is theoretically possible.

Precautions:
- Vaccination must be done before symptoms appear and as soon as possible after exposure as vaccination after rash appears will not affect the severity of the disease; vaccination is done by scratching the skin with a small needle on the upper arm, leaving a characteristic pox scar.
- Contact precautions should be used, which includes the use of gowns and gloves to enter the room and keeping the patient in a private or cohorted room.

Chickenpox

Varicella zoster ("chickenpox") is a common childhood illness, though it can cause severe illness and complications such as encephalitis and bacteremia in adults. It is highly contagious, and can be spread 2 days before the appearance of a rash until the point where all lesions are crusted over. Signs and symptoms include the following: incubation 11-21 days; runny/stuffy nose, cough, sneezing, 24-48 hours later, rash with small blisters of variable size usually beginning on head and chest, spreading to limbs, reddened skin, fever. Diagnosis is based on physical exam, can confirm with blood test if necessary. Treatment includes:
- Patient must be kept in isolation. If the patient scratches the lesions they will spread.
- Severe cases: acyclovir or infusion of immunoglobulin
- Immunization available; important, because once a child has had varicella, they can develop shingles later in life. However, cannot catch varicella twice.
- Symptom management: calamine lotion, cool oatmeal or baking soda baths, trim fingernails and have child wear gloves; Tylenol or Advil/Motrin for fever (do not give aspirin, which may cause Reye syndrome).

Common Household Safety Concerns

There are several areas of the standard American household that can pose dangers to families and small children. Listed below are some common household issues (including multiple foodborne illnesses) that the nurse should be aware of and educate patients regarding.

Falls

The following are risk factors for falls and interventions:

- Orthostatic hypotension: Rise and move slowly; stand in place for several seconds; walk short distances
- Urinary frequency or incontinence: bedside commode; assist to bathroom, bladder training, frequent toileting
- Weakness: physical/occupational therapy; call for help; monitor tolerance, gait belt, assistive devices
- Current medications: sedatives, hypnotics, tranquilizers, narcotic analgesics, diuretics; bed in low position, side rail up on one side or half rails maintained
- Monitoring devices/bed alarms: use if available

Fire Safety

RACE is an acronym for fire safety:

- **R**escue – remove all patients from area of danger
- **A**ctivate alarm - pull fire alarm/call 9-1-1
- **C**onfine the fire - close doors to unit/place.
- **E**vacuate/Extinguish (NFPA/OSHA fire safety) - Use PASS for fire estinguisher
  - Pull
  - Aim at the base of the flames
  - Squeeze the trigger
  - Sweep – use a sweeping motion across the flames.

Ergonomics

Ergonomics is the study of preventing workplace injury and stress. In nursing, it refers to the way in which a nurse can prevent injury to self and others due to the stressors and strains required in the nursing field. Some important ergonomic principles include:

- Body Mechanics: The body should be kept in proper alignment during tasks, with a wide base of support and center of gravity low. Use larger muscles (buttocks, thighs, shoulders) for activities rather than smaller when possible. Avoid twisting or jerking movements. Maintain 90° angle in elbows and knees when sitting, elbows at the side, with back straight and looking straight ahead.
- Lifting: Use appropriate transfer devices; use as many people as necessary. Manual lifting should be avoided. Bend at the knees, tighten core, and keep weights close to the body – never bend or twist when lifting.
- Repetition: Avoid repetitive movements/stressors and use proper safety equipment when needed (earplugs for loud noises, etc.).

Carbon Monoxide Poisoning

Carbon monoxide poisoning occurs when people breathe in carbon monoxide, usually related to industrial or household accidents or suicide attempts. Carbon monoxide binds to hemoglobin 200 times more readily than oxygen, and once the carbon monoxide binds to hemoglobin (creating carboxyhemoglobin), the hemoglobin can no longer bind to or transport oxygen, resulting in hypoxemia. Signs and symptoms vary depending on percentage of saturation. At 10%, patients may complain of headache and nausea. At > 20%, patient becomes increasingly weak and confused with alterations in mental status. At > 30%, patient may have dyspnea, chest pain, and increased confusion. When the level continues to increase, patient may experience seizures, coma, and death. Skin color may be cyanotic, pink, or bright cherry red (but not a reliable sign); realize that pulse oximetry may read 100%, but patient is severely hypoxic. Diagnosis is based on evaluation of symptoms and situation and carboxyhemoglobin level per CO-oximeter. Patient should be administered 100% oxygen with non-rebreather mask. Hyperbaric oxygen treatment is utilized for some patients with severe symptoms.

First Aid for Seizures
Seizure disorders are broadly categorized as partial seizures (which begin locally) or generalized seizures (which are bilateral and symmetrical and may be convulsive or non-convulsive):

- Partial seizures include simple partial (with motor, sensory, and/or autonomic symptoms but without impaired consciousness), complex partial (with cognitive, affective, psychosensory, and/or psychomotor symptoms, as well as impaired consciousness), or partial secondarily generalized.
- Generalized seizures include seizures that are bilateral and symmetric without local onset and may be convulsive or non-convulsive. These seizures include tonic-clonic, tonic, clonic, absence (petit mal), atonic, and myoclonic seizures, as well as unclassified seizures.

First aid for a seizure includes ensuring privacy and providing supportive care, such as easing the patient to the floor and providing padding to protect the head. Side rails should be raised and pillow removed if the patient is in bed. The patient should be placed on one side with the head flexed so the tongue does not block the airway. The patient should **not** be restrained or a padded tongue-blade inserted between the teeth.

Norwalk Family of Virus Infections
Viral gastroenteritis, more commonly known as food poisoning, has at its root a member of the Norwalk family of viruses. It is a preeminent cause of illness in the United States, occurring mostly during winter months. It is estimated that Norwalk viruses are behind about a third of all viral gastroenteritis cases, and the only viral illness reported to a greater extent is the common cold. Though not permanent (people can become reinfected), half the population over 18 develops immunity because it gradually increases with age.
Norwalk gastroenteritis is transmitted through drinking water or foods that have been contaminated with human feces, water being the most common source of outbreaks. Eating raw or insufficiently steamed clams and oysters that come from polluted beds makes for a high risk of Norwalk virus infection. But other foods, not just shellfish, may be contaminated by food handlers. Illness usually comes on about 24 to 48 hours after eating or drinking. The disease is self-limiting, lasting between 24 and 60 hours, and is mild. It is characterized by diarrhea, nausea, vomiting, and abdominal pain. Treatment is supportive.

Prevention includes the following:
- Eat thoroughly cooked foods
- Wash hands, disinfect common areas.

Entamoeba histolytica infections
Amebiasis (or *amoebiasis*), the infection caused by *E. histolytica*, can last for up to 4 years with no symptoms, some gastrointestinal distress, or dysentery, complete with blood and mucus. Potential complications include pain from ulcers or abscesses, and, rarely, intestinal blockage. The amoeba's cysts survive, especially under moist conditions, in water, soils, and on foods. They result in infections when they are swallowed; they excyst to the trophozoite stage in the digestive tract, with the possibility of other tissues being invaded. Ingestion of

- 22 -

one viable cyst, it is thought, is enough to cause an infection. Amebiasis is transmitted primarily by fecal contamination of drinking water and foods, and also through direct contact with dirty hands or objects. Because sexual contact may also transmit the disease, AIDS/AIDS-related complex (ARC) patients are very vulnerable. Fatalities are infrequent. Treament includes supportive care and rehydration.

Prevention includes the following:
- Wash hands, drink clean drinking water, wash fruits/vegetables.
- Close mouth when swimming/avoid swallowing pond water.

Gram-negative Clostridium botulinum infections
The heat-resistant spores of *Clostridium botulinum* can produce a deadly neurotoxin in poorly processed foods, with most of the outbreaks reported annually in the United States (from 10 to 30) associated with home-canned foods. Occasionally, though, commercially produced foods are at fault—canned meat products, canned vegetables, and canned seafood products are the most frequent sources. The organism and its spores occur widely in soils as well as stream, lake, and ocean sediments, intestinal tracts of fish and mammals, and in the gills and viscera of crabs and other shellfish. It also appears in honey, which is definitely linked to infant botulism but not in any cases involving adults. Foods are not involved in the botulism sometimes found in wounds; it results when *C. botulinum* infects a wound, producing toxins that travel via the bloodstream to infect other parts of the body. Treatment includes supportive care and antitoxin.

Prevention includes the following:
- Heat canned foods for 80°C for 10 minutes or longer to destroy spores
- Never feed infants younger than 1 year raw honey
- Difficulty breathing/muscle rigidity—report immediately!

Gram-negative Campylobacter jejuni infections
While seldom deadly, *Campylobacter* is the most common cause of diarrhea in the United States. Of some 100,000 who contract it yearly in the United States, only about 100 die. It can sometimes occur in outbreaks, and there may be long-term consequences of infection. Some people may develop arthritis following campylobacteriosis. Others may develop Guillain-Barré syndrome, which is a rare autoimmune disease that affects nerves throughout the body, beginning several weeks after the diarrheal illness. Paralysis may last several weeks and usually requires intensive care. As many as 40% of Guillain-Barré syndrome cases in this country may be triggered by campylobacteriosis, usually as a result of eating or handling raw or undercooked poultry meat. An outbreak in 1988 was caused by milk that had been improperly pasteurized. Treatment is as follows:
- IV fluids/electrolytes, supportive care.
- Should resolve in a week; may prescribe antibiotics

Prevention includes the following:
- Cook meat thoroughly, use separate cutting boards for meat/vegetables, wash hands before and after handling raw meat.
- Wash hands after petting animals/before eating

<u>E. coli</u>
Escherichia coli (E. coli), the coliform bacteria most abundant in the colon and normally innocuous, can upon acquiring a virulence factor, cause enteric infections such as traveler's diarrhea. This can lead to osmotic diarrhea by inhibiting uptake of salt. It can also cause hemolytic uremic syndrome (HUS), making possible acute renal failure as well as urinary tract infections such as cystitis and pyelonephritis, neonatal meningitis, respiratory infection, and bacteremia. Particularly bad strains can produce hemorrhagic colitis with severe cramping and bloody diarrhea. The illness, usually self-limited, lasts for an average of 8 days. Treatment includes:
- Fluid resuscitation – IV fluids and electrolytes
- Antibiotics are discouraged, due to the germ's resistance; urinary tract infections can be treated with trimethoprim/sulfamethoxazole or ampicillin, and meningitis with third-generation cephalosporin (ceftriaxone).

Prevention includes:
- Cook meat thoroughly and wash all vegetables before eating.
- Wash hands after petting animals/before eating.

<u>Cryptosporidium parvum infections</u>
Severe watery diarrhea marks intestinal *cryptosporidiosis*, while tracheal cryptosporidiosis causes coughing and mild fever, and sometimes severe intestinal distress. They are both caused by a single-celled obligate intracellular parasite. Herd animals (cows, goats, sheep) and humans may be infected with the *Cryptosporidium parvum* sporocysts, which are resistant to most chemical disinfectants. Drying and the ultraviolet portion of sunlight are deadly to them. Presumably, one organism in infected food touched by a contaminated food handler can initiate an infection. Incidence is high in child day care centers where food is served. Another possible source of human infection is raw manure that has been spread over garden vegetables, but large outbreaks invariably have contaminated water supplies as their source. Up to 80% of the population has been infected with cryptosporidiosis. There is no effective treatment, and the severe watery diarrhea is often a contributor in the death of AIDS victims; invasion of the pulmonary system may also be fatal. Treatment includes supportive care and rehydration.

Prevention includes the following:
- Wash hands
- Clean drinking water
- Wash fruits/vegetables.

<u>Giardia lamblia infections</u>
Giardia lamblia is a parasite and the causative agent of giardiasis, the most frequent source of non-bacterial diarrhea in North America. Ingestion of 1 or more protozoan cysts may bring on diarrhea within a week; however, for most bacterial illnesses, at least thousands of organisms may have to be consumed to produce illness. Illness normally lasts for 7-14 days, but there are cases of chronic infections lasting months to years. Chronic cases, both those with defined immune deficiencies and those without, are difficult to treat.
Giardiasis most frequently results from drinking contaminated water, though outbreaks have been traced to food contamination, and it is impossible to rule out contaminated vegetables eaten raw as sources of infection. It is more prevalent in children, possibly

because many adults seem to have a lasting immunity after infection. It can also spread through anal sex. Treatment includes:

- Supportive care: rehydration
- Medications: metronidazole, tinidazole, nitazoxanide if severe.

Prevention includes:

- Wash hands, clean drinking water, wash fruits/vegetables.
- Close mouth when swimming/avoid swallowing pond water.
- Practice safe sex.

Gram-positive Listeria monocytogenes infections

Listeriosis, caused by *Listeria monocytogenes*, finds expression in encephalitis, meningitis (or meningoencephalitis), and septicemia. It is also a factor in intrauterine or cervical infections in pregnant women. (It can result in stillbirth or spontaneous abortion.) Onset to GI symptoms may take more than 12 hours, whereas the time to serious forms of listeriosis may range from a few days to 3 weeks. For infections during pregnancy, the mother usually survives. It has been associated with consuming raw or badly pasteurized milk, raw meats of all types, ice cream, and uncooked vegetables. Cheeses, raw and cooked poultry, fermented raw-meat sausages, and raw and smoked fish are thought to be other sources. Particularly concerning is the fact that it can grow in refrigerated foods. Listeriosis is effectively treated with penicillin, ampicillin, or trimethoprim/sulfamethoxazole.

Prevention includes the following:

- Date all refrigerated items and do not use past expiration/best-by dates.
- Cook meat thoroughly; wash hands before and after preparation.

Rotavirus infections

Rotaviruses, transmitted by the fecal-oral route, are spread most commonly by dirty hands. Commonly found in day care centers, pediatric and geriatric wards, and family homes, they may also be found in uncooked food contaminated by infected food handlers. Sanitary measures adequate for bacteria and parasites seem to be ineffective in controlling rotavirus; a similar incidence of infection is observed in countries with both high and low health standards. Those with severe diarrhea who do not get quick access to fluid and electrolyte replacement may die; otherwise, recovery from infections is usually complete. Childhood mortality due to rotavirus is relatively low in the United States, with an estimated 100 cases/year, but approaches nearly a million cases per year worldwide. Of childhood cases of severe diarrhea that require hospitalization, about half can be attributed to group A rotavirus. Treament includes supportive care and rehydration.

Prevention includes the following:

- Wash hands, drink clean drinking water, wash fruits/vegetables.
- Close mouth when swimming/avoid swalling pond water.

Shigella infections

The illness caused by *Shigella (shigellosis)* accounts for less than 10% of the reported outbreaks of foodborne illness in the United States, at an estimated 300,000 cases. Infants, elderly patients, and those in poor health are susceptible to the most severe symptoms of the disease, but all humans are susceptible to some degree. Fatalities may be as high as 10%-15% with some strains. Shigellosis is a very common malady suffered by individuals with AIDS. The organism is frequently found in water polluted with human feces. Infection, which requires as few as 10 cells, depending on age and condition of the host, is characterized by abdominal pain, cramps, diarrhea, fever, vomiting, blood, pus, or mucus in stools. The usual medium is food contamination, usually through the fecal-oral route, as a result of unsanitary food handling. Treatment includes supportive care and rehydration.

Prevention includes the following:
- Wash hands, drink clean drinking water, wash fruits/vegetables.
- Close mouth when swimming/avoid swallowing pond water.
- Practice safe sex.

Vibrio cholerae serogroup O1 infections
Unsanitary conditions pollute waters, providing the breeding grounds for *Vibrio cholerae*, the bacterium responsible for epidemic cholera. Ingested viable bacteria attach to the small intestine and produce cholera toxin. Dehydration and loss of essential electrolytes bring death. While formerly responsible for mass epidemics, with today's medical advances, supportive care means the illness is generally self-limiting. Treatment includes the following:
- Rehydration, either intravenously or orally, with a solution containing sodium chloride, sodium bicarbonate, potassium chloride, and dextrose (glucose).
- Antibiotics such as tetracycline have been shown to shorten the course of the illness.

Prevention includes the following:
- Ensure water is clean before drinking: avoid drinking stale water or water from outdoor streams/ponds
- Increased risk with seafood.

Hepatitis A
Hepatitis A is a systemic viral infection (short incubation type hepatitis) that involves the liver. Hepatitis A is extremely contagious and caused by an RNA enterovirus. It is transmitted via the fecal-oral route or paternally. It is most often found in areas of poor sanitation and overcrowding, though epidemics from contaminated food and water also occur. The period of communicability extends from early in the incubation period to about a week after the development of jaundice. Most cases resolve within 3 weeks and there are seldom fatalities. Signs and symptoms include sudden onset of fever, malaise, nausea, anorexia, abdominal discomfort, jaundice, enlarged liver (hepatomegaly), dark urine, transient pale stools, upper right abdominal quadrant pain, and fatigue. Diagnosis is based on blood work - hepatitis A antibodies. Treatment is as follows:
- Supportive; rest, fluids, nutrition.
- Patient education should include education on the disease and disease process, education on hygiene, handwashing, vaccinations to prevent hepatitis A; educate the individual to cover broken or open skin; avoid sexual contact and food preparation.

*Hepatitis E, which has symptoms similar to Hepatitis A, has a fatality rate of 20% among pregnant women.

Reporting Incidences or Irregular Occurrences During Nursing Care

Incident reporting should take place anytime there is a situation in which patient/employee safety is actually or potentially compromised. While many nurses may hesitate to complete incident reports due to fear of punitive action, it is important to realize that incident reporting is a critical component of quality improvement and safety. Incident reports should be filled out as quickly as possible after the occurrence, to ensure the report is accurate and devoid of omissions. The nurse should use simple and precise language to describe what occurred, and should not include opinions or theories related to the event. When reviewing incident reports, the circumstances and precipitating factors of the incident should all be analyzed to see where the break(s) from policy occurred, or if there needs to be new policy written to avoid future incidents of the same kind.

Security plan

A security plan is a plan that is set in place to help guide the actions of employees in case of a breach in security at a healthcare facility. All employees must be educated and comfortable with their facilities plan, in order to facilitate the safety of staff and patients alike. The security plan usually has several components:

- Security workers: Most facilities have securities guards who patrol the campus and help maintain patient and visitor safety. If a patient/visitor threatens violence or becomes combative, security should be called immediately.
- Silent Alarms: Most units have "silent alarms", which are usually buttons or switches underneath the secretary's desk or in some other discreet location. These are pushed in the case of a threat to security in which a call cannot safely be made.
- Locked units: Certain units in the hospital (such as Mother/Baby, critical care units, psychiatric floors, etc.) are locked and require an access code to enter.
- "Do Not Acknowledge": Certain patients may be deemed as "do not acknowledge", meaning that the nurse cannot give out any information regarding these patients, including acknowledging the patients' presence in the facility. Examples include psychiatric patients, victims of crime, celebrities, and others. If someone calls asking about the patient, it is appropriate and ethical for the nurse to state "I do not have any information regarding a patient with that name".
- Over-head Announcements: Many facilities have different codes that they may call overhead to alert staff of emergences/safety threats.

Health Promotion and Maintenance

This domain is defined by the NCSBN as "providing and directing nursing care of the client that incorporates the knowledge of expected growth and development principles, prevention and/or early detection of health problems, and strategies to achieve optimal health." This section includes outlines for the growth and development from birth to old age, including healthcare and screening involved in these age groups.

Women's Health

Menstrual Cycle Phases

The menstrual cycle is a three-phase cycle in which a woman's body prepares for pregnancy. The days listed are based on a typical 28-day cycle, but it is important to realize that the days can vary based on cycle length and hormone levels of the individual woman.

1. Menstruation (day 1-6): During the menstrual cycle, the woman experiences decreased levels of estrogen and endometrial tissue detaching, resulting in 3-7 days of vaginal bleeding.
2. Proliferation Phase (day 7-14): During the proliferation phase, the woman will experience endometrial thickening, peak levels of estrogen, and decreased body temperature. This phase ends with ovulation
3. The Luteal Phase (day 14-28): The luteal phase of the menstrual cycle consists at first of increased uterine vascularity, and preparatory signs of implantation. However, if no fertilized ovum implants, the levels of estrogen and progesterone levels begin to decrease, resulting in pale endometrial tissue, vasoconstriction of the spiral arteries, rupture of the blood vessels, and the stromal cells of the uterus become filled with blood as the body prepares for menstruation.

Ovulation

Ovulation is the release of an egg (ovum) from the ovaries, generally occurring on day 14 of the typical menstrual cycle. The ovarian cycle consists of the follicular phase, during which follicle-stimulating hormone (FSH) and luteinizing hormone (LH) begin to be excreted in increasing amounts, causing the maturation of one or more of the graafian or ovarian follicles. When fully mature, the ovarian follicle ruptures and expels the ovum or female egg into the fallopian tube. This event is known as ovulation. If implantation occurs, the ovum will continue to grow and the corpus luteum will secrete estrogen and progesterone to maintain pregnancy. Otherwise, the corpus luteum disintegrates and the levels of progesterone and estrogen will steadily decrease, signaling menstruation to occur.

Some signs and symptoms of ovulation may include:
- Increased watery vaginal discharge
- "Ferning" pattern of vaginal mucous/saliva.
- Sharp, unilateral abdominal pain (called *Mittelschmerz*, "lightning pain")
- Increase in basal body temperature (BBT)
- Slight mid-cycle spotting.

Irregularities Associated with Menses

The following are common irregularities associated with menses:
- Amenorrhea is characterized by a lack of or uncharacteristic pause of menses.
- Dysmenorrhea is characterized by painful menses.
- Hypomenorrhea is characterized by a menses of short duration.
- Menorrhagia is characterized by an extensive menses.
- Oligomenorrhea is characterized by infrequent menses/ cycle length greater than 35 days.
- Polymenorrhea is characterized by abnormally frequent menses.
- Anovulatory cycle is characterized by a menstrual cycle in which a woman does not ovulate.

Endometriosis

Endometriosis is the occurrence of endometrial tissue in areas other than the uterine cavity, such as peritoneal surfaces, fallopian tubes, lymph nodes, ovaries, or bowels. Endometriosis can occur in a woman at any age. It is theorized to be caused by retrograde menstruation (flow of menstrual blood backwards through fallopian tubes), but exact cause is not known. Family history, PID, abnormally shaped uterus, and woman without children are at greater risk. Signs and symptoms include dyspareunia (painful intercourse), dysmenorrhea, dyschezia (difficult production of stool), pelvic and low-back pain (acute or chronic), premenstrual spotting, spontaneous abortion, and infertility. Diagnosis is based on pelvic US, laparoscopy, and pelvic exam. Treatment includes:
- Pain medications: NSAIDs,
- Hormone Therapy: OCPs, medroxyprogesterone injection, Gn-RH agonists/antagonists, danazol (risk of birth defects)
- Surgery: to remove endometrial tissue or radical hysterectomy.
- Lifestyle Modification: regular exercise, drink fluids, heating pads/warm baths.

Pap smear

A Pap smear is an exam that checks for changes in the cells of a woman's cervix. It is performed by a gynecologist during an annual exam. It is important for all women to have an annual Pap smear if they are sexually active or older than 18 years. The test is key to catching cervical problems and cancers early, allowing prompt diagnosis and treatment. The woman should avoid sex, douching, tampons, and the use of vaginal suppositories 24-48 hours before the test. There are no firm contraindications for a Pap smear, but it may be avoided during pregnancy, menstruation, or in patients with existing cervicitis until treated. On the day of the exam, the woman is placed in the lithotomy position, with her legs in stirrups. The doctor will then insert a speculum without lubricant into the woman's vagina, and open it up. A small brushing of the cells of the cervix is then taken to send to the laboratory. There the cells are tested for infection, abnormalities, and/or cancer.

Vaginitis

Vaginitis is a condition in which there is inflammation of the vagina. This most often occurs after menopause, but hormonal changes, medications (antibiotics, steroids, OCPs), STIs, IUDs, and douches/bubble baths can increase risk. Signs and symptoms include pain with intercourse, vaginal itching/pain/discharge, and vaginal irritation after intercourse. Diagnosis is based on pelvic examination, blood work (hormones), and lab evaluation of vaginal secretions. Treatment includes the following:

- Treat underlying cause: antibiotics for infections, removal of IUD, cease use of allergens, etc.
- Atrophic vaginitis: caused by low estrogen levels; hormone therapy and use of vaginal lubricant
- Lifestyle modification: do not use douches/sprays, practice safe sex, use sufficient lubricant for comfort.

Bacterial vaginosis

Bacterial vaginosis (BV) is a bacterial infection of the vagina, which can be caused by several different types of organisms. BV occurs when hydrogen peroxide–producing lactobacilli of the normal flora of the vagina are replaced by anaerobic bacteria, causing an increase in the pH of the vaginal secretions. Common causes of bacterial vaginosis include multiple sexual partners, frequent sex, douching, and the use of intra-uterine devices to avoid pregnancy. Symptoms include white/gray vaginal discharge, "fishy"/foul smelling discharge, pain with intercourse and vaginal itching/irritation. Diagnosis is based on gynecological exam and microscopic examination of vaginal secretions. Treatment includes:

- Metronidazole (Flagyl) or other antibiotics: oral
- Clindamycin 2% cream: vaginal suppository
- Lifestyle modification: stop douching, condoms during sex, feminine hygiene education

Trichomoniasis

Trichomoniasis is one of the most common sexually transmitted infections (STIs), caused by a species of the genus *Trichomonas*. Trichomoniasis can be found in both women and men. Those at highest risk of trichomoniasis are those with multiple sexual partners and those who have unprotected sexual intercourse with infected individuals. Signs and symptoms include excessive vaginal discharge, genital irritation, difficult urination (dysuria), odor, painful sexual intercourse, suprapubic pain and discomfort. Diagnosis is based on genital exam and microscopic examination of secretions. Treatment includes:

- Metronidazole (Flagyl): treat all sexual partners.
- Abstinence from sex to deter transmission until treatment is complete and patient is symptom free.
- Sex education

TSS

Toxic shock syndrome (TSS) is an infection of Staphylococcus aureus or another organism that ultimately causes shock and organ failure. It is generally associated with super-absorbent tampons, contraceptive sponges and diaphragms, but can also be related to recent surgery, infected wounds, or a viral infection. While more common in woman, TSS can affect both genders and all ages. Signs and symptoms include:

- Seizures, headaches, hypotension, fatigue, multiple organ involvement, fever, nausea, vomiting
- Progress to shock and kidney failure.

Diagnosis is based on evaluation of vital signs, urinalysis, blood work, CT scans, x-ray, and depends on organ involvement. Treatment includes:

- IV antibiotics
- Vassopressors if hypotensive and fluid resuscitation
- Dialysis if renal failure develops
- Surgery to remove necrotic tissue
- Teaching: change tampons frequently, and use lowest absorbancy.
- Wear pads at night. If had TSS, patient cannot use tampons or internal devices because TSS can occur again.

PID

Pelvic inflammatory disease (PID) is an infection of the fallopian tubes, uterus, or ovaries. It is commonly caused by an STI (generally chlamydia or gonorrhea), though it can be caused by intrauterine devices, childbirth/miscarriage, or abortion. Often, PID is asymptomatic; it is usually not diagnosed until fertility or pain problems are seen. Those with multiple sexual partners, recent IUD insertion, or a history of PID/STI are at an increased risk. Signs and symptoms include:

- Pain in pelvic region or with intercourse, discharge, fever, nausea, painful urination, irregular menstruation
- Untreated can lead to ectopic pregnancies, infertility, and chronic pelvic pain.

Diagnosis is based on pelvic exam, laparoscopy, ESR, endometrial biopsy
WBC count, pregnancy test, or cultures for infection. Treatment includes:

- Antibiotics: oral, or IV if severe infection. Partner should come in for testing and be treated as well.
- Surgery: could require drainage of abscess, or hysterectomy if severe.
- Lifestyle modification: abstinence until cleared from infection, safe sex, regular STI testing, don't douche, wipe front-to-back.

Obstetrics/Labor & Delivery

Birth rate, infant mortality, and maternal mortality

Birth rate is the number of babies born alive per 1,000 individuals in a population during a specific period of time (normally 1 year). Infant mortality is the number of babies who die per 1,000 live births in a population during a specific period of time (normally 1 year). Maternal mortality is any death of a woman during pregnancy or that occurs within 42 days of the termination of a pregnancy per 100,000 live births.

Signs of pregnancy

Signs and symptoms of pregnancy are as follows:

- Presumptive signs:
  o Delayed menstruation
  o Nausea and vomiting; 2-8 weeks after conception
  o Tender or swollen breasts; 1-2 weeks after conception
  o Feeling exhausted or "sleepy"; 1-6 weeks after conception,

- o Backaches/Headaches
- o Food cravings
- o Frequent urination; 6-8 weeks after conception
- Probable signs:
  - o Chadwick's sign: a bluish discoloration of the vaginal tissue, caused by venous congestion; ~6 weeks
  - o Hegar's Sign: softening of the uterus; ~6 weeks
  - o Goodell's Sign: softening of the cervix; ~6weeks
  - o Abdominal enlargement
  - o Positive pregnancy test (blood or urine)
- Positive signs:
  - o Fetal movements felt by examiner (ballottement); 16-22 weeks after conception
  - o Doppler of fetal heart beat; 10-14 weeks
  - o Fetal outline on x-ray
  - o Ultrasound examination of fetus: 4-6 weeks

High-risk Pregnancies

High-risk pregnancies are pregnancies in which some physiological condition causes an increased risk of injury to mother and baby. Maternal conditions that increase this risk include:
- Diabetes mellitus: severity of effects on infant affected by severity of disease. Hypoglycemia is one major risk in infant, and can occur in infant after birth within 1.5-4 hours.
- Drug abuse: narcotics readily cross placenta; will see symptoms of withdrawal in infant after birth.
- Smoking: Low Birth Weight (LBW) and low APGAR scores in infant; smoking in the home increases risk of SIDS, respiratory infections, and developmental delays in childhood.
- Alcohol use: leads to fetal alcohol syndrome (FAS); infant will show cognitive and physical impairment; facial dysmorphia. This is a leading cause of preventable intellectual disability.
- Maternal infection – especially in early pregnancy

*TORCH is a helpful mnemonic to remember the infections that can be vertically transmitted from mother to fetus/embryo, causing marked birth defects.
- Toxoplasmosis
- Other viruses
- Rubella
- Cytomegalovirus
- Hepatitis A and B

> **Review Video: TORCH Syndrome**
*Visit **mometrix.com/academy** and enter **Code: 734704***

Pelvic Structure

The various types of pelvic structures of women are explained below:
- Gynecoid pelvis: A gynecoid pelvis is characterized by a round inlet, and is the most often seen type of pelvic structure.
- Android pelvis: An android pelvis is characterized by a heart-shaped inlet, and is the normal male pelvis.
- Anthropoid pelvis: The anthropoid pelvis is characterized by an oval-shaped inlet.
- Platypelloid pelvis: A platypelloid pelvis is characterized by a transverse oval inlet, and is often noted as a flat pelvis.

Nagel's rule

Nagel's rule is a method used to calculate a woman's due date, or Estimated Date of Delivery (EDD). It is crucial to remember that the steps of this rule must be completed in order for the result to be accurate.
EDD = 1st day of last menstrual period + 1 year - 3 months + 7 days

Weight Gain During Pregnancy

Proper diet and adequate weight gain during pregnancy are essential for good health of the mother and optimum development of her baby. The appropriate total weight gain during a pregnancy depends on several factors, including mother's pre-pregnancy weight and age. A woman who is of average weight is encouraged to gain somewhere between 25-30 pounds during pregnancy. Underweight women need to gain a bit more weight, and overweight women will need less. It is generally not advised for an overweight woman to try to lose weight, especially late in the pregnancy, as this could harm the baby. For a pregnant woman of a healthy weight, the expected weight gain should be approximately 2.5-5 lb in the first trimester (12 weeks), and then approximately 1 lb/wk in the second and third trimesters.

Gestational Diabetes

Gestational diabetes (GDM) is defined as glucose intolerance of variable degree with onset or first recognition during the present pregnancy. Pregnancy results in an elevation in serum estrogen, progesterone, and many other hormones. These hormones form as a catalyst for insulin production, causing an increase in insulin during the early months of pregnancy. However, during the last months of pregnancy, there is a rise in cortisol and glycogen. This will cause insulin resistance to occur. The result of all this is hypoglycemia in early pregnancy, followed by hyperglycemia in later months. It can be screened by drawing a 1-hour glucose level following a 50 g glucose load, but is definitively diagnosed only by an abnormal 3-hour oral glucose tolerance test (OGTT) following a 100 g glucose load. For the mother with GDM, there is a higher risk of hypertension, preeclampsia, urinary tract infections, cesarean section, and future diabetes. For the infant, there is the potential for problems such as macrosomia, neural tube defects, neonatal hypoglycemia, hypocalcemia, hypomagnsemia, hyperbilirubinemia, birth trauma, prematurity syndromes, and subsequent childhood and adolescent obesity.

Hyperemesis Gravidarium

Hyperemesis gravidarum (HG) is a severe and intractable form of nausea and vomiting in pregnancy. The peak incidence is at 8-12 weeks of pregnancy, and symptoms usually resolve by week 16. Interestingly, nausea and vomiting of pregnancy is generally associated with a lower rate of miscarriage. HG is a diagnosis of exclusion, since the cause remains unknown; however, extreme nausea and vomiting may be related to elevated levels of estrogens or human chorionic gonadotropin. These patients need to be monitored, as severe dehydration and metabolic imbalances can develop. Signs and symptoms include nausea and vomiting, weight loss, dehydration, decreased skin turgor, and postural changes in BP and pulse. Diagnosis is based on physical exam, CMP, and tests to rule out other causes. Treatment includes:
- Medications: oral/IV antiemetics: ondansetron, promethazine (off-label), Diclegis, etc.; IV fluids/electrolyte replacement for dehydration.
- Lifestyle Modification: frequent small meals and sips of fluid, increased protein may help, eating before getting out of bed.

Preeclampsia

Preeclampsia is a condition characterized by an increase in blood pressure caused by pregnancy. If not promptly recognized and treated, it can lead to *eclampsia*, a condition that is very dangerous for mother and baby. Risk factors include first pregnancy/pregnant with multiples, history of previous preeclampsia, obesity, increased maternal age, and history of other conditions such as diabetes, HTN, or renal disease. Symptoms include abnormal and rapid weight gain, hypertension, protein in the urine, headaches, peripheral edema, nausea, anxiety, and decreased urine output. Tests include urinalysis, blood pressure, daily weight, and complete blood cell count. Treatment includes:
- Medications: antihypertensives may be used.
- Frequent monitoring: worsening preecampsia will indicate need for hospitalization and possible delivery
- NOTE: HELLP syndrome is an acronym/syndrome that indicates preeclampsia is worsening and/or leading to eclampsia. The acronym discusses the main symptoms of this disorder:
    o H - hemolysis
    o EL - elevated liver enzymes
    o LP - low platelet count

Eclampsia

Eclampsia is a condition in which seizures occur during pregnancy due to abnormally high blood pressure, which can result in severe neurological compromise and death. It is a progression of untreated/uncontrolled preeclampsia. Signs and symptoms include:
- Severe hypertension, upper right quadrant pain, sudden weight gain, vision changes, severe headache, seizures, abdominal pain, proteinuria
- Progression of signs and symptoms of preeclampsia

Diagnosis is based on elevated liver function tests (AST/ALT), vital signs, and urinalysis. Treatment includes:

- Medications: Magnesium sulfate IV*, antihypertensives
- Seizure precautions, bedrest; immediate delivery of infant may be only cure.
- *NOTE: BURP is a helpful mnemonic to assist you to remember the symptoms of magnesium sulfate toxicity:
  - Blood pressure - decreased
  - Urine output - decreased
  - Respiratory rate - decreased
  - Patellar reflex - absent

Umbilical Cord & Possible Complications

The umbilical cord is a maternofetal vessel that serves as a pathway for oxygen and nutrients to be passed between the fetus and mother during the intrauterine period. The umbilical cord should measure 55 cm in length and contain two arteries and one vein; the acronym "AVA" is often used to remember this (artery-vein-artery). The nurse should be aware of the following anomalies that can occur during birth related to the umbilical cord:

- Prolapsed cord: The cord is delivered prior to the presenting fetal part. May result in cord compression.
- Cord compression: A cease in flow of blood and oxygen between the mother and fetus.
- Missing vessels: Congenital artery absence can cause fetal anomalies and problems with gestational age.
- Rips or tears in the cord: Due to lack of Wharton's jelly (the natural protective mechanism of the cord). Causes hemorrhages and fetal heart rate irregularities.
- Shortened cord: May lead to umbilical hernia, abruptio placenta, and cord rupture.
- Extensive cord: Increased risk of nuchal cord and knots in the cord that decrease blood and oxygen supplies.
- Nuchal cord: Cord wrapped around baby's neck. May require emergency cesarean delivery to prevent strangulation if severe.

Placenta & Possible Complications

The placenta is a fetomaternal organ, meaning that it is an organ that is shared by mother and child. The function of the placenta is the exchange of nutrients, waste, blood, and oxygen between the blood of the fetus and the mother. The placenta continues to function throughout the birthing process until the umbilical cord is cut and/or the baby takes his first breath. However, there are certain complications that happen in relation to the placenta of which the nurse should be aware:

- Abruptio Placenta: An early and unexpected break of the placenta from the intrauterine wall during pregnancy or labor. This causes blood flow/oxygenation to the baby to cease, causing fetal demise and possible maternal hemorrhage if not caught early.
- Placenta Previa: Placenta previa is an altered position of the placenta, traditionally on the lower uterine wall or covering the cervical os. This can cause the placenta to be delivered before the child, resulting again in hemorrhage and fetal demise. The treatment is cesarean delivery and no vaginal exams.

- Retained Placenta: After birth, parts of the placenta may still be retained inside the uterus. This places the mother at a greatly increased risk of hemorrhage and infection, and must be dealt with immediately if caught.

Abruptio placentae

Abruptio placentae (ie, placental abruption) refers to separation of the placenta from the uterine wall. The exact cause of abruptio placentae is not known; potential causes include smoking, ingestion of alcohol, trauma, multiple pregnancies, and maternal hypertension. It is important to catch this condition early; vaginal bleeding is not always present, and the mother can hemmorhage before diagnosis is made.

Classification:
- Class 0: Asymptomatic - diagnosis is made retrospectively by finding an organized blood clot or a depressed area on a delivered placenta.
- Class 1: Mild – absent to mild vaginal bleeding, slightly tender uterus
- Class 2: Moderate - Moderate to severe uterine tenderness. Maternal tachycardia with orthostatic changes in BP and heart rate, fetal distress
- Class 3: Severe - very painful tetanic uterus, maternal shock, coagulopathy, fetal death

Signs and symptoms include sharp, stabbing pains in uterus, tender on palpation, rigid/board-like uterus, and drop in H&H. Diagnosis is based on physical exam of abdomen/uterine palpation, CBC, and ultrasound. Treatment includes oxygen, fluids, lateral position, bedrest, and emergency C section for fetal distress. ***No pelvic examinations***

Stages & Landmarks of Fetal Development

Fetal development takes 40 weeks from fertilization to birth.
- Pre embryonic phase: Fertilization – Week 2: rapid growth and cellular replication to form embryonic membranes and germ layers
- Embryonic phase: Week 3-12 - Embryo developing tissue that will distinguish the various organs, development of external features.
- Week 8: Embryo has the appearance of a human.
- Week 13-16: Fetal heartbeat and movements discernible.
- Week 16-20: Fetal movements felt by mother ("quickening"); gender discernible at this time.
- Week 24: Development of alveoli in the lungs.
- Week 25-28: Fetal lungs can facilitate gas exchange.
- Weeks 29-32: Fetal bone and central nervous system development.
- Week 37: The fetus is considered to be full term at 37 weeks.

Fetal lung development

Embryonic and fetal lung development is a continuous process that begins during the embryonic stage.
- Embryonic stage (weeks 3-7): Two lung buds develop from endoderm of the foregut, and the trachea and main bronchi begin to form.
- Pseudoglandular stage (weeks 7-16): Airway branches form until they reach a pattern similar to those in the adult by the end of the period. Cartilage and smooth muscle also begins forming about the airways. Primitive lung lobules are evident.
- Canalicular stage (weeks 16-24): Capillary networks form. Gas exchange units form. Epithelial cells differentiate. Pulmonary arteries and veins develop along the branching airways. The air-blood barrier forms that could support air exchange.
- Saccular stage (weeks 28-35): Epithelial cells thin, terminal saccules form, and surfactant production occurs.
- Alveolar stage (weeks 36-40 weeks): Alveolar formation begins (and continues after birth) and air spaces expand. Lungs support gas exchange.

Cardiovascular changes in neonates shortly after delivery

The birthing process brings about a marked change in the circulatory system of the newborn. During fetal development, blood is routed from the mother to the infant through the placenta. Upon birth, however, the first breath of the infant causes maximum inflation of the lungs. The resulting resistance stimulates increased blood flow to the pulmonary veins. Then, as blood begins to return from the pulmonary veins into the left atrium, the pressure in the right atrium decreases. The pressure in the right atrium is additionally decreased related to a marked drop in blood supply after the clamping of the umbilical cord. The clamping of the umbilical cord also causes the ductus venosus to close, resulting in the circulation of blood to the liver. The resulting change in arterial pressure will cause the foramen ovale (a hole between the left and right atria) to close within the first 2 hours following birth. The ductus arteriosus then closes as the flow of blood is rerouted into the pulmonary artery instead of the aorta.

Amniocentesis

Amniocentesis is the removal of some of the fluid surrounding the fetus for analysis. Fetus location is identified by US prior to the procedure. Using ultrasound, a long needle is inserted into the womans abdomen, and some fluid is aspirated and sent to a laboratory for testing. Results may take up to a month to come back. Amniocentesis is used to diagnose spina bifida, Rh compatibility, immature lungs, and Down syndrome. Potential complications include infection, miscarriage, bleeding, fetal harm, and oligiohydramnios.

Oligohydramnios/Polyhydraminos

Oligohydramnios is a condition in which there is a lack of sufficient amniotic fluid in the placenta surrounding the baby. This is concerning, as low levels of amniotic fluid can cause fetal abnormalities, miscarriage, and labor complications. Oligohydramnios can be caused by fetal kidney disorders, a ruptured amniotic sac, and possibly NSAID use; however, it is generally unknown as to what causes the condition. Treatment may include amniotic fluid infusions, fluids for the mother, and bedrest. Polyhydramnios is an abnormally high level of amniotic fluid that can cause premature labor/rupture of membranes, fetal abnormalities, and fetal death. It can be caused by hydrops fetalis, multiple fetus development, anencephaly, or other problems that would cause the fetus to have swallowing difficulty/excess urination. The treatment could include medication to reduce fetal urination, removal of fluid, along with bedrest/symptom management. However, treatment is often not indicated.

Chorionic villus sampling

Chorionic villus sampling is the removal of placental tissue from the uterus for analysis during early pregnancy. The advantage of chorionic villus sampling is that it can be performed earlier than amniocentesis, and is used to diagnose Tay-Sachs disease, Down syndrome, and other genetic disorders. Considerations are as follows:
- Ensure woman is well hydrated and able to lie completely still during test.
- Contraindicated rarely in conditions such as retroverted uterus or poor fetal positioning.
- Possible complications include infection, miscarriage, and bleeding.
- May want to have support person with her during procedure.

For the procedure, the woman is supine and abdomen is cleansed and prepped with a sterile drape. Using ultrasound, a long needle is inserted into the womans abdomen, and cells are aspirated to be sent to the lab. Risks include infection, miscarriage, and bleeding; this test can also be performed transvaginally. The woman may experience some cramping during the procedure.

Down syndrome

Down syndrome, also sometimes referred to as trisomy 21 syndrome, is an abnormality with chromosome 21 that results in an individual having 47 chromosomes instead of 46. This results in several physiological and cognitive abnormalities. Maternal age greater than 35 years, family history, and a previous child with Down syndrome are all known risk factors for this condition. Infants with Down syndrome will have difficulty feeding and develop frequent respiratory infections. Many children with Down syndrome also have heart defects, and have an increased risk of Alzheimer disease and leukemia later in life. Signs and symptoms include intellectual disability, slanted eyes, flattened nasal bridge, small low-set ears, thick, fissured tongue, low muscle tone, short fingers, and Brushfield spots on the iris. Diagnosis is based on physical exam, karyotype test, and neonatal screening -not definitive. Treatment is as follows:
- No cure; ensure family has adequate support
- Education on health risks – ensure early recognition and treatment of infections
- Education: many people with Down syndrome can live normal lives.

Induced Labor

While formerly common practice, today it is rare that a doctor will choose to induce labor unless it is considered medically necessary for the health of mom and baby. Induced labor may occur in the following situations:
- Eclampsia/HELLP syndrome
- High serum creatinine levels
- Premature rupture of membranes (PROM)

- Thrombocytopenia
- Abnormal fetal growth
- 2 weeks past due date

Signs and Symptoms of Impending Labor

The following are signs and symptoms of impending labor:
1. Lightening: Also called engagement. Occurs when fetus moves into position for birth. Maternal breathing is easier after lightening, since it relieves pressure on the diaphragm. Other symptoms include lower extremity pain, pressure and leg cramping, a noted increase in the amount of pelvic discomfort and pressure felt, bilateral lower extremity edema related to the decreased return of blood flow to the heart.
2. Nesting: A subjective sign; the mother to be may experience a renewed energy. She may begin to clean and organize the baby's things, and have a sense of urgency to accomplish tasks before the baby arrives.
3. Braxton Hicks contractions: Consist of the irregular, discontinuous uterine contractions that should subside with rest. Braxton Hicks are termed "false labor" if the contractions are consistent. A vaginal exam may be required to differentiate between Braxton Hicks and true labor.
4. Cervical changes: As labor approaches, the cervix thins (called effacement) and the cervical os will begin to dilate.
5. Bloody show: The mucus plug that develops over the length of the pregnancy is released as the cervix thins. Once the presence of bloody show is evident, labor will proceed within 24 to 48 hours.
6. Rupture of membranes: When the bag of amniotic fluid that contains the fetus ruptures, labor traditionally results within 24 hours.

Stages of Labor

The stages of labor are as follows:
- Stage I: Starts with the beginning signs of labor and concludes at the time the cervix reaches a dilatation of 10 cm. Stage I labor consists of the latent phase, the active, and the transition phases.
  o Latent phase (cervix 1-3 cm; contractions 30-45 seconds/5-30 minutes apart): characterized by routine contractions and rupture of the membranes;
  o Active phase (cervix 4-7 cm; contractions 45-60 seconds/3-5 minutes apart): characterized by increased strength and frequency of contractions
  o Transition phase (cervix 8-10 cm; contractions 60-90 seconds/ 30 seconds-2 minutes apart): characterized by strong, frequent contractions and pressure in pelvis; anxiety and a sense of helplessness may be present.
- Stage II: Begins with complete dilatation and concludes with the birth of the baby. Fetal descent and crowning (baby's head becomes visible) takes place. As this stage progresses, the fetus changes position to accommodate birth. These changes of position are known as flexion, internal rotation, extension, restitution, external rotation, and expulsion.
- Stage III: Placenta seperates from the uterine wall / delivery of the placenta.
- Stage IV: Includes the first 4 hours post labor, in which the mother's body begins to return to its pre-pregnant state.

Variations Heard During Fetal Heart Rate Monitoring

During labor and delivery, it is common practice to monitor the fetal heart rate (FHR). The heart's rate and rhythm give the practitioner key information about the condition of the fetus. The following variations may be heard during fetal heart rate monitoring:
- Accelerations: The heart rate jumps up at random times during labor; also known as "variability" and is a normal and reassuring sign.
- Early decelerations: Slight dip in FHR at the beginning of contractions; due to head compression and is a reassuring sign.
- Late decelerations: A gradual decrease in fetal heart rate of 10-30 bpm, followed by a gradual return. They occur following a contraction, and signal decreased fetal oxygenation/ uteroplacental insufficiency.
- Variable decelerations: Random dips in fetal heart rate unrelated to contractions, with an abrupt onset and return. Variable decelerations are caused by umbilical cord compression. If they are rare and accompanied by variability, there is generally no cause for concern. However, persistent, deep, and long-lasting variable decelerations are nonreassuring.

*Interventions for late and variable decelerations are as follows:
1. Turn mother on her left side and apply manual pressure to baby's head
2. Apply 10L oxygen via facemask and stop oxytocin if infusing.
3. Call the MD.

> ➢ **Review Video:** <u>Fetal Heart Rate</u>
> *Visit **mometrix.com/academy** and enter **Code: 553173***

Fetal Tachycardia

Potential causes of fetal tachycardia are:
- Fetal hypoxia
- Maternal fever
- Hyperthyroidism
- Maternal or fetal anemia
- Drugs: atropine, hydroxyzine, terbutaline
- Chorioamnionitis
- Fetal heart arrhythmias
- Prematurity

Apgar score

The Apgar score is a universal tool used to determine the condition of the newborn at the time of birth. The Apgar score is taken 1 minute and 5 minutes after birth, with scores ranging from 0-10. Infants delivered by cesarean birth (C-section) will get an additional score 15 minutes after birth. The factors that make up the Apgar score include:
- Heart rate: 0, absent; 1, slow or below 100; 2, > 100
- Respiratory effort: 0, absent; 1, slow and irregular; 2, good, vigorous crying
- Muscle tone: 0, flaccid; 1, some extremity flexion; 2, active motion
- Reflex irritability: 0, none; 1, grimace; 2, vigorous cry

- Color: 0, pale blue; 1, body pink, extremities bluish; 2, completely pink

*Can be remembered by **APGAR**: **A**ppearance (color), **P**ulse (heart rate), **G**rimace (reflex), **A**ctivity (muscle tone), and **R**espirations.*

Variations in Coloring of Newborns

Healthy newborns have a characteristic pink flush to the skin. Any variation of this may indicate problems within the body.
- Ruddy (red) hues: increase in red blood cell concentration to the area; decreased amount of subcutaneous fat.
- Cyanotic at rest/pink during activity: may have a congenital defect known as choanal atresia (a blockage between the nose and pharynx).
- Cyanosis when crying: may signal cardio or pulmonary problems
- Pale: anemia; decreased fluid volumes.
- Acrocyanosis: transient, not normally a cause for concern; indicates normal pink coloring with bluish hands and feet.
- Harlequin sign: one side of the newborn's body red, other white; the result of vasodilatation, usually dissipates within a few hours.
- Jaundice: yellowish color noted at birth; caused by breakdown of red blood cells. Dissipates within the first 24 hours of birth; prolonged jaundice indicates liver dysfunction.

Newborn Reflexes

Common newborn reflexes include:
- Babinski: Toes should hyperextend if side of sole of foot stroked from heel to ball of foot.
- Blinking: Eyes should close if light flashed in eyes.
- Moro (startle): Infant should extend limbs and neck symmetrically and then pull back in response to loud noise or jolt.
- Palmar grasp: Infant should grasp finger if palm stroked.
- Rooting: Infant should open mouth and turn to the side of touch when the infant's cheek is stroked.
- Sucking: Infant should suck if mouth touched. Reflex may be weak in premature infants.
- Tonic neck (fencing): With infant lying flat and the head turned to one side, the infant should flex limbs on opposite side and extend limbs on the side to which head is turned.
- Trunk incurvation: With infant prone, stroking down one side of spine (1 inch from spine) should result in the pelvis turning to stroked side.
- Tongue extrusion: Infant should push tongue out of mouth if tip of tongue touched.

> ➢ **Review Video: Tonic Neck Response**
> *Visit **mometrix.com/academy** and enter **Code: 421866**

Prophylactic Measures

According to many state's laws, there are two different prophylactic (preventative) treatments that are given to all newborns delivered in the hospital setting.
1. Vitamin K shot: This is an intermuscular injection that provides a boost of vitamin K to the infant to prevent hemmorhage. At birth, the infant has little or no bacterial flora within the gastrointestinal tract that produce vitamin K, thus most newborns are deficient. Vitamin K is crucial to blood clotting, so this injection helps prevent hemmorhage and the resulting injury.
2. Antibiotic Eye Ointment: Newborns are also given prophylactic eye ointment to prevent blindness caused by exposure from the mother's vaginal tract to *Neisseria gonorrhoeae*. This ointment is given even if previous STI screening of the mother is clear. In order to be most effective, the ointment should be deposited directly in the lower conjunctival sac of both eyes shortly after birth.

Meconium Aspiration Syndrome

Meconium Aspiration Syndrome (MAS) is a syndrome caused by fetal asphyxia or intrauterine stress. It occurs when stress causes the relaxation of the anal sphincter of the infant, resulting in passage of meconium into amniotic fluid. This fluid is then breathed in by the infant, causing respiratory distress and compromise. Signs and symptoms include green-tinged skin/mucus of newborn; tachypneic; hypoxic; depressed; grunting; retractions; nasal flaring; hypothermic; hypoglycemic; hypocalcemic, quickly leads to respiratory failure. Treatment includes the following:
- Immediate suction, intubation and ventilator likely
- Broad-spectrum antibiotics to prevent infection likely
- Immediate transfer to Neonatal Intensive Care unit for monitoring.
- Surfactant replacement therapy
- Prevention:*Key*⋯→ Close monitoring for signs of fetal distress; caesarean delivery if indicated; suctioning as soon as head is through birth canal and chest still compressed to prevent inspiration of meconium may be effective, though not currently recommended.

Hypothermia

When infants are born, their thermoregulation system is still immature. This means that infants are especially susceptible to heat loss and subsequent hypothermia. There are generally four different types of heat loss that an infant can experience:
- Conduction is the flow of heat energy through direct contact from regions of warmer temperature (infant) to regions of cooler temperature (cold surfaces touching skin)
- Convection is the movement of heat by currents in the medium (such as wind [draft blowing over child's skin])
- Radiation is when heat is lost to cool objects near but not in contact with the infant (walls of crib, nearby objects)
- Evaporation occurs after bathing the infant or other times when water on the infant's skin evaporates, taking heat with it

Prevention includes the following:

- Do not place the infant's bare skin in contact with cool surfaces such as an uncovered table or tile flooring
- Protect infant from drafts from windows/air conditioning vents
- Keep temperature in nursery reasonably warm
- Dry infants thoroughly and quickly after baths/when wet.
- Note: Never cover infants with blankets during sleep (increased risk of SIDS)
- Skin-to-Skin contact is encouraged to promote heat regulation

Jaundice/Icterus

Jaundice/icterus (physiologic) is common in neonates after 2 days and is evident when bilirubin reaches 5 to 7 mg/dL. Jaundice should be assessed with transcutaneous or serum bilirubin measurements.

- Early onset/Breastfeeding-associated: Occurs within 1 week and relates to insufficient intake—the infant does not ingest enough colostrum, which helps expel meconium because of its laxative effect.
- Late-onset milk jaundice: Occurs after days 3 to 5 and may last up to 3 months. Cause is unknown but treatment is at least 8-12 feedings per day.
- Non-physiologic hyperbilirubinemia: Usually evident within first 24 hours and may result in acute bilirubin encephalopathy, leading to kernicterus (brain damage resulting from bilirubin in brain tissue). May result from hemolytic disease, infection, hypothyroidism, biliary atresia, and other congenital abnormalities.

The most common treatment for jaundice is phototherapy with the infant placed under fluorescent lights with eye coverings in place and wearing only a diaper. The bilirubin in the skin absorbs the light and converts into a water-soluble form that can be excreted in the urine.

Immune System of Neonates

Newborns are born with lower levels of immunity than typical adults. The alterations of the newborn's immune system make him/her vulnerable to infection and disease processes because the immune system does not readily recognize insidious bacteria. This is related to decreased levels of immunoglobulins and a decreased reaction of the complement system. Overall, this means that the newborn will not have the S&S of an infection found in an adult.

The following are signs a newborn may exhibit that indicate possible infection:
- The most reliable sign of infection or an infectious process in the neonate is hypothermia or an abnormally low body temperature.
- Poor feeding
- Difficulty breathing/periods of apnea
- Low heart rate
- Malaise
- Increased irritability, relentless crying
- Changes in skin color/jaundice

Aortic Coarctation

Aortic coarctation is a birth defect in which the aorta has a narrowed point of variable severity. This leads to serious reduction in cardiac output, and can cause complications if not recognized and treated. These patients are at a greatly increased risk of stroke, heart failure, aortic or cerebral aneurysm, and aortic dissection. Signs and symptoms are as follows:

- Infants: irritability, poor feeding, S&S of heart failure, diaphoresis
- Adults: nose bleeding, fainting, dyspnea on exertion, headaches

Diagnosis is based on marked blood pressure difference between arms and legs, ultrasound, echocardiogram, CT, MRI, ECG, chest x-ray, and cardiac catheterization. Treatment includes:

- Infants only: prostaglandin E to keep ductus arteriosus open (allows bypass of the narrowed areas)
- Blood pressure medications (before surgery)
- Balloon angioplasty/stenting
- Open heart surgery

Circumcision

Circumcision is the surgical removal of the prepuce (epithelial tissue sometimes termed "foreskin") from the tip or head of the penis. Formerly, circumcision was common practice and thought to reduce the risk of penile cancer and STIs in males and their female partners. However, there is debate as to whether these benefits are true. It is also a religious practice of the Jewish culture, being performed by their priest on the eighth day following birth. However, in the hospital, circumcision is an optional procedure, and usually takes place a few days after birth. This procedure should not be performed in infants with an increased risk of bleeding, those with hypo/hyperspadias, or medically unstable/premature infants. There is a small risk of infection or bleeding. For the procedure, the head of the penis is anesthezised and the child is restrained. A ring/clamp is attached to the end of the penis, and the foreskin is removed. The penis is coated with petroleum jelly and wrapped in loose guaze. It should heal within a week. The nurse should educate the parents that while some bleeding should be expected, any increased redness, foul-smelling or purlulent discharge, or fever in the infant should be reported immediately.

Newborn Assessment

The head-to-toe assessment of newborns is explained as follows:

- Head/Face: Circumference 32-38 cm. Sutures palpable with small separations noted. Anterior fontanel diamond-shaped and 4-5 cm and soft. Posterior fontanel triangle-shaped 0.5-1 cm. Molding may result in overriding sutures. Note caput succedaneum (crosses suture lines) or cephalhematoma. Facial features symmetrical.
- Chest: Circumference 2-3 cm less than head circumference. Chest movements during respirations symmetrical. Note sternal retraction, periods of apnea.
- Abdomen: Rounded and soft with bowel sounds. Note distention, masses, and abdominal wall defects. Umbilical cord should have 3 vessels.
- Genitalia: Females—labia majora cover clitoris and labia minora. Male—testes should be within scrotal sac, rugae on scrotum, and urinary meatus at the end of the penis.

- Back: Anus present and open. Back closed and no abnormalities felt in vertebral column.
- Extremities: Equal in size and shape, bilateral movements, flexed, good muscle tone, gluteal and thigh creases equal, two transverse palm creases, and feet in normal position.
- Vital signs: Axillary 36.5°C to 37.3°C, heart rate 120 to 160 bpm when awake and not crying, respirations 30 to 60 per minute with symmetric chest movement and clear breath sounds, BP 65-95/30-60 mm Hg.

Lochia

After labor, a woman will have continuous discharge as the uterus sheds the pregnancy lining and returns to its original state. This discharge is known as lochia, and may last 5 to 6 weeks.
- Lochia Rubra: Occurs 1-3 days postpartum; heavy flow, bright red and may have clots.
- Lochia Serosa: Occurs 3-10 days postpartum, appears brown-pink.
- Lochia Alba: Starts around postpartum day 10, lasting for 2-6 weeks; it is yellow in color

Postpartum Depression

Postpartum depression (PPD) is an episode of depression related to the birth of a child. PPD may begin during pregnancy, but onset is most common within the first 2 weeks to 3 months after delivery, although it may occur up to 1 year after. The cause is not clear but risk factors include first pregnancy; history of depression, alcoholism, or mental disorder; low self-esteem; hormonal imbalances, marital difficulties; lack of sleep; and chronic stress. Signs and symptoms include depressed mood with loss of emotional response and inability to respond with pleasure to the infant. Some patients may express dislike or hatred for the infant. Sleep disturbance and fatigue is common. Patients may feel anger, anxiety, or shame. Ensure the safety of the infant even if that means removing the infant from the mother's care. Patients may need psychotherapy and medications, such as SSRIs or TCAs, as well as emotional support of family and friends.

Sheehan syndrome

Sheehan syndrome is hypopituitarism caused by uterine hemorrhage during childbirth. The blood loss, hypotension, and resulting hypoxemia cause the pituitary gland to cease to function. The onset of symptoms may be rapid, or take years to develop. Sheehan syndrome is more commonly seen in underdeveloped countries. Signs and symptoms include amenorrhea, fatigue, unable to breast-feed baby, anxiety, decreased BP, hair loss, hypothyroidism, and decreased libido. Diagnosis is based on CT/MRI scan of pituitary gland, blood levels, and pituitary hormone stimulation test. Treatment includes:
- Life-long hormone therapy to replace lost hormones; may include levothyroxine, estrogen, growth hormone, and corticosteriods
- Prevention: early recognition and treatment of blood loss in post-partum period.

Rubin's Theory of Postpartum Phases

Reva Rubin discusses and theorizes the biopsychosocial experience of childbirth. The postpartum phases according to Rubin include:

1. Taking in: First 2 to 3 days following labor. This is a time in which the mother begins to claim her baby, and regenerate herself from childbirth. This is a period of rest and acquaintance for the neonate and the mother. The nurse should encourage the mother to reflect and verbalize her labor and delivery experience during this time.
2. Taking hold: Day 3 to Week 2. The mother begins to feel more autonomous and require less assistance from those around her, dominating the care of the infant. The mother's own bodily functions should be returning to normal during this period. Mothers in the "taking hold" phase are very sensitive to the care of the infant and insist they want everything to be done right. The nurse should praise the mother during this phase if they have the opportunity, and should educate the family on offering praise to new mothers.
3. Letting go: Week 2-3. The mother begins to see the infant as a separate entity from self. Until this point the mother may have felt guilt when separated from her infant and may grieve over this separation. The "letting go" phase is a time of returning to pre-pregnancy norms.

Breastfeeding Benefits

The following are health benefits of breastfeeding for mom and baby:
- Enhanced immune system and resistance to infection
- Breast milk contains antibodies to help protect infants from bacteria and viruses; this also helps with response to immunizations
- A mother's milk is nutritionally complete, perfectly balanced for baby's growth and development.
- Most babies find it easier to digest breast milk than formula.
- Nursing burns calories, making it easier to lose pregnancy weight. Immediately after birth, breastfeeding causes the uterine to clamp down, helping prevent hemorrhage.
- Breastfeeding lowers the risk of breast and ovarian cancers.

Mastitis

Mastitis is a common infection and inflammation of the breast due to bacteria, often *S. aureus*. Risk factors for mastitis include sudden cessation of breastfeeding, poor hygiene, prior colonization with *S. aureus*, and broken skin on the breast. It is important to note that doctors often recommend that a mother continue to breastfeed, despite the infection. Symptoms include fever, nipple pain/discharge, breast pain/swelling, and pain with breastfeeding. Diagnosis is based on physical examination, culture of breast milk, and rarely mammogram to rule out more serious cause of inflammation (breast cancer). Treatment consists of:
- Medications: oral antibiotics, pain relievers (Tylenol/Ibuprofen)
- Lifestyle Modification: moist heat, breastfeed often/change positions frequently, rest, increase fluids, wash nipples with plain water and allow to air dry to prevent cracking/drying.

Hypocalcemia in Newborns

Hypocalcemia is defined as a serum calcium level of less than 7.0 mg/dL in an infant. The normal range is 7.0-8.5 mg/dL. It can be of either early or late onset; either way, hypocalcemia should be recognized and treated immediately to prevent potential complications. High levels of phosphate can also cause hypocalcemia, due to the inverse relationship of phosphorus and calcium in the body. Early-onset hypocalcemia appears in first 24-48 hours. It is generally temporary and resolves on its own. It is most common in preterm/SGA infants, hypoxic infants, or infants born to a diabetic mother. Late-onset hypocalcemia appears after 3-4 days of life; also known as cow's milk-induced hypocalcemia or neonatal tetany. It is common with intestinal malabsorption, hyperinsulinemia, hypoparathyroidism, hypomagnesemia, or with phosphate enemas. Signs and symptoms of hypocalcemia are as follows:

- Jittery
- Long QT interval
- Apnea
- Cyanosis
- High-pitched cry/ neuromuscular irritation
- Abdominal distension

Treatment includes:

- Correction of underlying cause: switch formula, treat hypoparathyroidism or hypomagnesia, and feed often.
- IV calcium gluconate 10%-very slowly
  - o monitoring heart and BP; also monitor for seizures
  - o IV site for infiltration: necrotic to tissues
- Monitor for signs of hypercalcemia such as vomiting or bradycardia

Assessment of pediatric vital signs

Pediatric vital signs vary according to the age of the child:

- Temperature: rectal, axillary, or tympanic temperatures should be taken on small children, with oral temperatures reserved for older children and adolescents. Temperatures vary from about 36.3°C to 37.6°C (oral). Axillary temperatures run about 1 degree less and rectal temperatures 1 degree more.
- Blood pressure: An appropriately sized cuff is essential to accuracy, and auscultation should be used for assessment. The pulse may remain audible from the systolic reading to 0, so the diastolic reading is the point the sound changes. BP varies widely by age and gender, increasing as the child ages. The nurse should refer to a blood pressure chart for specific ranges.
- Heart rate: Heart rate should be assessed by auscultation with the child at rest if possible; heart rate increases in response to stress. Newborns, 100-150; infants to 2 years, 80-120; ages 2-6, 70-110; ages 6-10, 60-95; and age 10-16; 60-85.
- Respirations: Newborns, 30-55; 1 year, 25-40; 3 years, 20-30; 6 years, 16-22; 10 years, 16-20; and 17 years, 12-18.

Pain Response & Physiological Needs in Infants and Children

Because of communication barriers, infants and young children respond differently to pain than adults. The nurse needs to be aware of these variations in order to effectively care for this population:

- 47 -

- Young infant's response to pain:
  - Generalized response of rigidity, thrashing
  - Loud crying/ facial expressions of pain (grimace)
  - Do not understand stimuli-pain relationship; FLACC scale
- Older infant's response to pain:
  - Withdrawal from painful stimuli
  - Loud crying /facial grimace,
  - Physical resistance; FLACC
- Young child's response to pain:
  - Loud crying, screaming
  - Verbalizations: "Ow," "Ouch," "It hurts"; Faces scale
  - Thrashing of limbs/attempts to push away stimulus
- School-age child's response to pain:
  - Stalling behavior ("wait a minute"); Faces or Numerical scale
  - Muscle rigidity
  - May use all behaviors of young child
- Adolescent:
  - Less vocal protest/motor activity; increased muscle rigidity
  - Verbalizes pain ("it hurts" or "you're hurting me"); Numeric scale

Hospitalization is a stressful time for infants and young children. It is not uncommon for them to experience stress and *regression*, a coping mechanism in which the child returns to previous developmental stage. The nurse needs to be cognizant of the child's specific needs to better anticipate problems arising from loss of control and to mitigate its effects:
- Infants' needs:
  - Trust, consistent loving caregivers, daily routines
  - Loss of Control: agitation, malaise/failure to thrive (FTT)
- Toddlers' needs:
  - Autonomy, daily routines and rituals,
  - Loss of control: regression, negativity, temper tantrums
- Preschoolers' needs:
  - Egocentric and magical thinking, imaginative play, creativity
  - Loss of control: May view illness/hospitalization as punishment for misdeeds; fear mutilation
- School Age' needs:
  - Independence and productivity, feeling of control over self.
  - Loss of Control: Fears of death, abandonment, boredom
- Adolescent needs:
  - Independence/ liberation, connection with peer group, information about condition (talk to as an adult)
  - Loss of Control: anger, frustration, feelings of isolation

Developmental Milestones

Developmental milestones in fine and gross motor abilities are as follows:
- By end 2 years old:
  - Fine motor skills - Able to build a block tower to height of at least 4 blocks, able to hold a crayon or pencil and scribble on paper, and able to throw a ball. Able to remove clothes.

- o   Gross motor skills - Able to run and climb and descend stairs.
- Ages 2 to 3 years:
  - o   Fine motor skills - Able to draw rudimentary forms, such as circles, and can pour liquids and start to dress self.
  - o   Gross motor skills - Able to kick, jump, and throw ball overhand.
- Ages 3 to 6 years:
  - o   Fine motor skills - Able to use scissors, draw multiple shapes, and draw a 6-part human (stick figure). Learning to tie shoes and can button clothes and brush teeth. Enjoys doing arts and crafts projects.
  - o   Gross motor skills - Can climb, ride tricycle, and throw overhand.
- Ages 6 to 12 years:
  - o   Fine motor skills - Does more complex craft project, plays cards and board games.
  - o   Gross motor skills - Rides 2-wheel bicycle and can jump rope, roller skate/ice skate.
- Ages 12 to 18 years:
  - o   Fine motor skills - Can write, draw, and manipulate tools easily.
  - o   Gross motor skills - Engages in sports activities, such as team sports.

Developmentally Age-Appropriate Toys

The following are the best toys for different ages of children:
- 0 to 3 months: Infants enjoy mobiles, mirrors, and music players.
- 3 to 6 months: Infant begins grasping toys, such as rattles and small stuffed animals.
- 6 to 9 months: Infant begins to mouth items, so enjoys teething toys and soft stuffed animals.
- 9 to 12 months: Infant starts to enjoy blocks, pop-up toys, push and pull toys, toys that make noises.
- 2 to 3 years: The child is more engaged in play and enjoys heavy paper or cloth books, stuffed animals, dolls, toy cars and trucks, large wooden puzzles, toys they can manipulate, paper and large crayons, and household items (pans, spoons, dishes).
- 3 to 5 years: The child enjoys manipulating things such as dolls, cars and trucks, doll houses, building materials (such as Legos) and blocks, pens, paper, glue, balls, and dress-up materials.
- 6 to 12 years: The child enjoys bicycles, jump ropes, puzzles, board games, craft projects, roller skates, skateboards, and electronic games.

Theories of Developmental Psychologists

Freud's psychosexual stages of development
Three forces in humans: 1) Id: - unconscious/pleasure; 2) Ego: conscious/ reality; 3) Superego: conscience/ideals
- Oral : Birth to 18 months : Weaning
- Anal: 18 months – 3 y : Potty Training
- Phallic: 3-6 y: Sexual discovery
- Latent: 6 y - puberty: Learning/pause in sexual learning
- Genital: Puberty through adulthood: Sexual Relationships

Erik Erikson's stages of psychosocial development
- Trust vs. Mistrust (birth - 1 y)
- Autonomy vs. Shame and doubt (1 - 3 y)
- Initiative vs. Guilt (3 - 6 y)
- Industry vs. Inferiority (~6 - 12 y)
- Identity vs. Role confusion (~12 - 18 y)
- Intimacy vs. Isolation (~19 - 35 y)
- Generativity vs. Stagnation (~35 – 65 y)
- Ego Integrity vs. Despair (~65 – death)

Jean Piaget's stages of cognitive development
- Sensorimotor/Intuitive (birth to 2 y)
- Pre-operational (2 - 7 y)
- Concrete operational (7 - 11 y)
- Formal operational (12 y - adulthood)

Developmental Stages & Milestones: Infants

An infant (0-12 months) is in a period of intense cognitive and physical development:
- Biologic development:
  - Weight Gain: tripled since birth
  - Height: birth length increased by 50%
  - Growth: Head-to-toe development (termed *cephalocaudal*)
- Motor development:
  - 2-3 months: grasping objects, lift head (prone), social smile
  - 4-6 months: rolling over, sitting up alone, bringing object to mouth; holding own bottle; recognizes mother, likes/dislikes.
  - 6-7 months: crawling, transfer objects between hands; may begin to imitate sounds; stranger anxiety, responds to name.
  - 9-10 months: "creeping," pincher grasp, prone to sitting; hand preference; says "mama" and "dada"; waves "goodbye"
  - 11-12 months: block tower of 2, walking, removing objects from containers; shakes head yes/no, 5-word vocabulary
- Cognitive development:
  - Piaget: Sensory Motor / Intuitive thought: only aware of what is happening directly around them. No understanding of relationship between events.
  - Erikson: "Trust vs. Mistrust"
  - Freud: Oral – Nursing/Weaning
- Vision development:
  - Birth to 4 months: Able to see patterns of light, dark, and shades of gray. Focus is mere 8 to 12 inches, resulting in mostly blurred vision.
  - 4 to 6 months: As babies learn to push themselves up, roll over, sit, and scoot, eye/body coordination develops as they learn to control their own movements in space. Normal visual acuity, or a child's sharpness of vision, has usually developed to 20/20 by the time the child reaches 6 months.
  - 6 to 8 months: Most babies start crawling during this time, further developing eye/body coordination. They learn to judge distances and set visual goals, seeing something and moving to get it. Depth perception should be developing around this time

- 50 -

- o 8 to 12 months: Babies can now judge distances well. Eye/hand/body coordination allows them to grasp and throw objects fairly accurately.

Developmental Stages & Milestones: Toddlers

The toddler years (12-36 months) is an intense period of exploration using all senses, temper tantrums, fierce independence (prefer finger foods to feed themselves; give choices), and ritualistic needs (need routine).
- Biologic development
  - o Weight Gain: slows to 4-6 lb/year (4x birth weight by 2 years)
  - o Height: 3 inches per year
  - o Growth is "step-like" rather than "linear"
- Maturation of systems
  - o Physiologic systems relatively mature at end of toddlerhood
  - o Upper respiratory infections, otitis media, and tonsillitis are common among toddlers
  - o Sphincter control - age 18-24 months (anal – potty training)
  - o Locomotion - improved coordination, between ages 2-3, fine motor development. Learns spatial relationships
  - o Improved manual dexterity, throws ball by age 18 months; push/pull toys the best; parallel play seen.
- Cognitive development
  - o Piaget: sensorimotor and preoperational phase = awareness of causal relationships between two events; trial and error.
  - o Erikson: "Autonomy vs. Shame and Doubt"
  - o Freud: Anal Stage – Potty Training

Developmental Stages & Milestones: Preschoolers

The preschooler (3-5 years) exhibits increased attention span and memory and is highly literal (uses language for mental symbolization). Their greatest fear is body mutilation, and they have poorly defined body boundaries and fear that if skin is "broken" all blood and "insides" can leak out. Use dolls and play therapy to explain procedures to preschoolers.
- Biologic development
  - o Weight: 4-5 lb/year.
  - o Height: 2-3 inches/year.
- Motor development
  - o Fine motor: refinement in eye-hand and muscle coordination, drawing, art work, skillful manipulation.
  - o Gross motor: walking, running, climbing, and jumping well established.
  - o Associative/cooperative play; imaginative playmates, enjoys dress up, imitation; dramatic play without rules.
- Cognitive development
  - o Piaget: Preoperative; no concept of time/conversation. Egocentric.
  - o Erikson: "Initiative vs. Guilt"
  - o Freud: Phallic - Oedipus (male)/Electra(female) complex (attached to parent of opposite sex)

Developmental Stages & Milestones: School-Aged Children

The developmental stages and cognitive and physical milestones of the school aged child (6–11 years) are as follows:

- Developing sense of self-worth; praise is vital to avoid feelings of inferiority. Detail-oriented. Wants to get things right.
- Enjoy competitive games, physical activities (bike riding, etc.). Often plays with same sex, creates clubs.
- Inquisitive: Asks many questions, wants to know how things work. Enjoys memorization.
- Biologic development:
  o Weight: gain ~5 lb/year
  o Height: increase ~2 inches/year
  o Adult teeth come in; muscular strength and physical skills increase
- Motor development:
  o Fine motor skills refined; can complete arts/craft projects without difficulty – adult level ~12 years. Dressing self/completely capable of self-care.
  o Gross motor –rapid increase in coordination/motor control.
  o Verbal: Can read simple sentences. Vocabulary – 2500 words
- Cognitive development:
  o Piaget: Concrete Operational – literal thinkers, but able to see other's viewpoints and discern different tenses; able to organize.
  o Erikson: "Industry vs. Inferiority"
  o Freud: Latent – focus on cognitive learning, pause in sexual exploits.

Developmental Stages & Milestones: Adolescents

Adolescents (12-18 years):

- Time of sexual maturation and social development
- Emphasis on social events: enjoy team sports, social outings, and connection with peers. Biggest fear is social rejection.
- Begin to view self as separate from parents, values autonomy; may manifest in periods of rebellion of parents' rules.
- Biologic development
  o Weight: gain 15-60 lb by end of adolescence
  o Height: 2-12 inches of increase by age 18.
  o Maturation of sexual organs: females - develop breasts and begin menses; males - enlargement and maturation of penis and testes. Other secondary sexual characteristics develop.
  o Body image highly important to adolescents.
  o Increased activity of sebaceous glands produces acne.
- Motor development
  o Emphasis on physical activities
  o May have some clumsiness in early teenage years
  o Adult-level motor control ~15 years of age.

- Cognitive development
  - Piaget: Formal operational: adult level reasoning, able to handle abstract thoughts; can hypothesize and use inductive and deductive reasoning.
  - Erikson: "Identity vs. Social Isolation"
  - Freud: Genital – sexual relationships developed.

Intellectual Disability

There are four levels of intellectual disability (formerly known as mental retardation):
1. Mild intellectual disability: IQ of 52 to 69; This individual will achieve a mental age of 8 to 12 years, can learn daily living activities, elementary-level communication skills, and be able to function with minimal vocational skills to provide self-care and maintenance.
2. Moderate intellectual disability: IQ of 36 to 51; This individual will achieve a mental age between 3 and 7 years, has noted developmental delays, shows simple communication skills, and can learn self-help skills.
3. Severe intellectual disability: IQ of 20 to 35 ; This individual will have the mental age of a toddler, marked developmental delay, and little or no communication ability. They can learn repetition related to activities. This individual must be supervised continuously with self-protective mechanisms in place.
4. Profound intellectual disability: IQ ≤19; This individual will have the mental age of an infant, obvious developmental delays in all aspects of life, and require total care.

Tanner Staging

Tanner Staging is used to describe sexual maturation of preadolescents and adolescents:
- Males - Stages of pubic hair and external genital development include:
  1. Preadolescent: no changes.
  2. Scrotum and testes begin to enlarge, pubic hair at base of penis.
  3. Penis lengthens, scrotum enlarges, and more darkly pigmented pubic hair.
  4. Penis continues to grow, pubic hair more extensive, scrotum more pigmented.
  5. Pubic hair spreads to thighs, scrotum enlarges, and penis extends to bottom of scrotum.
- Females:
  - Stages of breast development :
    1. Only nipple raised above chest.
    2. Breast budding.
    3. Breast and areola enlarge.
    4. Areola enlarges and may form a secondary elevation.
    5. Full breasts with pigmented areola and projecting nipples.
  - Stages of pubic hair
    1. No pubic hair.
    2. Soft downy hair along labia majora.
    3. Sparse dark hair along the labia majora.
    4. Heavy coarse pubic hair about labia majora.
    5. V. Adult distribution of pubic hair extending laterally and superiorly.

- 53 -

Sexual Maturation in Adolescent Females

Sexual maturation in girls begins between the ages of 9 and 13. During this time, a woman will reach her peak height. The first sign of puberty in girls is the development of breast tissue. Other signs include:
- Appearance of pubic hair
- Increase in vaginal discharge (physiologic leukorrhea)
- Menarche: occurs approximately 2 years after breast buds. The average age of menarche is about 12½ years, but can occur any time between the ages of 10 and 15. While it is still unknown what exactly causes menstruation to begin, it is theorized that it is related to body fat percentage, with some genetic and nutritional components.

Nursing interventions include the following:
- Sexual education, with stress on birth control methods and normal menstruation.
- Nurse should suspect the need for further follow-up if no breast development by age 13 or no menarche within 4 years of onset of puberty.
- Ensure proper nutrition, emphasizing iron to prevent menarche-related anemia and calcium for bone health.

Sexual Maturation in Adolescent Males

Sexual maturation and puberty begin in boys between the ages of 10 and 14. During this time, a male will reach 20% to 25% of lean body mass and gain up to 50% ideal adult body weight. Boys often experience "growth spurts," which refer to general increase in growth of skeleton, muscles, and internal organs, which reaches peak at ~14 years of age. The first noted change signaling the beginning of sexual maturation is testicular enlargement accompanied by thinning, reddening, and increased looseness of the scrotum. Other signs include:
- Appearance of pubic and facial hair
- Voice changes
- Gynecomastia: temporary breast enlargement and tenderness may occur, ceasing after 2 years
- Ejaculation occurs more frequently, either spontaneously as a "wet dream" or via self-stimulation

Nursing interventions include:
- Sexual education, including ejaculation to allay embarrassment and fears regarding newfound sexuality
- Ensure proper nutrition, emphasizing protein for increased rate of growth

Breast Self-Examination

Breast self-examination should begin when patients are in their 20s and should ideally be performed monthly after menses when breasts are less tender (on day 5 to 7 with day 1 the first day of menses) or at any time in the month for postmenopausal women. Patients should begin by examining the breasts in a mirror to note any changes, such as skin dimpling, contour changes, discolorations, skin retractions, or nipple discharge. They should note any venous prominence, nipple inversion, or peau d'orange (orange peel appearance of tissue). Any abnormalities should be reported to their physician. The patient should palpate the breast when in supine position with the arm on the side examined extended above the head. The patient may use a circular, wedge, or vertical strip palpation pattern. If patients have had previous breast surgery, they should be advised to examine remaining breast tissue and the chest wall for any nodules or changes. Males who are at risk of breast cancer should also be advised to do monthly breast examinations.

Testicular Self-Examination

Testicular self-examination should begin during adolescence and should be carried out monthly, usually after a warm shower or bath because the scrotal tissue is more relaxed. The patient should hold the penis to the opposite side of the testes being examined. Steps include:
- Palpating the testicles with both hands to determine if they are smooth and uniform in size, shape, and consistency. It is not uncommon for one testis to be longer or larger than the other, but changes should be noted.
- Rolling the testes gently horizontally back and forth (thumb on top and fingers below) to feel for any abnormalities, such as lumps.
- Rolling the testes gently vertically in the same procedure as above.
- Using the index finger, palpate the epididymis, which is a cordlike structure superior and posterior to each testicle, and the spermatic cord on both testes.

Patients should be advised to report any changes, swelling, or lumps.

Normal Physiological Changes Experienced By Older Adults

With age, the human body begins to slow down, and the metabolic processes become slower and less effective at repairing age-related damage. The following are expected changes in the physical assessment of the older adult:
- Neurological: Decreased acuity of hearing/vision/smell; some mild memory loss, especially short-term memory, is common.
- Cardiac: Decreased elasticity of heart and blood vessels; anemia.
- Pulmonary: Decreased lung capacity. Weakened cough/gag reflex.
- Gastrointestinal: Decreased taste, peristalsis, and digestive enzyme production. Dry mouth. Increased occurrence of constipation; increase of fat-muscle ratio.
- Genitourinary: Decreased bladder capacity; genital atrophy.
- Integumentary: Decreased skin elasticity; dry skin common.
- Musculoskeletal: Decreased bone density, decreased balance and muscle strength. Increased fat-muscle ratio.

"Everything slows and decreases, except for fat."

Developmental tasks of older adults

Erikson's Psychosocial Theory of Development states that the older adults (65 years and older) are in the stage of "Ego Integrity vs. Despair." The older adult is adjusting to new situations including economic, social, familial, and sexual changes that occur with age. If the older adult comes to a place of accepting the aging process and looking back on their life with a feeling of accomplishment and gratefulness, they have completed the task of ego integrity. However, if he/she fails to accomplish this task, the person will experience despair. Common fears of the older adult include death, becoming a burden to their family, inability to care for themselves, and loss of self among others.

Menopause

Menopause is the permanent termination of the menstrual cycle, considered a normal process of aging. Menopause may also be caused by ovarian failure or hysterectomy; however, traditionally menopause begins on its own around age 50 for most women. Signs and symptoms include cessation of menstruation, insomnia, hot flashes/night sweats (vasomotor instability), and mood changes such as nervousness, irritability, anxiety, and depression. Due to the lack of estrogen production, women also often experience atrophy of the urogenital epithelium and surrounding skin. Diagnosis is based on age, physical exam, and blood hormone levels. Treatment includes:
- Medications: hormone replacement therapy (HRT) if desired
- Symptom management: fans/light clothing for hot flashes, counseling for mood swings, vaginal lubricant for painful coitus.

Levels of Disease Prevention

Levels of disease prevention include:
- Primary: The goal is to prevent the initial occurrence of a health problem, such as a disease or injury, through activities such as immunizations, smoking cessation, fluoride supplementation of water, promotion of seat belt use, and use of child car seat restraints. Interventions are often aimed at the general public or large groups of people.
- Secondary: The goal is to identify diseases or conditions quickly and provide prompt intervention for treatment and prevention of further disability through such activities as BP screenings, breast and testicular self-examinations, hearing and vision screenings, mammography, and pregnancy testing.
- Tertiary: The goal is to assist those who already have disease or disability to prevent further progress of the disease and to allow people to achieve the maximum quality of life through activities such as support groups, counseling, diet and exercise, stress management, and supportive services.

Childhood Immunization Schedule

Vaccines are one of the first lines of defense against infectious diseases in the community. Study the following graph carefully to understand the current vaccine schedule recommended for all children in the U.S by the CDC.

Note: Remember that live vaccines should never be given to those that are immunocompromised, and an egg allergy is a contraindication to the flu vaccine.

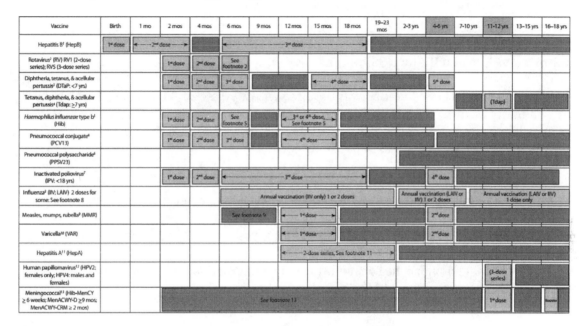

Vaccine	Birth	1 mo	2 mos	4 mos	6 mos	9 mos	12 mos	15 mos	18 mos	19–23 mos	2-3 yrs	4-6 yrs	7-10 yrs	11-12 yrs	13–15 yrs	16–18 yrs
Hepatitis B[1] (HepB)	1st dose	←——— 2nd dose ———→			←———————————— 3rd dose ————————————→											
Rotavirus[2] (RV) RV1 (2-dose series); RV5 (3-dose series)			1st dose	2nd dose	See footnote 2											
Diphtheria, tetanus, & acellular pertussis[3] (DTaP: <7 yrs)			1st dose	2nd dose	3rd dose		←—— 4th dose ——→					5th dose				
Tetanus, diphtheria, & acellular pertussis[4] (Tdap: ≥7 yrs)														(Tdap)		
Haemophilus influenzae type b[5] (Hib)			1st dose	2nd dose	See footnote 5		3rd or 4th dose, See footnote 5									
Pneumococcal conjugate[6] (PCV13)			1st dose	2nd dose	3rd dose		←——— 4th dose ———→									
Pneumococcal polysaccharide[6] (PPSV23)																
Inactivated poliovirus[7] (IPV: <18 yrs)			1st dose	2nd dose	←——————————— 3rd dose ———————————→							4th dose				
Influenza[8] (IIV; LAIV) 2 doses for some: See footnote 8					Annual vaccination (IIV only) 1 or 2 doses						Annual vaccination (LAIV or IIV) 1 or 2 doses		Annual vaccination (LAIV or IIV) 1 dose only			
Measles, mumps, rubella[9] (MMR)					See footnote 9		←—— 1st dose ——→					2nd dose				
Varicella[10] (VAR)							←—— 1st dose ——→					2nd dose				
Hepatitis A[11] (HepA)							←——— 2-dose series, See footnote 11 ———→									
Human papillomavirus[12] (HPV2: females only; HPV4: males and females)														(3-dose series)		
Meningococcal[13] (Hib-MenCY ≥ 6 weeks; MenACWY-D ≥9 mos; MenACWY-CRM ≥ 2 mos)							See footnote 13							1st dose		Booster

From: http://www.cdc.gov/vaccines/schedules/downloads/child/0-18yrs-schedule-bw.pdf

Nutritional Assessment

Nutritional assessments are the first step in determining a well-balanced diet that will promote optimal nutrition, body function, and healing processes. A nutritional assessment is performed for patients when there is a suspicion of nutritional imbalance/a change in health status that will require a change in dietary habits. If done correctly, a nutritional assessment will provide information on the amount of vitamins and minerals an individual is consuming on a routine basis; this information is then evaluated and compared with what is required to function with or without the individual disease processes the patient has. Nutritional assessments can be done quickly by reviewing a client's history during the initial assessment. If a more in-depth nutritional history is required, a practitioner may ask the individual to track dietary intake over a period of several days with a food diary or other tool, then go over the information with the client at a subsequent visit. If further evaluation is desired, a blood test may give a better clinical picture. Serum albumin (not weight) is the best clinical indicator of nutritional status (malnourishment). This means a person can be overweight/obese and still be considered malnourished.

BMI

Body mass index (BMI) is a method of measurement that includes the height and weight of an individual to help determine his/her nutritional status. The body mass index is determined by dividing the weight in kilograms by the height in meters squared. The preferred range for BMI for the adult is 18-25 kg/m². A BMI of ≤18 is considered underweight; a body mass index of greater than 25 designates the individual as overweight. A body mass index of ≥ 30 is considered obese.

$$BMI = \frac{mass_{kg}}{height_m^2} = \frac{mass_{lb}}{height_{in}^2} \; x \; 703$$

USDA's MyPlate and Dietary Guidelines

In 2011, the USDA's Food Pyramid was replaced with MyPlate. MyPlate consists of a picture of a dinner plate divided into four sections. Vegetables and grains each take up 30% of the plate, while fruits and proteins each constitute 20% of the plate. There is also a representation of a cup, marked Dairy, alongside the plate.

The USDA's guidelines can be easily summarized:
- To maintain or improve weight, individuals need to preserve a balance between exercise and food consumption.
- Individuals should choose to consume a diverse diet high in grains, fresh fruits, and vegetables.
- Diets that minimize the consumption of sodium, sugars, fats/cholesterol, and alcohol are recommended.

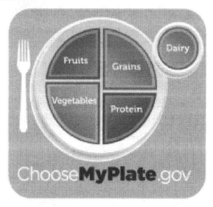

Dietary Standards

Dietary standards are a set of guidelines in which an individual can understand essential nutrients, food consumption, and the relationship they possess. Not only do dietary standards increase understanding of foods and their nutritional values, they offer a mechanism of comparison. The *Recommended Dietary Allowances (RDAs)* are a set of standards the federal government mandates that each individual needs on a daily basis to maintain balanced and adequate nutrition. *Reference Dietary Intake (RDI)* is a combination of recommended daily allowances and mechanisms of risk reduction for diseases such as coronary artery disease, obesity, cancer, and osteoporosis. The dietary standards of RDA and RDI are used today with meal preparation for military personnel, groups such as WIC (Women, Infants, and Children), and meals on wheels programs throughout the country.

- 58 -

Food groups & Recommended Daily Servings

The following are the five main food groups and the recommended daily serving for each:
- Grains (6-11 servings) - Foods in this category include rice, cereals, breads, and pasta.
- Fruits (2-4 servings) - Foods in this category include apples, bananas, grapes, and oranges.
- Vegetables (3-5 servings) - Foods in this category include green beans, corn, potatoes, and lettuce.
- Proteins (2-3 servings) - Foods in this category include beef, legumes, chicken, fish, turkey, and pork; also includes eggs and nuts.
- Dairy (2-3 servings) - Foods in this category include milk, cheese, and yogurt.

Other foods/added fats
Foods in this category include soda, candy, and processed snack foods. There is no recommended daily allowance for these foods; the USDA recommends they be limited as they generally have no nutritional value.

Nutrients

Nutrients are generally divided into six categories: carbohydrates, vitamins, proteins, minerals, lipids (fats), and water. Nutrients are further classified as either essential or nonessential, which refer to the body's ability to produce the needed nutrient. For example, essential nutrients are nutrients that must be obtained through diet. These essential nutrients are required by the body on a daily basis for growth and health maintenance. Nonessential nutrients are those nutrients the body is capable of producing on its own. The following are function of nutrients:
- Lipids (fats), Proteins, and Carbohydrates: provide energy for body functions, aid in tissue growth.
- Vitamins: perform in a catalytic role to promote the use of nutrients for energy.
- Water and Minerals: Tissue repair and function; body temperature regulation.

The following are the four main types of nutrients required by the human body and age-related concerns with these nutrients:
- Carbohydrates: 1 gram = 4 calories; Minimum recommended daily intake is 50-100 g/day. At least 50% of total calories should come from complex carbohydrate sources. Daily recommended fiber intake is 20-35 grams; fiber needs increase with aging to combat the constipation that often accompanies the slowing of the GI tract.
- Protein: 1 gram = 4 calories; 1-1.8 g pro/kg body weight per day for healthy adults; 12%-14% of total calories; increased need with disease processes/wound healing. Elderly patients are usually deficient.
- Fat: 1 gram = 9 calories; No more than 30% of total calories. Fats are needed for the transport of fat-soluble vitamins (A, D, E, and K). Fat digestion is inhibited with aging.

- Vitamins/Minerals: Elderly patients need higher levels of vitamin C and D; controlled exposure to sunlight when possible will help with absorption. Vitamin B12 (cyanocobalamin) needs also increase; this is because the intrinsic factor in the stomach needed to absorb B12 decreases with age (supplementation prevents pernicious anemia). Patients should eat vitamin B12–rich foods, such as lean red meat, chicken, and skim milk.

> ➤ **Review Video: Proteins**
> Visit *mometrix.com/academy* and enter *Code: 507186*

Vitamins

Vitamins are a type of nutrient required by the body for proper growth and metabolism. Water-soluble vitamins are those vitamins that the body cannot store, and need to be replenished on a daily basis. Water-soluble vitamins include all the B vitamins and vitamin C. A key fact to remember about water-soluble vitamins is that because they are excreted easily by the body/not stored, they need to be consumed regularly in order for the body to have an adequate supply.

Sources: Citrus, tomatoes, cantaloupe, potatoes, green leafy vegetables, pork, liver, and enriched breads and cereals

Vitamin	Major Functions	Found in
A	eyes, skin, immune system	dark green or orange fruits and vegetables, milk
B6	producing RBCs, brain/nerve function	spinach, beans, nuts, eggs, red meat, fish
B12	producing RBCs, nerve function	eggs, milk, chicken, red meat, fish
C	teeth, bones, skin	spinach, tomatoes, berries, citrus fruits
D	bones, absorbing calcium	milk, egg yolk, sunlight
E	protects cells from damage, involved in function of RBCs	nuts, grains, oils, green vegetables
Folic Acid	protects against heart disease, essential for cell health, fetal CNS development	fruits, dark green vegetables

Potassium

Potassium (K) is a key intracellular ion that is involved in the electrical and metabolic functions of the cell. The acceptable serum level of potassium is 3.5-5 mEq/L. It assists in the regulation of the acid-base balance and water balance in the blood and the body tissues, as well as in protein synthesis from amino acids and in carbohydrate metabolism. In addition, it is needed for the proper functioning of nerve cells, in the brain and throughout the body; it is especially key to the conduction pathways in the heart. In patients with kidney disease or on potassium-sparing diuretics, potassium is retained and can sometimes reach dangerously high levels. These patients will generally need to limit the amount of potassium in the diet.

Sources: Vegetables, including broccoli, peas, lima beans, tomatoes, potatoes (especially their skins), and leafy green vegetables such as spinach, lettuce, and parsley, contain potassium. Fruits that contain significant sources of potassium are citrus fruits, apples, bananas, and apricots. Fish such as salmon, cod, flounder, and sardines are also good sources of potassium. Various other meats also contain potassium. Salt-substitutes, orange juice, and black licorice are sources unusually high in potassium.

Sodium

Sodium (Na) is a key extracellular ion involved in multiple body functions. It is vital in maintaining proper fluid balance in the body, and helps maintain nerve function in the brain. Because high levels of sodium cause fluid to be retained in the body, patients with congestive heart failure, hypertension, liver disease, cirrhosis, or kidney disease should be on strict sodium-restricted diets as prescribed by their doctor.

Sources: Occurs naturally in most foods. The most common form of sodium is sodium chloride, which is table salt. Milk, beets, and celery also naturally contain sodium. Most seasonings, processed foods, and "fast foods" are extremely high in sodium, and should be avoided.

Nutritional Issues in the Adolescent Population

Adolescence is a time of accelerated growth and development, and thus brings with it different nutritional needs. The following are some of the common nutritional issues seen in this population:
- Undernourishment: Puberty can as much as double an adolescent's need for iron, calcium, zinc, and protein. Particularly for females, iron and calcium are crucial. Girls are more susceptible to iron deficiency at menarche due to blood loss. Also, maximum bone mass is acquired during the teen years, so the amount of calcium deposited determines risk of osteoporosis later in life.
- Obesity: related to an excess intake of calories. BMI equal to or greater than the 95th percentile for age and gender is considered overweight and should be investigated further. Obesity is found in all income, racial, and ethnic groups and both genders.
- Eating Disorders: May effect as many as 1/3 of adolescents in the United States. S&S include recurrent dieting when not overweight, distorted body image, BMI below the 5th percentile, use of laxatives, emesis after meals (may see stained teeth, throat irritation), starvation.

Infectious Mononucleosis

Infectious mononucleosis, sometimes called "the kissing disease," is a viral infection caused by the Epstein-Barr virus. Infectious mononucleosis characteristically occurs in young adults and most often is transmitted via saliva. Those at increased risk of infectious mononucleosis include students (both high school and college) and those with impaired immunity. Signs and symptoms include generalized lymphadenopathy, sore throat/pharyngitis, dysphagia, fever, chills, splenomegaly (enlarged spleen), headache, anorexia, nausea/vomiting, and generalized malaise/extreme fatigue. Diagnosis is based on blood work (antibody test/WBC) and physical exam.

Treatment includes:
- Rest : avoid contact sports, strenuous lifting / any other rigorous activity due to splenomegaly (risk of rupture)
- Antipyretics/mild analgesics for fever/discomfort
- Saltwater gargles/cool drinks and smoothies for sore throat/dysphagia
- Steroids possibly prescribed depending on severity
- Educate on prevention: do not share drinks; spread by oral contact, can be spread by person who is asymptomatic

Adolescent Pregnancy

Adolescent/teen pregnancy is defined as pregnancy in which the woman gives birth before the age of 20. Teenage pregnancies are considered high risk, as they have an increased incidence of poor outcomes for mom and baby. Common complications include:
- Bleeding: Likely to signal spontaneous abortion. *If a woman presents with bleeding and abdominal pain, the provider MUST rule out ectopic pregnancy.
- Ectopic pregnancy: Highest rate of mortality in teens; increased risk with history of intrauterine device, pelvic inflammatory disease/surgery or previous ectopic pregnancy.
- Prolonged labor: Labor may be prolonged in younger teens due to fetopelvic incompatibility, meaning the head of the fetus is too large to pass through the mother's pelvis. This is especially prevalent in pregnant mothers aged 12-16, due to their smaller stature and incomplete growth. This age group is at a greatly increased risk of cesarean delivery.

Prevention is as follows:
- Teaching abstinence as ideal.
- Educate on methods of birth control: condoms for younger teens, oral contraceptives for older adolescents.

Drug Use during Pregnancy

The use of drugs during pregnancy is extremely detrimental to mother and fetus. This is because the use of cocaine and other stimulant drugs causes systemic release of epinephrine and norepinephrine, resulting in vasoconstriction. This includes the arteries and veins in the umbilical cord. A decreased blood supply means a decrease in the amount of nutrients and oxygen to the fetus, causing impaired growth and intellectual disability. Women who continue to abuse drugs during pregnancy have an increased risk of abruptio placenta, abortion in the first trimester, growth limitations, premature, and non-living births. Babies who are born to mothers who ingest drugs have a tendency to have lower Apgar scores/neurological problems (often evidenced by a shrill, piercing cry), irritability, increased startle reflexes, and an increased risk of sudden infant death syndrome (SIDS).

Gram-positive *Neisseria gonorrhoeae*

Sexually transmitted *Neisseria gonorrhoeae* is a disease with horrific side effects if left untreated. While the organism is unable to survive dehydration or cool conditions, it is easily passed by sexual transmission from infected individuals and from mother to infant. Signs and symptoms are as follows:
- Asymptomatic during early infection.
- Males: urethritis with dysuria and purulent discharge.
- Female: purulent vaginal discharge and bleeding, pelvic inflammatory disease—this can lead to sterility, chronic pelvic pain, and ectopic pregnancy.

Diagnosis is based on laboratory examination of vaginal/seminal fluids. Treatment includes:
- Antibiotics: ceftriaxone, ciprofloxacin, etc (penicillin [PCN] resistant)
- Monitor for: endocarditis, meningitis, septic arthritis
- Prevention: sex education/condoms, antibiotic eye drops prevent mother-baby transmission.
- Chlamydia should be treated concurrently with gonorrhea using tetracycline or erythromycin.

Lifestyle Choices

Lifestyle choices are the choices that a person makes regarding how they live their life. While many of these choices do not affect one's health, some have a profound impact on a person's state of being throughout their lives. The following are considered basic examples of positive and negative lifestyle choices in regards to health:
- Positive lifestyle choices:
  - Exercise – increases bone-density, decreases chances of obesity, heart disease, diabetes.
  - A diet rich in fruits and vegetables – increases overall health, decreases risk of cancers and numerous diseases.
  - Preventative care – yearly physicals, follow-up with primary care physician; can help detect problems early and prevent complications.
- Negative/harmful lifestyle choices:
  - Use of illicit drugs/excessive drinking – increases risk of multiple diseases and complications; many drugs are addictive, even from first use. Can harm unborn children and others.
  - Smoking – known to cause cancers and other diseases, including Buerger's and COPD.
  - Exposure to high-stress environments – increases risk of heart attack and stroke; while unavoidable in some scenarios, patients should be referred to stress management techniques and counseling as needed.

Teaching Patients with CAD

The following are crucial educational points to discuss with patients diagnosed with Coronary Artery Disease (CAD) and their families:
1. Definition and causes of CAD
   - A buildup of plaque causing narrowing of vessels in heart
   - Modifiable vs. Nonmodifiable Risk Factors: genetics, family history, diet, exercise, smoking.
2. Signs and symptoms of an impending MI
   - Chest pain/pressure, radiating to neck/jaw, shortness of breath, sweating, nausea/vomiting – go to ER!
3. Signs of Heart Failure
   - Report swelling in legs, sleeping in recliner, difficulty breathing with activity – could be signs of heart failure.
4. Prescribed Medications
   - Take all medicines as prescribed! Medications for blood pressure, cholesterol, clot prevention, and aspirin common.
5. Cardiac Diet
   - Limit salt (canned and processed foods) and high-fat foods.
6. Lifestyle Modification
   - Immediatley stop smoking and use of any illegal drugs.
   - Low-impact exercise routine (30 minutes a day of an activity such as walking).

Teaching Patients with COPD

While chronic obstructive pulmonary disease (COPD) is a chronic disease, the quality of life of these patients can be greatly impacted by their adherence to the medical regimen. Crucial teaching points for these patients and their families are:
1. Smoking Cessation
   - Cause of disease, constricts bronchioles, and damages lungs further.
   - Support group, nicotine patch, and other helpful therapies.
2. Nutrition
   - Increased caloric needs since work of breathing in increased.
   - Frequent small meals throughout the day work best to decrease fatigue.
3. Breathing exercises
   - *"Cough and Deep Breath"*- Take 2-3 deep breaths into abdomen, and while exhaling the third, cough 2-3 times. This helps open lungs/move secretions.
   - *"Pursed Lip Breathing"*- Have patient take deep breaths in through nose, and force air out through pursed lips. This opens alveoli – "smell the cake, now blow out the candles!"
4. S&S of infection
   - Report increase in sputum, green/brown/rust-colored sputum, increased dyspnea, fever, chills, and racing heartbeat right away.
5. Oxygen safety
   - Never smoke in home with oxygen tank; replace before empty. Do not use more than 2-3 liters due to hypoxic drive to breathe.

Teaching Patients with Diabetes Mellitus

The severity of the effects of diabetes is greatly impacted by the care these patients take in managing their disease. The following are crucial educational points to discuss with the diabetic patient and their families:
1. Signs and symptoms of hypoglycemia/hyperglycemia.
   - "Cold & Clammy? Get some candy!"; irritability is often first sign.
   - "Hot & Dry? Sugar is high!"
2. Sick day rules:
   - Check sugar more often, stay hydrated.
3. Procedure for giving insulin injections:
   - Injection Sites: arm, abdomen, inner thigh: must rotate!
   - Use of syringe: ensure no air bubbles, use sharps container
4. Proper medication storage:
   - Do not store insulin in the refrigerator
   - Label with date/time; expiration date (generally 28 days)
5. Diabetic diet:
   - Count carbohydrates, avoid excess simple carbs/ add protein.
   - Refer to registered dietitian if needed
   - Check sugar before meals; eat more carbs if increased activity
6. Proper care of skin and feet.
   - Inspect feet daily with mirror, always wear diabetic shoes.
   - Do not cut own nails – go to podiatrist.

Techniques of Physical Assessment

A thorough and accurate physical assessment is the most important skill that a nurse performs, as it will determine the plan of care and help diagnose issues or complications that the patient may be having. There are four basic parts of physical assessment:
- Inspection: Looking at the body area, assessing for symmetry and the presence or absence of normal features. Assess features bilaterally, noting size, color, odor, sounds, or any deviations from expected findings.
- Palpation: Placing your hands on the patient, palpating to determine softness, irregularities in texture, abdominal masses, edema, or other abnormalities. Palpation ranges from light (1-2cm) to deep (4-6cm), depending on what area of the body is being assessed. Remember to wear gloves when palpating mucous membranes.
- Percussion: While not normally required in a nurses' daily assessment, percussion involves tapping ones fingers against a body part and listening to the sound. This can determine fluid build-up or thickness of underlying tissue. Percussion may also be used to determine tenderness.
- Auscultation: This is listening to the patient's heart, lung or bowel sounds using your stethoscope. Ensure the environment is quiet, and the stethoscope is clean and fits into your ears. Expose the area you are listening to, and use firm pressure with the diaphragm for high-pitched noises and light-pressure with the bell for low-pitched sounds.

*Note: For an abdominal assessment, auscultate before palpation and percussion, as these can alter the presence of bowel sounds in the patient.

Psychosocial Integrity

This domain is defined by the NCSBN as "providing and directing nursing care that promotes and supports the emotional, mental, and social wellbeing of the client experiencing stressful events, as well as clients with acute or chronic mental illness." This section contains information regarding common psychological issues affecting patients, including abuse, therapeutic communication, cultural communication, and psychological disorders.

Abuse

Child abuse is the intentional harm, either psychological or physical, of a child. The nurse's role is to identify, assist with treatment, and aid in the prevention of abuse and neglect. It is the nurse's duty to report suspected neglect/abuse to appropriate authorities; however, do not approach the abuser directly. Private interviews and asking, "Do you feel safe?" are common diagnostic tools for abuse; also a thorough physical exam. The most common signs and symptoms includes:
- Bruises, especially those in multiple stages of healing or on the central part of the body.
- Burns with clear borders, such as immersion or cigarette burns.
- Fractures, especially spiral or rib fractures.
- Lacerations and abrasions may appear on the mouth, gums, around the eye area, and in the genital region.
- Bite marks, fingernail scratches, and puncture wounds.
- Head trauma may present with bulging fontanelle, cranial suture separation, hematomas and broken vessels in the eyes, bleeding from the ears, and decreased or impaired hearing.

Psychological signs:
- Aggression and/or pulling back.
- Express fear with the home environment and/or the individual who is abusing them.
- Display no emotion/attachment with parents.
- Avoid eye contact, show signs of rigidity when they are approached, inappropriate responses to painful procedures.

The following are characteristics of victims of spousal/partner abuse:
- Feelings of failure as a mother, wife, or caregiver; feel as if they deserve abuse.
- Accept the abuse as a normal healthy relationship; denial.
- Do not have close family relationships or friendships; social isolation.
- Low self-esteem; show lack of independence in decision-making skills.
- Express fear or anxiety related to confronting or upsetting the abuser.
- Have conflicting stories related to injuries; the spouse dominates the questioning and unexplained injuries present.

Note: It is very appropriate for the nurse to first interview a couple, and then do a single interview with the individual they feel is being abused. Also, remember that victims of abuse often are in denial. The best thing to say to an abused woman: "You don't deserve to be treated in this manner."

The following are warning signs of sexual abuse/assualt:
- Detailed and overly sophisticated understanding of sexual behavior in young children.
- Regressive behavior (e.g., excessive clinginess in preschool children or the sudden onset of soiling and wetting)
- A child may appear disconnected or focused on fantasy worlds
- Sleep disturbances and nightmares
- Marked changes in appetite
- Fear states (e.g., anxiety, depression, phobias, obsession)
- Overly compliant behavior such as extensive grooming behaviors
- Parentified/adultified behavior (e.g., acting like a parent/spouse)
- Delinquent or aggressive behavior
- Poor or deteriorating relationships with peers
- Sudden inability to concentrate in school/deterioration in school performance
- Unwillingness to participate in physical/recreational activities, especially if this is due to symptoms of physical discomfort
- Truancy/running away from home
- Drug/alcohol abuse

Note: These signs are not diagnostic; must look at overall clinical picture before making a judgement.

Barriers to Effective Communication

Barriers to communication exist when the nurse is unable to effectively communicate the wants, needs, and desires of the patient, as well as to effectively discuss and explain the care and rational for the care needed. Barriers to communication may include:
- Minimization of concerns/belittling the patient or concerns
- Offering false reassurance/approval to the patient
- Rejecting individuals
- Choosing sides: the patient, the family, or the physician
- Placing blame on external factors or patient /family
- Conflicting opinions from the patient or family, giving advice
- Minimal feedback to questions – one word answers, cutting off
- Shifting the focus of concern
- Using medical terminology/jargon
- Offering unrealistic ideation or ignoring patient's concerns.

To fix these common barriers, the nurse needs to speak honestly and openly with the client about health concerns and treatments. The nurse should use language that is easy to understand, and take time to listen to all the patient's concerns and questions. Open-ended questions and open body language reinforce the nurses' concern for the patient. Never offer opinions and false reassurances to patients, and always speak positively of others.

Empathy

Empathy is the process of understanding another person by identifying with his/her situation, rather than seeing it from an outside perspective. It involves putting oneself into another's shoes and seeing the situation as the affected person does. When used in a helping relationship, the counselor can utilize empathy by trying to see the client's viewpoint and consider the situation from the client's perspective, rather than the counselor's. Empathy comprises two stages:

1. The first stage is experiencing the same emotions as the affected person. An example of this might be when a counselor cries with a client who is experiencing significant emotional pain.
2. Stage two of empathy involves realistically looking at the situation from the other person's point of view. An example of this situation might be when a counselor listens to the client and examines his own reaction by considering how he might feel in the same situation.

Active Listening

Attributes of active listeners include conveying warmth and respect, and offering acceptance of the client. The nurse must:

- Acknowledge all behavior of the client and realize it has meaning.
- Set boundaries and abide by them when taking part in a conversation.
- Do not lead the client in a direction; allow client to direct conversation as appropriate.
- Give ample time for expression.
- Ask questions related to the topic of discussion.
- Body language: maintain eye contact, and face the client, lean in as listening intently, nod, smile, and frown to show agreement or disagreement.

The nurse must be aware of his or her own experiences and how they can alter the relationship with the client. If a nurse feels she is unable to adequately care for a client related to the nurse's past experience, she must relay this information to her superiors.

Contracting with Clients

A contract is a type of agreement drawn up between people that is done to promote action and possible reward. A counselor may use a contract with a client who wants to change a behavior; for example, a client may express frustration about making rash decisions that significantly affect his personal life. As part of a contract, a counselor may require that the client agree to consult with a family member or professional before making any decisions that will affect his finances, family life, or health. The contract is drawn up with specific terms and signed by the client. The three characteristics of a good contract are:

1. Feasible - the contract should be written in such a way that the client can actually perform the terms.
2. Specific - leaving little room for interpretation.
3. Retractable - in that the client can decide that he/she does not want to meet the terms.

Learner Readiness

Learner readiness is the term used to describe whether the person being educated is willing to receive and implement the information given. The client, family, or support person will not learn, retain, or be able to repeat the material if they are not at a point in the care in which they are ready to learn. It is important to document the level of learner readiness in the chart to prevent the nurse from being liable if the patient is readmitted or noncompliant with care. The nurse may also assist in identifying barriers to learning and addressing those barriers to enhance the learning process. Barriers to learning can include terminal diagnosis, cognitive disability/injury, denial of health problems, and low educational/reading level.

Methods to increase learning include:
- Use visual aids, videotapes, and clearly written handouts.
- Ensure material is appropriate to patient learning level.
- Encourage family participation.
- Limit what is taught during each session.
- Put special emphasis on the needs of the patient after the patient goes home, rather than just focusing on the here and now.
- Allow time for questions and answers.

Coping Mechanisms

Coping mechanisms (also known as defense mechanisms) are ways that an individual responds to increased stress or a crisis in order to process the event and maintain their psychological integrity. Coping mechanisms are considered a healthy response to stress; however, disproportionate or exclusive use of one coping mechanism over others is considered unhealthy. Coping mechanisms include:
- Compensation: Making up for a perceived weakness by exaggerating a different feature
  John is failing math, but becomes an all-star basketball player.
- Conversion: Changing psychological stress into a physical problem
  John gets nauseated before his midterm in math.
- Denial: Refusing to accept an unpleasant reality
  John refuses to study for his math test, thinking he will probably pass it.
- Displacement: Directing anger at situation at another person/object.
  John screams at his little sister after his parents chide him about his math test.
- Dissociation: Separating the emotions from an event/situation.
  John jokes and laughs with his friends about failing his class and repeating the grade.
- Fantasy: A conscious creation of an alternate reality as an escape from unpleasant feelings.
  John fantasizes about playing basketball during math class.
- Identification: Assimilating feelings/actions of a desired person
  John buys expensive shoes endorsed by his favorite basketball player.
- Introjection: Unconsciously assimilating behaviors external to one's self.
  John swears at his opponents during an intense game, as he has heard his father do before.

- 69 -

- Projection: Ascribing undesirable feelings, motivation, and behaviors to another person.
  John states that his teacher just hates him, and doesn't want him to pass the class.
- Rationalization: Deciding that undesirable feelings or actions are bearable and satisfactory.
  John decides that math is not an important subject, and he doesn't need to pass it
- Reaction Formation: Feelings and motives are completely opposite of actions and behavior displayed
  John skips and whistles as his goes into math test, stating math is his favorite subject.
- Regression: A retreat back to an earlier stage of comfort
  John begins to hang out with younger kids and avoid his older friends.
- Repression: Unconscious amnesia regarding unpleasant circumstances and feelings
  John completely forgets to attend his math tutoring session at school.
- Restitution: Trying to alleviate subconscious guilt regarding an event
  John gives extra effort in English class to impress his parents.
- Sublimation: Converting unacceptable behaviors into acceptable ones
  John uses his obsession with basketball to participate in an after-school program for troubled youth.
- Substitution: Decision to change a negative attitude into a more positive emotion.
  John decides that while math is not his favorite, he really likes English.
- Suppression: Choosing not to think or dwell on an unpleasant experience or emotion
  John refuses to talk about his failing math grade with his siblings.
- Symbolization: Using a physical object to represent an internal emotion or idea
  John burns his math book at the end of the semester.
- Undoing: An attempt to alleviate conscious guilt regarding a negative event.
  John apologizes to his parents for failing math and promises to try harder in the future.

Substance Abuse

Substance abuse, which includes the abuse of alcohol, prescription drugs, and illegal drugs, is a major problem in the United States. Of the 14% of adults who admit to dependence at sometime in their life, half have experienced the problem during the last year. More than 3 million teenagers have a problem with alcohol. There is a strong connection between drinking and teenage problems such as suicide, early sexual activity, and driving accidents. Abuse of alcohol and drugs affects not just the addict, but family members, friends, and coworkers as well. Characteristics include low self-esteem, anxiety, sexual problems, suicidal impulses, fear of failure, and social isolation. The Substance Abuse Subtle Screening Inventory (SASSI) can be used to detect indications of addiction. Since addictions are both physical and mental, successful treatment must involve both. With certain substances, hospitalization and medications will be required to treat acute withdrawal symptoms. For long-term recovery, one effective treatment method is a 12-step program coupled with individual, group, and family counseling. It is especially important that counseling involve the family. Behavior modification and social learning theory can be used effectively in a residential program.

A common danger with substance abuse is the risk of withdrawal. Delirium tremens (DT) is a potentially fatal form of ethanol (alcohol) withdrawal. Symptoms may begin a few hours after the cessation of ethanol, but may not peak until 48-72 hours. Physicians and nurses must recognize that the presenting symptoms may not be severe and identify those at risk of developing DT. Signs and symptoms include tremors, agitation/irritability, insomnia, nausea/vomiting, hallucinations, confusion, and seizures. Diagnosis is based on patient history, symptoms, and blood alcohol levels. Treatment includes:

- IV sedation; IV midazolam or lorazepam
- Close monitoring; generally in ICU during acute withdrawal; may require restraints if they become violent with hallucinations.
- Teaching: Drinking cessation- join support group such as Alcoholics Anonymous.
- Must ask patient the time of last drink, and realize symptoms may not manifest for 6-48 hours.

Forensic Nursing

Victims of crime

Victims of crimes vary widely, from those with emotional distress to those with life-threatening injuries, so it is especially important to follow protocols for care. A complete detailed history of the injury sustained and any trauma should be taken, documenting carefully with direct quotations and objective observations, avoiding subjective observations that might not hold up in court. Clothing, which may contain evidence, should be carefully removed and placed in separate bags. A head-to-toe physical examination should be carried out, and injuries should be carefully noted and photodocumentation taken if possible with the patient's consent. If the police have not been notified prior to the patient's admission for care, then a report may need to be filed, depending on the state laws and the type of injuries. For example, gunshot wounds generally must be reported to the police, while physical assaults, such as with domestic violence, may or may not require reporting.

Rape victims

Rape victims need to sign a consent before examination with a rape kit and can refuse any part of the examination. Patients should remove clothing while standing on a clean sheet or drape, placing each item of clothing into a separate paper bag. Female patients should receive a baseline pregnancy test and be offered emergency contraceptive prophylaxis (for up to 120 hours). Patients should be offered antibiotic prophylaxis for sexually transmitted infections and counseled about HIV prophylaxis. Drugs used to facilitate rape may be detected for up to 96 hours. Blood tests are done for the first 36 hours after a drug-facilitated rape and urine tests after that time. The assault should be carefully documented, using direct quotations. Patients often want to shower and should be advised when they will be allowed to do so. Toluidine dye may be applied to the labia and perineal/perianal areas to help identify superficial lacerations before a vaginal examination. Photo documentation should be completed following protocols.

Suicide

Suicide is among the most frequent causes of death in the United States, and the third most common causes of death in 10-14 year olds, and second among 15-34 year olds. The risk of suicide is increased in men over 50 years, those with mental illness, gay/lesbian youth, and those of Native American or Alaskan descent. While males are more likely to commit suicide than females, the attempt rate is higher among females. Counselors should be aware of support groups, have a crisis plan, and involve the community when working with at-risk clients. Warning signs of depression and anger, experiencing loss or rejection, talking about suicide, planning and securing the means to commit suicide, and giving away possessions. A sudden, unexpected uplift in mood is considered a red flag, as it may indicate the person has finalized a plan; educate family and caregivers to look out for this. Suicide precautions include the following: locked windows and stairwells, breakproof glass and mirrors, break away shower heads/wall railing, plastic flatware, no cords of any kind, no belts, sharps, razors, matches or cigarettes, frequent observation or 1 to 1 care, communicate therapeutically, make a behavior contract, restraints if ordered, medications if ordered, monitor and restrict visitors.

Cultural Health Considerations

The following are cultural health considerations:
- Proxemics (space considerations): Cultures vary in the amount of personal space they require, and people may feel uncomfortable if others stand too close or too far away. North Americans and Northern Europeans tend to want the most space and may feel uncomfortable if someone stands within arm's length. Latin Americans, Asians, Middle Easterners, and Southern Europeans often feel comfortable standing very close to others.
- Eye contact: While direct eye contact is a cultural norm in North America and many European countries, it may be considered aggressive by some cultures and disrespectful by others. African Americans, Native Americans, Asians, and Mexicans often avoid eye contact to show respect.
- Time: While punctuality is considered the norm in the United States, time is much more flexible in many cultures, so some people, such as Latin Americans and Mexicans, may consider time in relation to day and night or before or after meals rather than by the clock.
- Complementary/Folk medicine: People from other cultures may utilize alternative medical systems (such as Chinese herbal medications), healers, meditation, manipulative or body-based therapies, or practices such as coining and cupping (which may leave distinctive bruising).
- Touch: There may be restrictions in touch between males and females in some cultures (such as Middle Eastern), and some in Asian cultures may be upset if the head is touched without permission because they believe the spirit resides in the head.
- Holiday/Religious observance: Patients may want to continue to observe cultural holidays or religious practices, such as eating kosher meals and fasting during Ramadan. They may have restrictions as to what they are able to do during religious days, such as ultra-conservative Jews on the Sabbath.
- Family hierarchy: In some cultures (Mexican, Asian, and Middle Eastern) decisions are made by the males or the head of the family rather than by the individual, so a wife, for example, may expect her husband to make decisions about her care.

Common Religious & Spiritual Influences on Health

A person's spiritual and religious beliefs can often have a pronounced impact on their health. While it is not the nurses' duty to try to change those beliefs, the nurse should be aware of them in order to respect the patient's wishes and give safe and effective care. This will always start with an assessment of the patient's beliefs: the nurse should ask the

- 72 -

patient if they have any religious or spiritual beliefs that they would like their health care team to be aware of, and then use open-ended questions to determine if there is anything that may potentially cause a spiritual conflict during the course of treatment. For example, if the patient is Jewish and wishes to abstain from pork, a note should be made to the dietitian. More commonly, a patient who is a Jehovah's Witness will often refuse blood products, so special planning will be necessary for these patients when they undergo surgery or other medical procedures. If a patient has religious/spiritual preferences, the nurse's responsibilities are to be respectful of the patient and to facilitate their preferences as much as possible while still providing excellent care.

End of Life Care

The nurse often plays a crucial role in end of life care. End of life care (also known as palliative or "comfort care") is care centered on providing patient ease as they transition into the end of life. There are few things the nurse should keep in mind when providing palliative care:

- Pain control: This is the #1 priority for palliative care patients. Adequate pain control in these patients often includes opioids and anxiolytics in high doses. For some nurses this may cause moral distress, as drugs at this level may shorten the life of the patient. However, the nurses' creed is to "first, do no harm"; thus, this practice is deemed ethical and compassionate for the patient.
- EENT: Dying patients will often require frequent suctioning due to increased secretions; the MD may even order a scopolamine patch to help dry up the excess saliva and mucous in the back of the throat that causes the characteristic "death rattle". These patients will also need the mouth swabbed frequently for comfort, and sometimes artificial tears to treat dry eyes.
- Positioning: Turn and support with pillows to increase comfort; it may help to elevate the head of the bed to facilitate breathing for the patient.
- Psychological: If the patient is still coherent and talking, allow them to verbalize their feelings about death and reminisce. Do not patronize or dismiss their concerns, but be honest regarding their condition and treatment options. Spiritual interventions are considered high priority during this time.

> ➤ **Review Video: Death Rattle**
> *Visit* ***mometrix.com/academy*** *and enter* ***Code:*** **882000**

Phases of Grief

Kübler-Ross is famous for her five phases of grief, the process that people move through when losing something important to them, including the loss of a loved one, successful job, or even body image changes. It is important to realize that Kübler-Ross taught that a person does not necessarily move through the stages in exact order, and may skip or regress to different stages. Children especially move through the phases faster than adults. The five phases (DABDA) are:

1. Denial: does not really believe loss has happened, talks as if nothing has changed. Family/caregivers may fear delirium; educate that this might be a normal part of grieving process.
2. Anger: upset about loss, may act out, exhibit previously unfelt aggression at the lost individual; may blame caregivers or others for loss.

- 73 -

3. Bargaining: trying to change results of loss/avoid consequences of loss; may ask God to change what happened.
4. Depression: loss of interest, may feel life is not worth living/fatalistic, withdraw from friends/family. Offer support, and do not try to prematurely pull out of grief.
5. Acceptance: come to terms with loss and able to cope, accepted consequences; back into a pattern of daily living.

Impaired/complicated grieving: when debilitating feelings of grief and sadness remain ≥ 6 months after event; requires medical intervention.

> **Review Video: Patient Treatment and Grief**
> Visit *mometrix.com/academy* and enter *Code:* **648794**

Support Systems

A large factor in a patient's recovery from illness is the patient's support system at home. This usually refers to the patient's friends and family members who are involved in the patient's life, and who will be largely involved in the patient's care. An adequate support system may require different levels of involvement depending on patient condition and situation; the nurse should assess:
- What are the patient's thoughts about their support at home? Is it adequate? Is the family in the home supportive and agreable with the care that is going to be required?
- What support systems have worked for the patient in the past? What has changed this time that might necessitate a different level of involvement?
- Will the patient require outside help, such as a support group (e.g. AA, group therapy sessions, etc.)?

Once the nurse has answered these questions, he/she should work closely with the case manager to get the patient the help they need to have a successful recovery.

Caregiver Strain

Signs and symptoms of caregiver strain:
- Caregiver appears anxious or depressed and easily irritated.
- Caregiver complains of fatigue and difficulty sleeping.
- Caregiver gets upset or lashes out excessively in response to irritating or stressful events.
- Caregiver complains of new ailments or of worsening health.
- Caregiver is forgetful and has difficulty concentrating or carrying through with activities.
- Caregiver is increasingly angry and resentful toward the patient.
- Caregiver no longer engages in leisure activities.
- Caregiver increasingly withdraws from outside relationships and social activities.
- Caregiver begins to neglect the patient and other responsibilities.
- Caregiver shows signs of compensatory behavior, such as excessive drinking, eating, or smoking.
- Caregiver neglects personal care and needs.
- Caregiver complains of feeling hopeless about future.

- Caregiver increasingly blames patient for things beyond patient's control.

Offer support/therapeutic listening; community support groups/social services for relief care. Notify social services if abuse is suspected.

Mental disorders

The following are types of mental disorders:
- Anxiety is a state of uneasiness or apprehension, which can cause physical tension. Severe anxieties or multiple anxieties, especially when they have comorbidity with another disorder, are abnormal behavior. Panic disorder, phobias, posttraumatic stress, and obsessive-compulsive disorder are examples of anxiety disorders. Medication, relaxation techniques, cognitive behavioral therapy, and exposure exercises are acceptable treatments for anxiety disorders.
- Somatoform disorders involve physical symptoms for which no specific physical cause is present. The disorders include hypochondria, somatization disorder, conversion, and pain disorder. Treatment is more management than cure and may or may not include medication.
- Dissociative disorders involve the breakdown of a person's perceptions of his environment, memory, or identity. Dissociative disorders include dissociative amnesia, dissociative fugue (flight), dissociative identity disorder (multiple personality) and depersonalization disorder. Psychotherapy and sometimes hypnosis are among the treatments for dissociative disorders.
- Mood disorders are conditions in which the person's prevailing mood is disturbed or inappropriate. The disorders include depression, anxiety, and bipolar syndrome. The mood disorders are the most common psychological illnesses. Treatment includes medication, counseling, disorder-specific.

Bipolar Disorder (Manic-Depression Disorder)

Bipolar disorder or manic-depressive disorder is a psychological condition in which the patient swings between depressive and manic episodes. These swings can be sudden or the phases can last for long periods of time:
- Depressive symptoms: chronic pain, decreased energy, loss of interest in activities, weight/appetite changes, excessive crying, suicidal thoughts and/or attempts, feelings of helplessness, changes in sleep patterns, social withdrawal.
- Manic symptoms: overly inflated self-esteem, decreased need for rest and sleep, irritability, distractedness, physical agitation/aggression, provocative or destructive behavior, increased talkativeness, excessive "high" or euphoric feelings, increased sex drive/energy level, denial, uncharacteristically poor judgment.

Treatment includes:
- Medication: Mood stabilizers (lithium), antipyschotics, anticonvulsants, antidepressants.
- Psychotherapy
- Teaching: stress medication compliance, increased risk of self-harm/suicide, feed finger foods and engage in nonviolent activities during manic phase.

Schizophrenia

Such dysfunctions as delusions, hallucinations, inappropriate emotions, disorganized speech, and inappropriate behavior make up the category of mental illness called schizophrenia. A person with schizophrenia may not have any outward appearance of being ill. In other cases, the illness may be more apparent, causing bizarre behaviors. Advanced paternal age, illegal drug use, family history, and autoimmune diseases increase a person's risk of developing schizophrenia. Signs and symptoms include social withdrawal; depersonalization (intense anxiety and a feeling of being unreal); loss of appetite; poor hygiene; delusions; hallucinations; paranoia; and disrupted or disturbed thought processes, perceptions, speech, and movement ("negative symptoms"). Treatment includes:

- Medications: antipsychotics (atypical preferred)
- Psychotherapy: individual and family therapy, social skills training, vocational rehabilitation.
- Teaching: stress medication compliance, support groups, increased suicide/self-harm risk.

Note: Schizophrenia is NOT multiple personality disorder.

Physiological Integrity

Basic Care and Comfort

This domain is defined by the NCSBN as "providing comfort and assistance in the performance of activities of daily living." This section includes assistive devices, effects of immobility, hygiene, and pain control.

Amputations

Types of amputations are as follows:
- Lower extremities—toe, metatarsal (mid-foot amputation), Syme (removal of foot at ankle), knee disarticulation (amputation through knee joint), below knee (BKA), and above knee (AKA).
- Upper extremities—digit, wrist articulation, below elbow (BEA), above elbow (AEA), elbow disarticulation, shoulder disarticulation, and forequarter amputation (removes a large portion of shoulder and the arm). Others include hemipelvectomy (removal of half of pelvis and all of legs), hemicorporectomy (removal of lower half of body with resultant colostomy and urinary diversion).

Postoperatively, patients must be carefully monitored for signs of shock or bleeding. Focus is on stump care to provide correct molding and prevent infection, pain control, emotional support, acceptance of change in body image, and mobility. Place patient in prone position several times a day to improve oxygenation and prevent contractures. Patients should have a clear understanding of prognosis and rehabilitation efforts needed. Patients may need to learn how to provide stump care and many need to be taught to use assistive devices and prostheses. Patients should understand pain control and be taught about phantom pain.

NG tube and NJ tube

NG/NJ tubes are long, thin tubes that are inserted through the patient's nose, throat, and esophagus down into the stomach/intestine for feeding or suction purposes. The length is determined by measuring from the tip of the nose, to the earlobe, to the end of the xiphoid process; in pediatric patients, measure to the umbilicus. It is critical to remember to check placement before feeding or giving medications through the tube, either by aspiration or checking pH of gastric contents. The initial placement will usually be verified with x-ray.

<u>NG tube (nasogastric)</u>
This tube ends in the stomach. For feeding, a smaller Dobbhoff or other brand of tube is used, and a pump or gravity feed may be used. Feeds can also be given in bolus or continuous amounts. Bolus feeds are often set up to mimic meals, given in three large amounts at separate times of the day. For patients needing extra calories, or for those who do not tolerate bolus feeds, continuous or overnight feeds may be used. Patients with intestinal blockage, severe vomiting, or a high risk of aspiration may benefit from suction via an NG/NJ tube.

NJ tube (nasojejunal)
Similar to an NG tube, the NJ tube passes through the stomach and into the jejunum. Because the end of the tube is in the jejunum instead of the stomach, NJ tubes can help reduce vomiting associated with reflux. Thus, a J tube is used when it is desired to bypass the stomach.

Ileostomy and colostomy

An ostomy is either a permanent or temporary artificial opening created to allow stool or other substances out of the body. An ileostomy occurs as the result of total removal of the colon and the rectum; the anus is sutured closed and an opening in the lower abdominal wall in the area of the ileum is formed to allow for fecal evacuation. A colostomy, however, is formed when the colon is routed to an opening in the abdominal wall forming an artificial opening for feces to be removed and collected. The anus is also sutured with a colostomy. A urostomy is the diversion of one or both ureters to an opening in the abdominal wall. The following should be taught to the patient:

- Avoid gas-producing foods, can use deoderizers.
- Stool from ostomy more formed than illeostomy (pure liquid).
- Ostomy should be healthy, pink, beefy color. Report pale color (could mean loss of blood flow to tissue) or dark red with irritation or drainage (infection).
- Change as directed; teach patient to cut wafer to correct size to prevent skin irriation.
- Body image disturbance is problem for these patients. Educate to alleviate fears and embarrassment.

Stress incontinence

Stress/urge incontinence is an involuntary leakage of urine due to a laugh, sneeze, urge to urinate, or activity that causes increased pressure on the bladder. It is generally due to urethral sphincter dysfunction. Increased age, childbirth, trauma, certain medications, and other factors may increase the risk of stress incontinence. Diagnosis is based on rectal exam, x-rays, pad test, urine analysis, PVR test, cystoscopy, pelvic exam, and prostate exam (men). Treatment includes:

- Medications - pseudoephedrine/phenylpropanolamine, estrogen, and other medications may help treat underlying cause.
- Physical therapy - Pelvic floor re-training; also biofeedback training.
- Lifestyle modification: fluid restrictions, can wear pads/briefs, teach Kegel exercises for strengthening.

Pressure ulcers

Pressure ulcers are ulcers that appear in areas of prolonged pressure on the human body. They are often the end result of pressure on overlying skin of bony prominences in patients who are debilitated or immobilized for any reason. "Bed sores," "decubital gangrene," "pressure sores," and "hospital gangrene" are all alternate names given to pressure ulcers. The most frequent location of pressure ulcers is the base of the skull, sacrum, elbows, ischial tuberosities/hips, and heels. The staging of pressure ulcers indicates their severity and helps mark the progress or regression of the wounds. They can be prevented by frequent turning, protecting bony prominences, shear precautions, and good nutrition.

The staging of pressure ulcers is discussed below:
- Stage One: skin may be cool to touch, does not blanch, and may be accompanied by pruritus and tenderness; skin intact.
- Stage Two: partial loss of skin thickness; epidermal and dermal involvement; may appear as a blister or abrasion.
- Stage Three: subcutaneous tissue involvement; can see yellow tissue (fat) in wound; may involve necrosis.
- Stage Four: tissue loss into layers of muscle and/or bone; widespread loss of tissue and broad tissue necrosis.
- Unstageable: full tissue loss across all layers; base of wound is covered in necrotic tissue, may appear yellow, green, or black; unable to see underlying structure.

Non-pharmacological interventions for pain

Non-pharmacological interventions are nursing interventions that decrease pain and discomfort in patients without the use of drugs. Listed below are some common interventions that may be seen:
- Heat/Cold: Usually requires a physician order; can be moist or dry. Be cautious as intense temperatures may cause burns or damage the skin. Always use a barrier between the source and the patient's skin, and instruct patients to never lay heating devices or sleep with them in use. Always maintain the prescribed temperature, and check the skin every 15 minutes. Heat/cold is contraindicated with sensory loss or cognitive impairment (diabetics, altered mental status, stroke patients, etc.).
- Music/Distraction: Multiple studies have shown that calming music or other forms of distraction can help to relieve mild pain and discomfort. Always remember to ask the patient's preferences, and keep the volume low so as not to disturb others. Remember that pain relieved by distraction does not indicate that the pain is not real.
- Mobility/Positioning: Early ambulation and increased activity as tolerated (e.g. up in the chair for meals) are interventions which can greatly increase patient comfort/decrease risk for complications during the hospital stay. For bedridden patients, active and passive ROM and frequent turning (every two hours) can increase comfort and decrease risk of bedsores.

Progression of Diet Types

For patients who are having severe nausea/vomiting, prolonged fasting, or other digestive difficulties, the doctor will often give a restricted diet order. Additionally, they will often include "Advance as Tolerated" order, which will allow the patient to progress through the types until their normal digestion is restored.
1. Nothing by Mouth (NPO): No food or liquids (including water or ice chips). Often before procedures; may be exception such as "sips and chips"), or "may give medications with small sips of water."
2. Clear Liquid Diet: Liquids that are clear and in liquid form at body temperature. This may include coffee (no creamer), gelatin, and broth.
3. Full Liquid Diet: Similar to clear liquid diet, with the addition of milk, soups, and other opaque liquids.

4. Pureed Diets: Foods that are smooth in consistency; often normal food items that have been blended. This diet is often seen in patients with chewing/swallowing difficulties.
5. Mechanical Soft Diet: A mechanical soft diet provides nutrition in the form of foods that require only a nominal amount of chewing.
6. Soft Diet: Foods that are easily digestible for the patient, such as bland food, white breads, or cooked vegetables. Soft diets are used when a patient is progressing from a clear to a regular diet.
7. Regular Diet: The term regular diet is for a diet that has no limits or needed modifications.

Personal Hygiene for Hospitalized Patients

In the midst of the chaos of special tests, doctor's rounds, and medication passes, it can be easy to forget the basic personal hygiene needs of the patient. While they may not seem to be a top priority, adhering to basic hygiene during patient care can reduce the risk of infection and have a positive effect on patient outcomes.

The following practices should be followed for every patient, as well as taught to those in an outpatient setting:
- Handwashing before meals/after using the bathroom (minimum)
- Oral care every day; every two hours if the patient is NPO/ventilated (prevents pneumonia); if the patient has dentures, these should be cleaned every night and given to the patient before meals.
- The patient should receive a full bath and linen change every day and when they are soiled; offer the patient lotion and deodorant at this time, as well as a clean gown.
- Toilet frequently and change incontinent patients every time they are soiled (check hourly and as needed). Educate female patients to wipe "front to back" to prevent UTIs.

Note: If the patient refuses any part of personal hygiene, be sure to document that it was offered and the patient was educated about its importance.

Rest and sleep during illness recovery

Good quality sleep is hard to come by for the hospitalized patient. While it may not be a high priority to the nurses, sleep and rest are key components to recovery in patients. Lack of sleep may lead to agitation, delirium, falls, and many other adverse events.

The following are interventions which the nurse may implement to promote rest and sleep in his/her patients:
- Turn down lights in the evening hours and offer personal hygiene before rest.
- Ensure the patient is positioned comfortably and linens/gown are clean and straightened.
- Keep the area around the room quiet at night, and limit loud talking/noises from the nurse's station.

- Cluster care: minimize disturbances to the patient by doing multiple tasks during one visit into the room. Work quietly and as quickly as possible to help the patient fall back asleep when finished.
- Realize some medications that promote sleep actually shorten or eliminate the REM cycle, preventing the patient from feeling well rested and mentally alert.

Note: While sleep is important, it must be noted that sleep and rest are not an valid excuse to avoid required nursing duties and checks. It may seem difficult to arouse a resting patient, but their safety comes first.

Pharmacological and Parenteral Therapies

This domain is defined by the NCSBN as "providing care related to the administration of medications and parenteral therapies." This section discusses the nurses' role in the administration and maintainence of pharmacological therapies.

Rights of medication administration

The Eight Rights of Medication Administration are as follows:
1. Right Patient
2. Right Medication
3. Right Dose
4. Right Route
5. Right Time
6. Right Documentation
7. Right to Education
8. Right to Refuse

Preventing Medication Errors

The following are nursing duties to prevent medication errors
- Checking the first five rights before medication administration against the medication administration record (MAR). These should be checked a minimum of 3 times each.
- Ensure the right patient by using three patient identifiers—this generally means checking the name, DOB, and medical record number (MRN) on the patient's armband with the MAR, and have the patient state name and DOB.
- The nurse should inform the patient what they are giving them and how it works, as well as expected side effects before administration; allergies should also be checked at this time.
- Realize that the patient has the right to refuse any and all medications. NEVER force a medication on a patient unless it is a safety issue.
- Sign off on **all** medications **after** they are administered.

Prefixes and suffixes used in pharmacology

The various prefixes and suffixes used in pharmacology that are helpful in identifying the classification of drugs are explained below:

Drug	Prefix/Suffix
ACE Inhibitor	*-pril*
Alpha-1 Antagonist	*-zosin*
Angiotensin Blocker	*-sartan*
Antifungal	*-azole*
Barbiturates	*-barbital*
Benzodiazepine	*-pam* OR *-lam*
Beta-2 Agonist	*-terol*
Beta Antagonist	*-olol*
Calcium Channel Blocker	*-dipine*
Cephalosporin	*Ceph-* OR *Cef-*
Fluoroquinolone	*-floxacin/-floxin*
H2 Antagonist	*-tidine*
Methylxanthine	*-phylline*
Penicillin	*-cillin*
Phenothiazine	*-azine*
Pituitary Hormone	*-trophin*
Protease Inhibitor	*-navir*
Sulfonamides	*Sulfa-*
Tetracyclines	*-cycline*
Thrombolytics	*-ase*
Tricyclic Antidepressant	*-ipramine*

Toxicity reversal agents and therapeutic drug levels

Toxicity Reversal Agents

Acetaminophen	N-Acetylcysteine
Alcohol withdrawal	Librium
Ammonia	Lactulose
Warfarin	Vitamin K
Digoxin	Digibind
Heparin	Protamine Sulfate
Iron	Deferoxamine
Narcotics	Naloxone

Therapeutic Drug Levels

Digoxin	0.5-2 ng/mL
Lithium	0.8-1.5 mEq/L
Dilantin	10-20 mcg/dL
Theophylline	10-20 mcg/dL
Warfarin	INR levels of 2-3 (A-fib, MI, DVT, PE)
Warfarin	INR levels of 2.5-3.5 (for mechanical heart valves)

Pharmacokinetics

Pharmacokinetics includes the absorption, distribution, metabolism, and elimination of drugs/medications. These processes must all take place during the course of drug therapy for the drug to be safe and effective. A helpful pneumonic for remember the four parts is "AD ME!":

- Absorption is the rate a drug leaves the site of administration and the extent of the drug's entrance into the cells. Absorption determines the *bioavailability* of the medication. This refers to the amount of drug available when it reaches its target destination or organ system.
- Distribution involves the mechanism of distribution of the drug throughout the body, sometimes involving carrier proteins.
- Metabolism: The breakdown of the drug, usually occurring in the liver. This results in metabolites, which can either be more or less potent than the parent drug, depending on mechanism of action.
- Excretion is the way drugs are eliminated from the body, generally taking place in the kidneys. This is an important concept, as impaired excretion can lead to increased serum levels and toxicity.

NEUROLOGICAL DRUGS

Cholinergics

The indication, mechanism of action, side effects, and important teaching points for cholinergic drugs are discussed below:

- Indications: treatment of myasthenia gravis, glaucoma (eye drops), post-op urinary retention and abdominal distention/atony.
- MOA: Mimic acetylcholine and bind to muscarinic receptors; also indirect-acting cholinergic drugs inhibit cholinesterase, which is the enzyme responsible for breaking down acetylcholine
- Activates para-sympathetic nervous system: "rest and digest"
- Medications: edrophonium, prostigmine, pilocarpine, bethanechol, carbachol
- Side Effects: low heart rate, GI spasm, increased salivation and diaphoresis.
- Teaching:
  - Hold pressure on canthus for 60 seconds to prevent systemic absorption of cholinergic eye drops.
  - Take 1 h before/2 h after meals (bethanechol)
  - Antidote for cholinergic OD: atropine
  - Do not give to patients with asthma, urinary or bowel obstruction, or gastric ulcers.
  - Toxicity: visual disturbance, bronchospasm, hypotension, cardiovascular collapse

Anticholinergics

Indications for anticholinergic use are as follows:

- Bradycardia
- Pre-op to reduce GI/respiratory secretions
- COPD treatment
- As anti-spasmodics

- 83 -

- Parkinson disease
- Motion sickness
- Pesticide poisoning.

MOA: Interrupt parasympathetic nerve impulses in the central and autonomic nervous systems; block acetylcholine. Medications include belladonna alkaloids, atropine, scopolamine, trimethobenzamide, cyclizine, dimenhydrinate, meclizine, etc. Side Effects include drowsiness, dry mouth, urinary retention, constipation, blurred vision, and decreased sweating. Patient should be taught the following:
- Can chew sugarless gum/suck on ice or sugar-free candy to help alleviate dry mouth.
- Avoid overheating: saunas, yard work in hot weather, etc; decreased sweating increases risk of heat-related illness
- Do not drive or perform other potentially dangerous tasks until you know how this drug will affect your vision
- OD symptoms: hallucinations, seizures, rapid heart rate, coma.

A way to remember the effects of anticholinergics:
- Can't spit: dry mouth
- Can't pee: urinary retention
- Can't poop: constipation
- Can't see: blurred vision

> **Review Video: Cholinergic and Anti-Cholinergic Drugs**
> Visit *mometrix.com/academy* and enter *Code: 770491*

Antiepileptic drugs/mood stabilizers

Indications:
- Seizures
- Neuropathies
- Headaches
- Bipolar disorder
- Muscle tremors

MOA: Depresses nerve cell excitation in the brain by altering ion movements into nerve cells; increases seizure threshold.
- Medications: carbamazepine, valproic acid, gabapentin
- Neurontin: diabetic nerve pain

Side effects include:
- Changes in behavior
- Hepatotoxicity and pancreatitis (valproic acid)
- Bone marrow depression (carbamazepine)

Teaching:
- Do not take carbamazepine with grapefruit (increases serum levels) or give valproic acid with carbonated beverages.
- Can reduce the effects of oral anticoagulants and oral contraceptives.
- Monitor serum levels of drugs, as well as liver function (divalproex sodium); platelets and hemoglobin (carbamazepine)

Phenytoin

The classification, mechanism of action, side effects, and key teaching points of phenytoin are discussed below:
- Indication: epilepsy/seizures
- MOA: Classified as a hydantoin (prototype: fosphenytoin); increases seizure threshold/decreased nerve cell excitability. Also works as cardiac antiarrythmic
- Side effects: drowsiness, confusion, dizziness; long term – gingivial hyperplasia, acne, hirshutism, osteoporosis
- Teaching:
  - IV: rapid administration can cause sudden cardiac arrest; Administer no faster than 50 mg/min and flush at same rate.
  - Will cause overgrowth of gums: use soft-bristled toothbrush and brush/floss often.
  - Weakens bones over time; vitamin D supplement may be needed
  - Educate teenagers especially on importance of compliance; also counsel on body image, as this medication can cause alterations in self-esteem due to unpleasant cosmetic side effects.
  - Toxicity: rapid eye movements (nystagmus), difficulty with speech, poor muscle coordination/tripping and falling, encephalopathy (neurological effects)

Barbiturates

The classification, mechanism of action, side effects, and key teaching points of barbiturates are discussed below:
- Indication: daytime sedation; insomnia; preop sedation and anesthesia; anxiety relief; anticonvulsant
- MOA: increase effect of GABA in CNS, reducing excitability and producing sedation.
- Medications: phenobarbital (prototype), secobarbital; *ends in -barbital*
- Side effects: respiratory depression, sedation, GI upset, hypersensitivity, angioedema, tolerance, psychological and physical dependence
- Teaching:
  - Do not take with alcohol; do not drive or operate heavy machinery until you know how this drug will affect you.
  - Decreases efficiency of oral contraceptives
  - Does not allow for REM sleep – this is the cycle of sleep where mental rejuvenation takes place; may result in increased agitation/decreased ability to deal with stress.
  - Can cause paradoxical excitement in children and elderly
  - Phenytoin and valproic acid may increase toxic effects.

- 85 -

Succinylcholine

The classification, indication, mechanism of action, side effects, contraindications, and teaching considerations of succinylcholine are discussed below:

- Indications: Given as adjunct to anesthesia or for orthopedic manipulation to ensure relaxation of muscles and to facilitate intubation.
- MOA: Prevents transmission of nerve impulses to certain muscles, resulting in muscle paralysis, by binding with cholinergic receptors at the motor endplates of nerves to produce depolarization and prevent repolarization. Skeletal muscle relaxant, depolarizing neuromuscular blocker, pregnancy risk category C.
- Side Effects: arrhythmias, hyperkalemia, respiratory depression, anaphylaxis, malignant hyperthermia, rhabdomyolysis, rash, postoperative muscle pain and rigidity, and increased intraocular pressure.
- Contraindications: angle-closure glaucoma, history (personal, family) of malignant hyperthermia, upper motor neuron injury, major burns, and penetrating eye injuries. Drugs should be used with caution in patients who are elderly or debilitated.
- Teaching: If patient has prolonged muscle stiffness, talk to patient and reassure him/her that symptoms will subside.

Atypical antipsychotics

The classification, mechanism of action, side effects, and key teaching points of atypical antipsychotics are discussed below:

- Indication: schizophrenia, bipolar
- MOA: Block the dopamine and serotonin receptors; increase levels.
- Medications: clozapine, olanzapine, and risperidone, aripiprazole, lurasidone, quetiapine, and others.
- Side effects: weight gain, high cholesterol, dry mouth, blurred vision, drowsiness, tremors; persistent/painful erection (ziprasidone).
- Teaching:
  o Because of the decreased instance of extrapyramidal effects, atypical antipsychotics are becoming more widely prescribed.
  o Suck on sugar-free candy/chew sugar-free gum for dry mouth.
  o Need lab tests regularly to avoid blood issues/check cholesterol.

Typical antipsychotics

The indication, mechanism of action, side effects, and important teaching points for typical antipsychotics are discussed below:

- Indication: schizophrenia, bipolar disorder, and other various psychoses
- MOA: Precise mechanism of action unknown; thought to work by affecting levels of dopamine and serotonin in the brain.
- Medications: Haloperidol (oral or IM injection), fluphenazine, chlorpromazine, perphenazine, and others
- Side effects: extrapyramidal symptoms, tardive dyskinesia (muscle twitching; strange, uncontrollable movements), serotonin syndrome (dangerously low levels of serotonin leading to coma and death)
- Teaching:

- o May take a few weeks to become effective; cannot stop taking suddenly.
- o This classification is cheaper than atypical antipsychotics. While there is an increased risk of side effects, it may be more desired financially when long-term treatment is indicated.
- o Report immediately: unusual muscle twitching, increased temperature or drooling, increased anxiety/agitation.

Lithium

The indication, mechanism of action, side effects, and important teaching points for lithium are discussed below:
- Indication: mania (bipolar disorder), mood stabilizer; also used in headaches, depression, and neutropenia
- MOA: Unknown; acts in central nervous system as mood stabilizer.
- Side effects: drowsiness, dizziness, confusion, poor memory
- Teaching:
  - o Serum lithium levels: 0.8-1.5 mEq/L; must check regularly.
  - o Critical to maintain an adequate level of sodium in diet: low-sodium diets lead to toxicity in these patients; also avoid overheating and excessive sweating to prevent sodium loss.
  - o Drink plenty of fluids to ensure adequate excretion.
  - o Do not take with haloperidol: encephalopathy could occur.
  - o Toxicity (report immediately): blurred vision, seizure, lack of appetite, N/V/D, ringing in ears, slurred speech, muscle weakness/decreased coordination, increased urination.

Benzodiazepines

The classification, indication, mechanism of action, side effects, and known contraindications of benzodiazepines are discussed below:
- Indication: agitation, anxiety, insomnia, seizures, alcohol withdrawal
- MOA: Decrease excitability in different areas of the brain, may interact with GABA receptors
- Medications: temazepam, diazepam; *ends in –lam or –pam*
- Side Effects: drowsiness, dizziness, headache, paradoxical excitement.
- Teaching:
  - o Do not drive/operate heavy machinery or use alcohol while on this medication.
  - o Cannot use if pregnant or have narrow-angle glaucoma.
  - o Risk of addiction and abuse.
  - o Overdose: decreased level of consciousness, decreased reflexes, coma, respiratory arrest.
  - o Antidote: flumazenil.

Tetracyclic/tricyclic antidepressants

The classification, mechanism of action, side effects, and key teaching points of tetracyclic/tricyclic antidepressants are discussed below:
- Indication: major depressive disorder; also used for migraine headaches, phobias, urinary incontinence, attention deficit disorder, ulcers, and diabetic neuropathy
- MOA: block reuptake of serotonin and norepinephrine
- Medications: amitriptyline, amoxapine, imipramine, nortriptyline, etc.
- Side effects: dry mouth, constipation/urinary retention, sedation, orthostatic hypotension, diaphoresis, weight gain, serotonin syndrome.
- Teaching: May take a few weeks to become effective
- Increased suicide risk with initial treatment/change in dose; monitor closely, especially with children and young adults (<25 y.).

Selective Serotonin Reuptake Inhibitors

The classification, mechanism of action, side effects, and key teaching points of selective serotonin reuptake inhibitors (SSRIs) are discussed below:
- Indication: depression, anxiety
- MOA: Inhibits the reuptake of serotonin in the brain, resulting in increased levels of serotonin available for use.
- Medications: citalopram, escitalopram, fluexetine, paroxetine, sertaline.
- Side Effects: N/V/D, dizziness, weight fluctuations, dry mouth, headache, agitation/nervousness, sexual dysfunction (decreased desire, erectile dysfuntion)
- Teaching:
  - Take with food/before bed to avoid stomach upset.
  - Takes several weeks to become effective.
  - Withdrawal symptoms if stop taking suddenly.
  - Serotonin syndrome: report increase agitation, tremors, sweating, confusion, rapid heart rate immediately.
  - St. John's wort can cause serotonin syndrome if taken with an SSRI.
- SSS is a helpful mnemonic to remember the adverse effects of SSRIs: Stomach upset, Sexual dysfunction, Serotonin syndrome.

MAO Inhibitors

The classification, mechanism of action, side effects, and key teaching points of MAO inhibitors are discussed below:
- Indication: depression, anxiety, Parkinson disease
- MOA: Inhibits monoamine oxidase, the enzyme that normally metabolizes norepinephrine and serotonin, making these neurotransmitters more available to the receptors.
- Medications: tranylcypromine sulfate, phenelzine sulfate, isocarboxazid, selegiline
- Side effects: dry mouth, headache, drowsiness, dizziness, N/V/D, constipation; weight gain, sexual dysfunction, paresthesia also possible.
- Teaching:
  - React with most medications: ask MD before starting any new medication or supplement.

- o Interact with tyramine (amino acid in food), causing dangerously high blood pressure; must avoid all foods with this substance, including:
  - Aged cheeses
  - Fermented products (soy sauce, miso/tofu, sauerkraut, draft beer, wine)
  - Cured meats
- o Serotonin syndrome: immediately report increased agitation, tremors, sweating, confusion, rapid heart rate

CARDIOVASCULAR DRUGS

Antiarrhythmics

The classification, mechanism of action, side effects, and key teaching points of antiarrhythmics are discussed below:
- Indication: Treatment of atrial and ventricular arrhythmias:
- MOA: Divided into 5 classes (Vaughan Williams):
  - o Class I: Sodium Channel Blockers
    - Ia: quinidine, procainamide, disopyramide
    - Ib: lidocaine, phenytoin, mexiletine
    - Ic: flecainide, propafenone, moricizine
  - o Class II: beta-blockers (prototype: propranolol HCl)
  - o Class III: Potassium Channel Blockers (amiodarone, sotalol, dofetilide)
  - o Class IV: Calcium Channel Blockers (verapamil, diltiazem (Cardizem)
  - o Class V: Variable Mechanism – adenosine, digoxin, magnesium sulfate
- Side Effects: varies by class; generally risk of new or worsening arrhythmias, loss of appetite, diarrhea/constipation, change in taste, photosensitivity
- Teaching: Monitor pulse while on these medications: report low heart rate or irregular rhythm to doctor.

Adenosine

The classification, mechanism of action, side effects, and key teaching points of adenosine are discussed below:
- Indication: acute treatment of paroxysmal supraventricular tachycardia; cardiac stress testing
- MOA: temporarily decreases the conduction of impulses through the AV node; "resets" heart rhythm. Effective against reentry tachycardias (when an impulse depolarizes an area of heart muscle and returns and repolarizes it) that involve the AV node.
- Side effects: facial flushing, shortness of breath, dyspnea, chest discomfort.
- Teaching:
  - o Patient MUST be hooked up to continuous heart monitor and the nurse should have the crash-cart nearby
  - o IV Push: given quickly (1-3 seconds); nurse should expect a pause in heart rate—looks like a flat line on the machine, followed quickly by return to normal rhythm.

- If being used for scheduled stress test, the patient should not have any caffeine for the 12 hours before the test, including coffee, chocolate, tea, colas, or medications with caffeine.
- Not a long-term solution to arrhythmias.

Alpha-adrenergic blockers

The classification, mechanism of action, side effects, and key teaching points of alpha-adrenergic blockers are discussed below:
- Indication: hypertension, BPH (benign prostatic hypertrophy), heart failure, Reynaud phenomena, pheochromocytoma, skin conditions
- MOA: interrupts the actions of the catecholamines at the alpha receptors, resulting in relaxation of the smooth muscle in the blood vessels and increased dilation of blood vessels.
- Medications: doxazosin, prazosin, terazosin; *ends in -zosin*
- Tamsulosin: BPH
- Side effects: orthostatic hypotension, headache, dizziness, nasal congestion, decreased libido/impotence
- Teaching:
  - "First-Dose Effect" – extreme drop in blood pressure with first dose; give at bedtime to avoid falls/injury.
  - Men: educate about possible sexual side effects and treatment options.
  - Do not stop taking abruptly – rebound hypertension could occur.

Beta-adrenergic blockers

The indication, mechanism of action, side effects, and important teaching points for beta-adrenergic blockers are discussed below:
- Indication: heart attacks, angina, hypertension, hypertrophic cardiomyopathy, and supraventricular arrhythmias
- MOA: Prevent stimulation of the sympathetic nervous system by inhibiting the action of catecholamines at the beta-adrenergic receptors; cardioprotective.
- Propranolol, metoprolol tartrate - *ends in -olol*
- Side effects: bradycardia, respiratory depression, arrhythmia, bronchospasm, hypotension, fatigue.
- Teaching:
  - "Xanax for your heart": protects heart from harmful chemicals released after heart attack; crucial to keep taking.
  - Check pulse – do not take if < 60, call your doctor.
  - Orthostatic hypotension: change position slowly to prevent dizziness and falls
  - Caution in diabetics: may block S&S of hypoglycemia

Calcium channel blockers

The classification, mechanism of action, side effects, and key teaching points of calcium channel blockers are discussed below:
- Indication: hypertension, arrhythmias, Raynaud disease, migraines, angina pectoris
- MOA: affect the movement of calcium into the cells, relaxes blood vessels, reducing cardiac workload.
- Medications: amlodipine, nifedipine, verapamil, diltiazem, nicardipine
- Ends in –dipine
- Side effects: hypotension, bradycardia, GI upset, edema, rash, flushing
- Teaching:
  - Monitor blood pressure and pulse; call doctor if unusually low.
  - May be more powerful when taken with other blood pressure medications.
  - Grapefruit juice may also potentiate effects.

> ➤ **Review Video: Calcium Channel Blockers**
> *Visit mometrix.com/academy and enter Code: 345329*

Digitalis glycosides

The indication, mechanism of action, side effects, and important teaching points for digitalis glycosides are discussed below:
- Indication: Heart failure, hypotension, supraventricular arrhythmias, paroxysmal atrial tachycardia
- MOA: Increases intracellular calcium at the cell membrane, thus increasing the force of the heart's contractions.
- "Positive inotrope, negative chronotrope"
- For arrhythmias, a loading dose is often given
- Medications: digoxin
- Side effects: bradycardia, headache, loss of appetite.
- Teaching:
  - Serum digoxin level: 0.5-2 ng/mL (very narrow therapeutic index)
  - Check pulse before administration (Nursing: apical)
  - Adequate potassium levels protect against toxicity. Ensure a diet that has a moderate amount of potassium, and do not take medications that would decrease levels (diuretics, steroids, theophylline, and amphotericin B) without potassium replacement.
  - Toxicity: visual disturbances (green and yellow halos around lights/double vision), nausea/vomiting, diarrhea – report immediately.

Nitrates

The indication, mechanism of action, side effects, and important teaching points for nitrates are discussed below:
- Indication: Acute angina, myocardial infarction, hypertension
- MOA: Dilates blood vesels, increasing blood flow to the heart and decreasing preload, afterload, and oxygen requirements of the heart.
- Medications: nitroglycerin, erythrityl dinitrate, isosorbide dinitrate, isosorbide mononitrate, pentaerythritol tetranitrate.

- Side effects: headache, hypotension, tachycardia
- Teaching
  - Nitroglycerin:
    - Lie down, and take 1 tablet under the tongue every 5 minutes until relief (max dose is 3 tablets in 15 min). If still no relief, call 9-1-1.
    - Store in dark container/protect from light; should feel a slight burning sensation under the tongue, means it is still working.
    - Can be given continuous IV infusion: monitor blood pressure closely, and titrate for pain relief/BP control.
  - Headache is common, means medication is working; can take acetaminophen for relief
- NEVER take nitrates/give nitrates to patient with history of erectile dysfunction on medications such as sildenafil (PDE5 inhibitors); can cause severe, irretractable hypotension.

Statins and fibric acid derivatives

Statins (HMG-CoA reductase inhibitors) are cholesterol-lowering medications. Commonly used statins include lovastatin, pravastatin, simvastatin, atorvastatin, cerivastatin, fluvastatin, and rosuvastatin.
- MOA: Statins reduce cholesterols levels by blocking the enzyme HMG-CoA reductase, which the liver requires to produce cholesterol.
- Side effects: GI disturbance, rash, headaches, blurred vision, ophthalmoplegia, fatigues, insomnia, constipation, diarrhea, nausea, and myalgia/myopathy.
- Patient teaching: Patients who experience myalgia/myopathy may progress to rhabdomyolysis, so they should be cautioned to immediately report any muscle pain. The medication should be used with caution with oral anticoagulants.

Fibric acid derivatives (fibrates) are cholesterol-lowering drugs that primarily affect triglycerides but may also lower LDL and total cholesterol.
- MOA: Fibrates activate lipoprotein lipase, an enzyme that breaks down cholesterol, cleaving triglycerides from LDL or VLDL and leaving just the lipoprotein behind.
- Side effects: nausea, vomiting, diarrhea, gall stones, acute appendicitis, impotence, dysuria, hematuria, dizziness, rash, pruritus, alopecia, vertigo, headaches, and eczema. Increased risk of rhabdomyolysis if given with a statin.
- Patient teaching: Fibrates may enhance the action of anticoagulants, increasing risk of bleeding. Patients should report adverse effects.

HEMATOLOGICAL DRUGS

Antiplatelets

The classification, mechanism of action, side effects, and key teaching points of antiplatelets are discussed below:
- Indication: prevent arterial thromboembolism in patients at risk of MI, stroke, and arteriosclerosis, maintain patency of stents
- MOA: Inhibit platelet aggregation.
- Medications: aspirin, persantine, clopidogrel, ticlopidine, pentoxifylline, cilostazol

- Pentoxifylline/Cilostazol: increases flexibility of RBCs, treats intermittent claudication with PAD.
- Side effects: bleeding, epigastric upset, dizziness, headache, neutropenia/agranulocytosis (ticlopidine).
- Teaching:
  o Along with lifestyle modification, will help prevent heart attack, stroke, stent occlusion.
  o Report signs of bleeding immediately.
  o Cannot be given to patients with hemorrhage, trauma, thrombocytopenia, or hemorrhagic stroke.

Aspirin

The indication, mechanism of action, side effects, and important teaching points for *aspirin (ASA)* are discussed below:
- Indication: analgesic, anti-inflammatory (gout), antiplatelet - prevention of MI and stroke
- MOA: Salicylate: prevents platelets from sticking together and forming blood clots.
- Side effects: increased bleeding, bruising, stomach upset
- Teaching
  o People at increased risks for bleeding should not use aspirin (e.g., hemophilia, severe liver disease, stomach ulcers)
  o Aspirin should NEVER be given to children ≤15 years old, due to risk of Reye syndrome (potentially fatal liver disease in presence of viral infection, exclusively in this age group).
  o Toxicity: dark, tarry stools (GI bleed); tinnitus (ringing in ears, metabolic acidosis)

Chemotherapy

Chemotherapy has been discussed as "bringing someone to the edge of death, to try and bring them back to life again." While this is a graphic description, it illustrates that fact that chemotherapy kills all types of cells in the body, normal and cancer cells alike. Normal cells usually recover when chemotherapy is over, so most side effects gradually go away after treatment ends, and the healthy cells have a chance to grow again. However, during chemotherapy, the patient should be prepared to experience any of the following side effects:
- Severe fatigue
- Nausea/Vomiting
- Pain and generalized aches
- Hair Loss (alopecia) including eyebrows and lashes
- Anemia and blood clotting issues (risk of hemorrhage)
- Infection prone – low white blood cell count
- Mouth and throat sores
- Diarrhea/Constipation
- Infertility (may be permanent)

The nurse should educate the patient on the importance of rest and adequate hydration during treatment, as well as on differing methods to help alleviate discomfort.

Immunosuppressants

The indication, mechanism of action, side effects, and important teaching points for immunosuppressants are discussed below:

- Indication: organ transplant rejection prevention, autoimmune disorders, some cancer drugs
- MOA: exact mechanism of action unknown; may disrupt RNA synthesis, inhibit T cells.
- Medications: azathioprine, cyclosporine, lymphocyte immune globulin (ATG), muromonab-CD3, and tacrolimus. Cyclophosphamide; steroids are also considered immunosuppressants
- Side effects: increased risk of infection, GI upset, increased blood pressure/cholesterol, insomnia, skin irritations, mood swings/insomnia
- Teaching:
  - Avoid contact with sick individuals; wash hands frequently, avoid crowds
  - Report fever, foul-smelling urine, reddened wounds, nausea/vomiting, or any other signs of infection right away.

Epoetin Alfa

The classification, mechanism of action, side effects, and key teaching points of *epoetin alfa* are discussed below:

- Indication: normocytic anemia in ESRD, anemia in cancer patients and patients with HIV, and other anemias.
- MOA: Stimulates RBC production in bone marrow
- Trade names: Epogen, Procrit
- Side effects: hypertension, headache, GI upset, cough, fever, generalized pain, insomnia, irritation at injection site, weight loss, blood clots, allergic reaction
- Teaching:
  - Subcutaneous Injection: store vials in refrigerator away from bright light; do not shake and do not reuse individual vials. Dispose of needles properly
  - May cause unsafe rise in hemoglobin or blood pressure; monitor both regularly.
  - May need to take iron supplements/vitamins due to increased demand of body while making more RBCs
  - May notice increase in energy due to resolved anemia; however, still need to attend dialysis since actual issue is not resolved.
  - Teach S&S of blood clots.

Folic acid supplements

The classification, mechanism of action, side effects, and key teaching points of folic acid supplements are discussed below:

- Indication: folic acid deficiency in alcoholism, pregnancy, liver/kidney dysfunction, prevention of neonatal neural tube defects.
- MOA: Supplement (vitamin B9); necessary for creation of blood in body
- Medications: folic acid, vitamin B9, FA-8, folacin, folate
- Side effects: bitter taste, GI distress, headache, hypotension, skin issues (itching, rash, flushing, hypoglycemia, insomnia, decreased zinc levels)

- Teaching:
  - o Large doses may counteract the effects of phenytoin, potentially leading to seizures.
  - o Found naturally in dark, leafy greens, fruits, organ meats, cereals, and tomato juice.
  - o Most effective in preventing neural tube defects in children if taken before pregnancy/during the first trimester. Woman seeking to become pregnant should begin taking a supplement with folic acid immediately.

Iron supplements

The indication, mechanism of action, side effects, and important teaching points for iron supplements are discussed below:
- Indication: iron deficiency anemia, low iron levels (pregnant women, toddlers, and teenage girls), hemmorhage, burns, hemodialysis
- MOA: mineral replacement; necessary component of blood (2/3 of iron in body)
- Medications: ferrous fumarate, ferrous gluconate, ferrous sulfate, iron sucrose, and iron dextran
- Side Effects: gastric irritation, dark stools; IV – allergic reaction, phlebitis, hypotension, orthostatic hypotension
- Teaching:
  - o Take with food to avoid gastric upset
  - o Vitamin C increases iron absorption: take with orange or fruit juice.
    - ▪ Absorption is reduced by antacids, coffee, tea, dairy products, eggs, whole grains; avoid 1 h before/2 h after
  - o Liquid: stains teeth; mix and drink through straw.
  - o Common cause of OD in chidren: keep away in locked cabinet.

Warfarin

The classification, mechanism of action, side effects, and key teaching points of warfarin (Coumadin) are discussed below:
- Indication: prevention of DVT/PE/stroke, atrial fibrillation, valve replacement
- MOA: inhibits clotting factors that rely on vitamin K (II, VII, IX, and X)
- Side Effects: bleeding, increased bruising, GI effects (nausea, cramps)
- Teaching:
  - o Monitor PT/INR: INR should be between 2-3 (a little higher for valve replacements)
  - o Avoid large doses of foods high in vitamin K (dark, leafy greens especially), as these inactivate warfarin's effects.
  - o Soft-bristled toothbrush, electric razor, avoid activities with high risk of injury; often taken in the evening before bed.
  - o May take a while to reach therapeutic levels, often "bridged" with heparin until INR is therapeutic.
  - o Antidote: vitamin K (phytonadione)

> ➤ **Review Video:** Warfarin: Most Popular Anticoagulant?
> *Visit **mometrix.com/academy** and enter **Code: 712643***

Heparin

The indication, mechanism of action, side effects, and important teaching points for heparin are discussed below:

- Indication: DVT prophylaxis, venous thromboemboli, atrial fibrillation, acute MI, used in lines and machines to prevent blood clotting (cardiopulmonary bypass, hemodialysis, etc)
- MOA:Inhibits conversion of prothrombin to thrombin, thus preventing clot formation (does not dissolve clots already present).
- Medications: heparin (IV or SQ), enoxaparin (SQ)
- SQ: abdomen @ 90-degree angle, do not aspirate or massage.
- Side Effects: bruising, increased risk of bleeding, thrombocytopenia, rash, fever, heparing-induced thrombocytpopenia (HIT); long-term use: hair loss and osteoporosis
- Teaching:
  o Monitor aPTT; theraputic when 1½ to 2½ times normal value.
  o SQ injection: go over injection sites and proper needle disposal
  o IV heparin infusion: titrated to achieve goal pTT, must continuously monitor and adjust according to hospital policy.
  o Do not take NSAIDs/aspirin: increased risk of bleeding
  o Use electric razor and soft-bristled toothbrush; avoid activities such as contact sports, ice skating, or anything that increases risk of falls or trauma.
  o Antidote: protamine sulfate (works in 5 minutes)

Thrombolytics

The classification, mechanism of action, side effects, and key teaching points of thrombolytics are discussed below:

- Indications: embolism, acute MI, ischemic stroke, PE/DVT
- MOA: Intravenous medication that dissolves clots by activating conversion of plasminogen to plasmin, which breaks apart fibrin particles.
- Medications: alteplase (TPA), streptokinase, anistreplase
- Side Effects: hemorrhage, allergic reaction, hematuria, hemoptysis, hematochezia, melena; hypotension, and dysrhythmias
- Teaching:
  o These medications are generally given in emergency situations to dissolve clots and prevent further damage in MI and stroke; however, they must be given within 4-6 hours of onset of symptoms.
  o Cannot give if patient has history of recent trauma, concussion/head bleed, surgery, post-partum, uncontrolled HTN, or abdominal bleed.
  o Report immediately signs of bleeding such as bleeding from IV or old puncture wounds, coughing up blood, nose bleed, or blood in urine or stools
  o Antidote: aminocaproic acid

> **Review Video: Anticoagulants, Thrombolytics, and Antiplatelets**
> *Visit mometrix.com/academy and enter Code:* **587118**

Antihistamines

The indication, mechanism of action, side effects, and important teaching points for antihistamines are discussed below:

- Indication: Acute allergic reactions, seasonal allergies, motion sickness, sleep aid
- MOA: Histamine 1 (H1) receptor antagonists compete with histamine for binding to the H1 receptor sites throughout the body but cannot displace bound histamine.
- Medications: diphenhydramine, chlorpheniramine, prochlorperazine, loratadine, hydroxyzine hydrochloride, and hydroxyzine pamoate
- Side effects: drowsiness, dizziness, dry mouth, nausea/vomiting, paradoxical excitement/agitation in children
- Teaching:
  - Do not drive/operate machinery until you know how these medications will affect you.
  - Since antihistamines cannot displace bound histamine, these medications are best when taken before symptoms appear/as soon as possible to prevent worsening.

Note: Loratadine may cause serious cardiac effects when taken with macrolide antibiotics (e.g., erythromycin), fluconazole, ketoconazole, itraconazole, miconazole, cimetidine, ciprofloxacin, and clarithromycin.

Antitussives

The indication, mechanism of action, side effects, and important teaching points for antitussives are discussed below:

- Indication: Used to treat a serious, nonproductive cough that interferes with a patient's ability to rest and perform ADLs; pneumonia, bronchitis, the common cold, and COPD; also for diagnostic procedures
- MOA: Suppress or inhibit dry, nonproductive coughing.
- Medications: benzonatate, codeine, dextromethorphan hydrobromide, and hydrocodone bitartrate.
- Narcotic antitussives (codeine and hydrocodone) are used to treat the intractable cough associated with lung cancer
- Side effects: nausea/vomiting, excitation, elevated temperature, increased blood pressure; narcotics may cause CNS depression.
- Teaching:
  - Do not take with productive cough; will prevent clearance of mucus from respiratory tract
  - Do not give to children younger than 6 years of age
  - These medications only provide symptom relief; do not "cure" anything. Drink plenty of fluids and get rest.

Decongestants

The indication, mechanism of action, side effects, and important teaching points for decongestants are discussed below:

- Indications: relieve the symptoms of swollen nasal membranes resulting from: hay fever, allergic rhinitis, vasomotor rhinitis, acute coryza, sinusitis, and the common cold
- MOA:
  - Systemic: stimulate the sympathetic nervous system to reduce swelling of the respiratory tract's vascular network.
  - Topical: same MOA, with quicker effects.
- Sudafed (pseudoephedrine), Sudafed PE (phenylephrine), Afrin (oxymetazoline),
- Side effects: anxiety/agitation, insomnia, increased blood pressure.
- Teaching:
  - Do not take nasal spray > 3 days (rebound congestion)
  - Increased CNS stimulation may occur when taken with other sympathomimetic drugs.
  - Do not take with MOA inhibitors or alkalinizing drugs.

Expectorants

The classification, mechanism of action, side effects, and key teaching points of expectorants are discussed below:

- Indication: chest congestion, upper respiratory infection, bronchitis, influenza, sinusitis, bronchial asthma, emphysema, and other respiratory disorders.
- MOA: Thin mucus so it is cleared more easily out of airways.
- Medications: guaifenesin
- Side effects: Nausea/Vomiting
- Teaching:
  - Drink plenty of fluids; will thin mucus further and make it easier to cough up.
  - Do not use for dry cough (ineffective); do not give to children younger than 6 years of age.

Methylxanthines

The indication, mechanism of action, side effects, and important teaching points for methylxanthines are discussed below:

- Indication: Used to treat breathing disorders, including asthma, chronic bronchitis, emphysema, and neonatal apnea.
- MOA: Relax smooth muscle of bronchioles, resulting in dilation of airway
- Medications: anhydrous theophylline, aminophylline, oxtriphylline, and theophylline sodium glycinate.
- Side effects: agitation, tachycardia, urinary frequency, gastrointestinal distress, seizures

- Teaching:
  - Smoking increases elimination, decreasing serum concentrations and effectiveness.
  - Avoid coffee, tea, chocolate, soda, and other foods or drinks containing caffeine, as these may result in additive adverse reactions.
  - Theophylline: therapeutic serum level is 10-20 mcg/dL

GASTROENTEROLOGICAL DRUGS

Antacids

The classification, mechanism of action, side effects, and key teaching points of antacids are discussed below:
- Indication: gastroesophageal reflux disease (GERD), heartburn, indigestion
- MOA: alkaline in nature, therefore is able to neutralize gastric pH
- Medications: aluminum hydroxide, calcium carbonate, sodium bicarbonate (baking soda), magnesium hydroxide (Milk of Magnesia), etc.
- Aluminum hydroxide - reduces phosphorus (ESRD)
- Calcium carbonate: supplement to prevent osteoporosis
- Side effects: rare; N/V/D; rebound increase in acid production
- Teaching:
  - Do not cure issue, simply help manage symptoms
  - Talk to doctor before use if you have kidney disease, foul-smelling and painful diarrhea, or have heartburn that lasts longer than 2 weeks.
  - Lifestyle modification: avoid spicy foods, stay upright for hour after meals, and avoid drinking large amounts of liquids with meals.

Bile acid sequestrants

The classification, mechanism of action, side effects, and key teaching points of bile sequestering drugs are discussed below:
- Indication: high cholesterol; especially in cardiac and diabetic patients.
- MOA: resins that trap bile acid in intestines and promote excretion through feces.
- Medications: cholestyramine (prototype), colestipol hydrochloride, colesevelam.
- Side effects: GI upset: constipation, nausea, heartburn, flatus, indigestion.
- Teaching:
  - Take other medications 1 h before/4 h after these drugs, as they can decrease absorption.
  - Comes as a powder: can mix with water or other foods.
  - Lifestyle modification: weight loss, low-fat diet, smoking cessation, and exercise are all effective ways to lower cholesterol.

Sucralfate

The classification, mechanism of action, side effects, and key teaching points of sucralfate are discussed below:
- Indication: gastric, duodenal and oral ulcers, GI bleed, stress ulcer prevention
- MOA: forms a protective barrier on the GI mucosa, high affinity for areas of ulceration; local acid neutralization.

- 99 -

- Side Effects: N/V/D, dry mouth, flatus, dizziness, rash.
- Teaching:
  o Must be given 1 h before/2 h after a meal.
  o Do not give within 2 h of other medications; will decrease absorption.
  o Decreased excretion in those with renal disease.
  o Lifestyle Modification: avoid spicy, highly acid foods, as well as NSAIDs or other medications that could irritate the stomach lining.

Histamine (H2) receptor antagonists

The classification, mechanism of action, side effects, and key teaching points of histamine H2 antagonists are discussed below:
- Indication: duodenal ulcers, GERD, esophagitis
- MOA: blocks histamine's stimulation of gastric acid secretion
- Medications: famotidine, cimetidine, ranitidine, and others.
- Side Effects: headache most common, also diarrhea, dizziness, rashes
- Teaching:
  o Take with a meal, often breakfast; can also take at bedtime.
  o Wait at least 30 minutes between taking H2 blockers and an antacid.
  o If required for more than 2 weeks, call doctor for further workup.
  o Lifestyle Modification: avoid spicy, highly acid foods, carbonated beverages, citrus fruit, as well as NSAIDs or other medications that could irritate the stomach lining.

PPIs

The classification, mechanism of action, side effects, and key teaching points of proton pump inhibitors (PPIs) are discussed below:
- Indication: heartburn, GERD, peptic ulcers
- MOA: Inhibits gastric acid production in the stomach.
- Medications: omeprazole, lansoprazole, esomeprazole, pantoprazole, and others.
- Side Effects: nausea, headache, diarrhea, constipation, flatulence, osteoporosis, hypomagnesia
- Teaching:
  o Take at least 1 hour before meals.
  o Does not provide immediate relief of symptoms.
  o May affect absorption of other drugs.
  o Pantoprazole sodium IV: dilute and push slowly over 2-3 minutes.
  o Lifestyle Modification: avoid spicy, highly acidic foods, as well as NSAIDs or other medications that could irritate the stomach lining.

Lactulose

The classification, mechanism of action, side effects, and key teaching points of lactulose are discussed below:
- Indication: hepatic encephalopathy (reduces blood ammonia levels), constipation.
- MOA: synthetic sugar that binds to ammonia in the blood, pulling it into colon to be expelled.
- Names: Enulose, Generlac, Constulose, etc.

- Side Effects: flatulence, bloating, diarrhea, hyperactive bowel sounds.
- Teaching:
  - Never hold dose due to diarrhea (means the drug is working)
  - Monitor patient's mental status and level of consciousness, ammonia levels
  - May raise blood sugar in diabetics: monitor closely.
  - Monitor patient for S&S of dehydration/fluid-electrolyte imbalance, especially elderly or pediatric patients.

Laxatives/stool softeners

The classification, mechanism of action, side effects, and key teaching points of laxatives/stool softeners are discussed below:
- Indication: constipation (treatment/prophylaxis), bowel surgery prep.
- MOA:
  - Osmotic: pulls in fluid; magnesium hydroxide (Milk of Magnesia)
  - Bulk-Forming: swell in water to form gel that increases bulk and softens stool, increases peristalsis; Metamucil, Citrucel, MiraLAX
  - GoLYTELY: potent laxative used for bowel prep; patient drinks gallon over several hours, until stools are clear.
  - Stool Softeners: reduce surface tension in the bowel increasing water absorption into stool; docusate (Colace).
- Side effects: diarrhea, nausea, fullness/bloating; Milk of Magnesia - hypermagnesemia, renal dysfunction.
- Teaching:
  - Dependence can develop, especially in elderly patients. Do not take unless needed; educate that it is normal for bowels to slow with age.
  - Lifestyle modification: increasing fluids, moderate exercise, eating high-fiber foods (prunes) are all ways to prevent constipation
  - Teaching - Do not strain for stools: can cause bradycardia and subsequent cardiac arrest secondary to vagal response.

RENAL/URINARY DRUGS

Anti-gout drugs/uricosurics

The indication, mechanism of action, side effects, and important teaching points for the medications used to treat gout are discussed below:
- Indication: treatment of acute and chronic gout.
- MOA: reduce the reabsorption of uric acid at the proximal tubules of the kidneys, increasing uric acid excretion in the urine.
- Medications: probenecid and sulfinpyrazone
- Other gout medications:
  - Allopurinol and febuxostat: xanthine oxidase inhibitors block enzyme necessary for production of uric acid.
  - Colchicine: treats acute attacks; prevent worsening of symptoms during initial uricosuric/xanthine oxidase inhibitor treatment.
- Side effects: GI upset, rash (allopurinol), headache

- Teaching:
  - o Must take these medications regularly to prevent attack.
  - o Do NOT take these medications during a flare-up if you were not taking them before, as they could worsen symptoms initially.
  - o Lifestyle Management: stay hydrated and avoid alcohol to decrease risk of flare-ups.

Potassium-sparing diuretics

The classification, mechanism of action, side effects, and key teaching points of potassium-sparing diuretics are discussed below:
- Indication: edema, diuretic-induced hypokalemia in patients with heart failure, cirrhosis, nephrotic syndrome, hypertension.
- MOA: blocks aldosterone, which leads to an increased excretion of sodium and water; conserves potassium and hydrogen ions; may be used in conjunction with other diuretics
- Medications: spironolactone (prototype), amiloride, and triamterene
- Spironolactone is used to treat hyperaldosteronism and hirsutism.
- Side Effects: frequent urination, stomach upset, rash, dizziness, headache, confusion, sexual dysfunction and gynecomastia (spironolactone), hyperkalemia
- Teaching:
  - o Frequent urination means drug is working, and should get better with time; take drug in morning to avoid nocturia
  - o Lifestyle modification: avoid foods high in potassium (potatoes, orange juice, etc.) and limit sodium
  - o Can cause hyperkalemia, especially when combined with ACE inhibitors.

Loop diuretics

The classification, mechanism of action, side effects, and key teaching points of loop diuretics are discussed below:
- Indication: HTN, fluid overload in heart failure, liver/kidney disease.
- MOA: blocks the resorption of sodium in kidneys, leading to increased excretion of sodium and water.
- Medications: furosemide (prototype), bumetanide, torsemide, ethacrynic acid
- Side Effects: hypokalemia, increased urination, dizziness, headache, N/V, diarrhea, hyperglycemia, blood issues, dehydration.
- Teaching:
  - o Furosemide IV: push slowly (~20 mg/min) to avoid kidey damage and hearing loss.
  - o Eat foods high in potassium to counteract loss; MD may prescribe supplement.
  - o Increased risk of digoxin toxity due to hypokalemia.
  - o Weigh daily, same time, naked, and before urination to determine effectiveness/spot early signs of heart failure.

> **Review Video: Diuretics**
> *Visit **mometrix.com/academy** and enter **Code: 431237***

ENDOCRINE DRUGS

Glucocorticoids

The indication, mechanism of action, side effects, and important teaching points for glucocorticoids are discussed below:
- Indication: replacement therapy in patients with adrenocortical insufficiency, immunosuppression, anti-inflammatory
- MOA: Also known as "steroids"; inhibit immune response by:
  - Decrease of leakage of plasma from the capillaries
  - Suppression of the migration of polymorphonuclear leukocytes
  - Inhibition of phagocytosis
  - Decreased antibody formation in injured or infected tissues
  - Medications: prednisone, cortisone, etc.; ends in –sone
- Side Effects: weight gain, emotional liability, acne, "moon face," "buffalo hump," increase blood sugar and bruising, increased risk of infection; osteoporosis over time.
- Teaching:
  - Monitor blood sugar closely, especially diabetic patients.
  - Increased risk of infection: wash hands frequently, avoid sick contacts, and stay hydrated.
  - Must taper dose when therapy is completed – sudden cessation can cause adrenal crisis.

Insulin

Prior to 1921, insulin-dependent diabetes was a fatal disorder. However, with the discovery of insulin, diabetic patients can lead close to normal lives. Insulin works as a gateway protein to allow glucose to enter the cells of the body for fuel. There are several different types of insulin, each with unique properties. The nurse needs to be aware of these, especially the peak time of the insulin he/she is administering, as the risk of hypoglycemia is greatest during that time.

Type	Names	Onset	Peak	Duration
Rapid acting	Humalog/ Lispro	5-15 min	1-2 h	2-6 h
Short Acting	Humulin/ Novolin	30 min	1-4 h	4-8 h
Intermediate/ Long Acting	NPH/ Ultralente	1-3 h	4-8 h	8-24 h
Long Acting	Lantus	1-2 h	No peak	16-24 h

Example: Samantha took her NPH insulin at 8:00 AM this morning. At what time should the nurse instruct her to be on the lookout for S&S of hypoglycemia?
Answer: Between noon and 4 PM.

- 103 -

<u>Correct method of mixing insulins</u>
Sometimes patients/caregivers will be required to mix long-acting and short-acting insulin to acquire the desired blood sugar stabilization:

1. Mix the insulin by gently rolling back and forth in the hands. Do not shake insulin or insulin products; air bubbles with alter dose.
2. Obtain syringe of appropriate size, draw up the same dose of air as insulin to be given.
3. Clean the tops of the insulin bottles with alcohol
4. Inject the cloudy insulin with the air equal to the dose of insulin to be given.
5. Inject the clear insulin with air equal to the dose of insulin to be given.
6. Draw up the desired dose of clear insulin.
7. Insert the needle again into the cloudy insulin and draw the desired dose.

Remember:
- "Clear before cloudy" – prevents contamination.
- **<u>Insulin is measured in units, and thus should ALWAYS be drawn up in insulin syringes; using any other type of syringe can lead to lethal medication errors.</u>**
- Insulin should be checked by two nurses prior to injection.

> ➢ **Review Video:** <u>Mixing Insulin</u>
> *Visit* ***mometrix.com/academy*** *and enter* ***Code: 388625***

Oral anti-diabetics

The indication, mechanism of action, side effects, contraindications, and teaching points of oral antidiabetics are discussed below:
- Indication: Treatment of hyperglycemia in type II diabetic patients.
- MOA:
  o Sulfonylureas: stimulation of insulin production in pancreatic B cells; glipizide, glyburide, chlorpropamide, tolazamide, tolbutamide; name generally ends in -ase
  o Biguanides: decreases liver production of glucose, promotes weight loss in obese patients; metformin.
  o Thiazolidinediones: facilitates glucose clearance; rosiglitazone.
  o Alpha-glucosidase inhibitors: slows absorption of glucose in intestinal tract; acarbose.
  o Meglitinide: increases insulin production; repaglinide.
- Side Effects: hypoglycemia, renal impairment; individual side effects with each drug.
- Contraindications: kidney dysfunction/recent IV contrast (metformin); must consult MD if drug is safe during pregnancy/breastfeeding.
- Teaching:
  o Patient should take regularly at same time every day.
  o Patient should ask MD about taking if scheduled for imaging test.
  o Weight loss, controlled diet, and regular exercise will help with blood glucose management.

DERMATOLOGICAL DRUGS

The skin functions to protect, regulate temperature, and offer immune responses, biochemical synthesis, and sensory detection. When the skin has been altered, it loses one or all of these abilities. Therefore, skin integrity is a nursing priority. Treatments for dermatological issues vary widely, but may include:

- Oral steroids; often used in adjunct therapy for skin conditions.
- Ultraviolent radiation: psoriasis.
- Sunscreens: prophylactic
- Vitamin D analogues, retinoids, and anthralin.
- Topical glucocorticoids: inflammatory conditions such as rash, pruritus, bullous disorders (e.g., herpes), collagen diseases such as systemic lupus erythematosus, and vasculitis.
- Antihistamines: rashes, allergic dermatitis

ANTIBIOTICS

Antibiotic therapy

The indications, common side effects, and teaching needed for *antibiotic therapy* are discussed below:

- Indication: Treatment and prophylaxis of bacterial infections
- Types:
  - Penicillins: end in –cillin.
  - Cephalosporins: cef-/ceph-; *cross-sensitivity with penicillins*
  - Tetracyclines: ends in -cycline
  - Aminoglycosides: ends in -mycin
  - Fluoroquinolones: ends in -floxacin
  - Sulfonamides: begins with sulfa-/ends in –azole.
- Side Effects: gastrointestinal distress, allergic reaction; some can cause nephro- and ototoxicity, photosensitivity.
- Contraindications: Do not take with alcohol or with known allergy.
- Teaching:
  - Take all prescribed doses until complete to prevent bacterial resistance and recurrent infection.
  - Take with food or milk to prevent stomach upset
  - If rash, swelling, or other signs of allergic reaction occur, stop taking and notify your doctor right away.
  - Wear sunscreen when going outdoors (tetracycline and quinolones).

Carbapenems

The classification, mechanism of action, side effects, and key teaching points of carbapenems are discussed below:

- Indication: mixed aerobic and anaerobic infections, as therapy for serious nosocomial infections, or infections in immunocompromised hosts.
- MOA: A class of beta-lactam; bind to cell wall interrupting growth.
- Medications: imipenem-cilastatin sodium and meropenem, ertapenem, doripenem

- Broadest spectrum possible in an antibiotic; broader than any other antibacterial to date.
- Side Effects: N/V/D; soreness/redness at injection site, headache, rash, fatigue, ringing in ears, paresthesias, secondary infections (candidiasis)
- Teaching:
  - Diarrhea is common, and could happen months after stopping medication; do not take anti-diarrheals without first consulting your doctor
  - Often given as an intramuscular injection
  - Report white coating over tongue, vaginal itching/discharge, and other signs of secondary infection.

Cephalosporins

The indication, mechanism of action, side effects, and important teaching points for cephalosporins are discussed below:
- Indication: Antibiotic used to fight infections, especially those in the respiratory and urinary tract, and skin and bone infections. Also used to prevent infections pre- and postoperatively.
- MOA: Bacteriocidal: inhibits cell-wall synthesis; begin in –cef/ceph
- First-generation: cefazolin, cephalexin; gram-positive organisms
- Second-generation: cefoxitin, cefuroxime; gram-negative organisms
- Third-generation: cefixime, ceftriaxone, cefotaxime; gram-negative and anaerobic organisms.
- Fourth-generation: cefepime; gram-positive and –negative organisms; widely effective
- Side Effects: gastrointestinal distress, nausea/vomiting, hypersensitivity (rash, itching, hives)
- Teaching:
  - Take all prescribed doses to prevent antibiotic resistance.
  - Take with food or milk to prevent GI distress.
  - Do not take with alcohol, as it can increase toxicity.
  - Cross-sensitivity with penicillin; use caution in these patients.

Lincosamides

The classification, mechanism of action, side effects, and key teaching points of lincosamides are discussed below:
- Indication: Bacterial infection; protozoal infections, toxoplasmosis, malaria, strep/staph, anaerobes, toxic shock syndrome (TSS)
- MOA: Bacteriostatic; very powerful; inhibits bacterial protein synthesis by interfering with ribosomes.
- Medications: lincomycin, clindamycin, pirlimycin
- Side Effects: gastrointestinal upset, pseudomembranous colitis, bitter taste (IV), dizziness, headache, neutropenia/thrombocytopenia, allergic reaction.
- Teaching:
  - Because of the potential for serious toxicity and pseudomembranous colitis, use is limited to a few clinical situations in which safer alternative antibiotics are not available.

- o Report diarrhea, bloody stools, abdominal cramps and fever immediately and do not take anti-diarrheals!
- o May block neuromuscular transmission and may enhance the action of neuromuscular blockers.

Macrolides

The classification, mechanism of action, side effects, and key teaching points of macrolides are discussed below:
- Indication: bacterial infections, H. pyloria (stomach ulcers), respiratory infections, otitis media
- MOA: bacteriostatic; inhibit protein synthesis, stopping bacterial proliferation
- Medications: azithromycin, clarithromycin, erythromycin
- Erythromycin: *Legionella pneumophila* and *Mycoplasma pneumoniae*
- Side Effects: severe GI upset (cramping and pain), N/V/D
- Teaching:
  - o Take with food to decrease GI upset
  - o Take all medication exactly as prescribed to prevent antibiotic resistance
  - o Do not take with theophylline: increases levels, increasing toxicity risk.

Sulfonamides

The classification, mechanism of action, side effects, and key teaching points of sulfonamides are discussed below:
- Indication: bacterial infection, especially UTIs; also pneumonia in AIDS patients.
- MOA: Bacteriostatic: stops manufacturing of folic acid by bacterial cells
- Medications: sulfisoxasole, sulfamethoxazole and trimethoprim (SMX-TMP); *prefix sulf-*
- Side Effects: urinary crystals, hypersensitivity, GI distress
- Teaching:
  - o Drink lots of water to help flush from kidneys and prevent stones (2,000-3,000 mL a day unless otherwise contraindicated)
  - o May increase the hypoglycemic affects of oral diabetic agents; be vigilant for S&S of hypoglycemia.
  - o High incidence of allergy; alert MD right away if signs of reaction occur.

Tetracyclines

The indication, mechanism of action, side effects, and important teaching points for tetracyclines are discussed below:
- Indication: broad-spectrum antibiotic; gram-positive and -negative aerobic and anaerobic bacteria; spirochetes; mycoplasmas; rickettsiae; chlamydiae; and some protozoa.
- MOA: Bacteriostatic – inhibits bacterial growth by inhibiting protein synthesis.
- Side Effects: gastric distress, photosensitivity, GERD
- Teaching:
  - o Do not take with milk; aluminum, calcium, and magnesium antacids reduce absorption.
  - o Do not give at bedtime. When patients lie down it often causes gastric reflux.

- o Can cause discoloration of the teeth of children, and fetuses when given to pregnant mothers.
- o Wear sunscreen; more susceptible to sunburns
- o Toxic: hearing loss, kidney dysfunction.

Fluoroquinolones

The classification, mechanism of action, side effects, and key teaching points of fluoroquinolones are discussed below:
- Indication: UTIs, upper respiratory infections, pneumonia, bone/joint/skin infections, gonorrhea, and others
- MOA: Bacteriocidal; alter DNA
- Medications: ciprofloxacin, levofloxacin, trovafloxacin, ofloxacin
- *Ends in: -floxacin or -oxacin*
- Side Effects: GI upset, photosensitivity, headache, vertigo/seizures
- Teaching:
  - o Take all medication exactly as prescribed
  - o Wear sunscreen and sunglasses when outdoors
  - o Take with food to minimize stomach upset; however antacids decrease absorption, as well as zinc and iron.

Anti-tuberculars

The classification, mechanism of action, side effects, and key teaching points of antitubercular agents are discussed below:
Indication: Treatment or prophylaxis if exposed to tuberculosis
- MOA: Alters DNA/RNA or lipid and nucleic acid synthesis; prevents growth of TB bacterium.
- Medications: isoniazid (INH; prototype), pyrazinamide (PZA), rifampin, rifapentine, rifabutin, streptomycin, ethambutol
- Side effects:
  - o Fever, liver dysfunction
  - o INH: hyperglycemia, rash, N/V, gynecomastia, peripheral neuritis
  - o Rifampin: orange-colored body fluids, inactivates oral contraceptives
  - o Ethambutol: retrobulbar neuritis, blindness
- Teaching:
  - o **Do not take alcohol with these drugs**: severe liver damage
  - o INH: take vitamin B6 to help with neuropathy, give before meals, and cannot take with phenytoin (toxicity)
  - o <u>Treatment can last > 2 years</u>; must stress compliance to prevent multi-drug resistant strains.
  - o Teach S&S of liver dysfunction: unusual bleeding, jaundice, fever, N/V, loss of appetite, numbness/tingling in extremities.

Antiviral drugs

The indication, mechanism of action, side effects, and important teaching points for antivirals are discussed below:
- Indication: Used to prevent or treat viral infections.
- MOA: Work by disrupting viral replication
- Acyclovir: herpes viruses and varicella-zoster virus
- Foscarnet: cytomegelovirus (CMV) retinitis in AIDS patients.
- Amantadine/rimantadine: Parkinson disease
- Ribavirin: nasal/oral: respiratory syncytial virus (RSV)
- Oseltamivir (Tamiflu): prophylaxis of influenza A or B, avian flu
- Others: ganciclovir, famciclovir, nelfinavir, zidovudine, didanosine, and zalcitabine.
- Side Effects: Vary widely; healthy cells often killed, so generalized malaise common
- Teaching:
  - Tamiflu – must be taken within 48 hours of onset of symptoms
  - No "cure" for viruses: simply control spread.
  - Viruses use the body's own cells to replicate, so antivirals kill body cells; this means side effects are often worse with these drugs than with antibiotics.

> ➢ **Review Video: <u>Viruses</u>**
> Visit ***mometrix.com/academy*** *and enter **Code: 735669***

Antifungals

The indication, mechanism of action, side effects, and important teaching points for antifungals are discussed below:
- Indication: systemic and local fungal infections, vaginal and oral candidiasis (thrush), ringworm,
- MOA: binds to sterols in fungal cell membranes and alters the permeability of the membranes.
- Medications: amphotericin B, fluconazole, nystatin, itraconazole, griseofulvin; most end in *-azole*
- Nystatin – "Swish and Swallow"; creams and mouthwash
- Fluconazole – fewer side effects than amphotericin B
- Side Effects: Headache, N/V/D, abdominal pain, rash. Amphotericin: fever, hypotension, malaise, join and muscle pain. Griseofulvin: blood dyscrasias.
- Teaching:
  - Monitor for severe side effects/allergic reactions.
  - Amphotericin B: pretreat with acetaminophen, antiemetic, and antihistamine for symptom management. Medication is light and time-sensitive: cover with foil and use within 24 h.
  - Prevention: keep skin clean and dry; avoid excessive moisture and tight clothes: fungi thrive in moist, warm environments. Yeast infections can also be a side effect of antibiotic use.

Blood Transfusions

While blood transfusions have saved millions of lives, there are still some inherent risks to giving blood. If you suspect a reaction, immediatley stop the blood transfusion (do NOT flush the line) and contact the doctor immediatley. The blood bag and the tubing will be sent down to the blood bank for inspection. There are several types of blood transfusion reactions: Remember AFH:

- **A**llergic: facial flushing, hives, rash, anxiety, wheezing, decreased BP
- **F**ebrile: high fever, headache, tachycardia, tachypnea, chills
- **H**emolytic: decreased BP, flank pain, increased respirations, hemoglobinuria, chest pain, anxiety, fever, tachycardia, chills

RBC Compatibility

DONOR								
RECIPIENT	AB+	AB-	B+	B-	A+	A-	O+	O-
AB +	YES	YES	YES	YES	YES	YES	YES	YES
AB-	NO	YES	NO	YES	NO	YES	NO	YES
B+	NO	NO	YES	YES	NO	NO	YES	YES
B-	NO	NO	NO	YES	NO	NO	NO	YES
A+	NO	NO	NO	NO	YES	YES	YES	YES
A-	NO	NO	NO	NO	NO	YES	NO	YES
O+	NO	NO	NO	NO	NO	NO	YES	YES
O-	NO	NO	NO	NO	NO	NO	NO	YES

> **Review Video: Blood Transfusions**
> Visit *mometrix.com/academy* and enter *Code:* **192415**

ID, SQ, and IM injections

The different types of injections are:
- Intradermal injections (ID)
  - Dermal layer of the skin; shallow, causes "bleb"; given into skin of inner forearm, or back, rarely chest.
  - Angle: 10°-15°
  - 27-30 g; ¼-3/8 inch length
  - ≤ 1 mL fluid: Mantoux test for TB exposure, allergy testing, etc.
- Subcutaneous injections (SQ)
  - Adipose (fat) tissue; upper, outer arm, the anterior thigh, and the abdomen
  - Angle: 45° (90° for insulin and heparin)
  - 25-28 g; 5/8 of an inch long
  - 0.5-1 mL of fluid; insulin, heparin, enoxaparin, etc.
- Intramuscular injections (IM)
  - Deep into muscle; ventrogluteal, vastus lateralis, or deltoid muscle
  - Angle: 90°
  - 23 g; 1-1½ inch length.
  - ≤ 3 mL of fluid; only 2 mL in deltoid.
  - MUST aspirate for blood prior to giving an IM injection to ensure medication will not be delivered intravenously.

- o Note: Dorsogluteal injections (into the upper, outer quarter of the buttocks) are now contraindiated due to risk of damage to the sciatic nerve. Do not use this site for injection.

Intravenous Fluids

Intravenous fluids are classified according to whether the total osmolality is the same as blood (isotonic), less than blood (hypotonic), or greater than blood (hypertonic):
- Isotonic fluids: These fluids expand extracellular volume because they diffuse rapidly from the blood into the ECF, so 3 L is needed to replace 1 L of blood. Isotonic fluids include dextrose 5% in water, normal saline, and lactated Ringer's solution (which is NS with potassium and chloride added).
- Hypotonic fluids: These fluids are used to replace cellular fluids and treat hypernatremia and hyperosmolar conditions. Excessive hypotonic fluids may result in hypotension, edema, and intravascular fluid depletion. Hypotonic fluids include 0.45% NS and sterile water.
- Hypertonic fluids: These fluids are used to treat hypovolemia and hyponatremia but may result in intravascular fluid volume excess, so they must be monitored very carefully. Hypertonic fluids include dextrose 10% in water, 3% saline, and 5% dextrose in NS. Solutions with concentrations of greater than dextrose 10% must be administered per central catheter.

Intravenous Access

Central venous access devices (CVADs) are lines used for intravenous access that are long, thick, and end in the superior or inferior vena cava. CVADs include tunneled and non-tunneled catheters, peripherally inserted central catheters (PICCs) and ports. Tunneled catheters and ports are placed surgically, and used when IV access will be needed for an extended period of time. PICCs and non-tunneled catheters can often be placed at the bedside in emergency situations, and are used for therapy that is expected to last days to weeks instead of months.

Nursing care guidelines
There are a few guidelines a nurse should be aware of when dealing with central venous access devices (CVADs):
- Central Line Associated Bloodstream Infections (CLABSI): CVADs greatly increase the risk of CLABSIs, which can be fatal. To prevent them, the nurse should maintain sterile technique when accessing the line. "Scrub the hub" for a minimum of 30 seconds before access and between uses. Change dressings weekly, using an occlusive chlorohexidine-impregnated dressing if available. Remove lines as soon as clinically possible.
- Medications: Because CVADs are significantly longer than peripheral IVs, medications may take longer to reach the patient. *ALWAYS* flush the first 5ccs at the same rate as the medication, as this will prevent the patient from receiving medications too quickly. TPN, pressors, and other potentially irritating or harmful medications should be given exclusively through central lines to avoid extravasation and tissue necrosis.
- Blood draws: When drawing blood from a port, remember to flush and waste the first 10 mL, as this may contain medication or be diluted. Always flush after

obtaining the sample with an additional 20 mL to avoid clotting off the catheter. If the catheter does become clotted, call the physician to obtain an orders for a thrombolytic agent.

Calculating Drip Rates of IV medications

A nurse will use the type of tubing, total time of infusion, and total volume of infusion to determine drip rate. Drip rate is always rounded to the nearest whole number: The formula is:

$$\frac{\text{Total volume infused} \times \frac{\text{drops}}{\text{mL}}}{\text{Total time of infusion in minutes}} = \text{drops per minute}$$

Example: The order is for 1 liter (1000 cc) of normal saline (NS) to be administered over 8 hours, with the use of an administration set that will deliver ten (10) drops (gtt)/cc. What will the drip rate be for this fluid?

$$\frac{1000 \times 10}{8 \times 60} = \frac{10,000}{480} = 20.8 = 21 \frac{gtt}{min}$$

Example: The order is for 2 liters (2000 cc) of 5% dextrose to be administered over 12 hours, with the use of an administration set that will deliver fifteen (15) drops (gtt)/cc. What will the drip rate for this be?

$$\frac{2000 \times 15}{12 \times 60} = \frac{30,000}{720} = 41.7 = 42 \frac{gtt}{min}$$

Note: Micro drip tubing delivers 60 drops/mL

> ➤ **Review Video:** <u>IV Drip Rates</u>
> *Visit **mometrix.com/academy** and enter **Code: 278763***

Complications Involving Intravenous Access Sites

While intravenous (IV) access sites are a valuable asset to nursing, there are some common complications that occur with their use. The nurse should assess for these every shift. Complications include:

- Infiltration: Infiltration occurs when the IV slips out of the vein and into the surrounding tissue. Common symptoms of infiltration include swelling, tenderness at site, decreased or no infusion rate, blanching of the skin and surrounding tissue, and the site may be cool to touch. Certain medications are necrotic to the tissues, so if infiltration occurs, the physician should be notified immediately.
- Phlebitis: Phlebitis is inflammation of a vein, sometimes caused by irritating solutions or prolonged age of the IV. Common signs of phlebitis include a red line along the vein, erythema, heat, edema, and tenderness.
- Accidental Removal: This occurs when a patient (or practitioner) accidentally pulls the IV out of the skin.

Treatment includes:
- Infiltration/Phlebitis: discontinuation of the IV, and application of warm compresses.

- Infiltration of necrotizing substances: injection of antidote into tissue; cool compress.
- Accidental removal: apply pressure to stop the bleeding with a sterile gauze, and cover with a bandage.

TPN

Total parenteral nutrition (TPN) is a form of nutrition that is maintained exclusively by intravenous routes. The purpose of TPN is to bypass the gastrointestinal system while still providing adequate calories and nutrition to the body. TPN is also used to maintain a positive nitrogen balance for healing as well as to replace lost electrolytes, vitamins, and minerals to the body. The administration of TPN is generally via a peripherally inserted central catheter (termed a PICC line), or any other type of central line (chest port, intrajugular central, etc); TPN should never be infused through a peripheral catheter, unless expressly ordered.

Nursing Considerations are as follows:
- These patients are at a considerably high risk of infection; TPN bag and tubing must be changed daily and any time a new bag is hung. Monitor patient for fever, chills, malaise, or other signs of infection.
- Hypoglycemia is another risk of TPN infusion: monitor blood glucose frequently. If TPN runs out before another bag can be obtained, run dextrose 10% in water until new bag is hung.
- **NEVER** run any other medications in the same line as TPN, and do not try to "catch up" infusion if delay occurs.

Pain Assessment

Assessment of pain is essential as part of overall evaluation and should be carefully documented, including the location, duration, and cause of the cause. Pain is categorized as:
- Acute: Usually associated with a specific injury or condition and lasting no more than 6 months. Acute pain usually responds to opioids, NSAIDs, or acetaminophen.
- Chronic: Constant or intermittent pain that lasts 6 months or longer. The cause of the pain may not be evident. Chronic pain is often very debilitating and is more difficult to control than acute pain because traditional pain medications are often ineffective. Patients may respond to complementary therapies (such as relaxation and acupuncture), local anesthetic agents, TCAs (such as amitriptyline), or anti-seizure medications (such as phenytoin).
- Cancer-related: May be acute or chronic and directly related to tumor growth or secondary to treatment. Pain control must be titrated to individual needs.

Assessment should include the characteristics of the pain, the intensity, the timing, the location, aggravating factors, alleviating factors, and the patient's response. Pain assessment/pain scales are as follows:
- Visual Analog Scale (VAS) (non-numeric): used to determine baseline pain.
- Numeric Pain Intensity (1 to 10 scale): for adolescents and adults to assess level of pain.
- Patient Comfort Assessment Guide: to assess pain status and pain relief, response to medications.

- Wong-Baker FACES: graphic depictions of pain through different facial expressions. Appropriate for children, non-English speakers, and some illiterate patients or patients with cognitive impairment. FACES has a pediatric version and an adult version.
- Brief Pain Inventory: assesses the effect pain has on activities.
- CRIES (crying, requires O_2, increased vital signs, expression, sleepiness): Assesses pain in neonates.
- FLACC (face, legs, activity, cry, consolability): appropriate for children to 3 years of age and older children with cognitive impairment.
- CPOT- Used in critical care settings (ventilated patients)
- Pain Assessment in Advanced Dementia Scale (PAINAD): appropriate for adults with cognitive impairment.

> ➤ **Review Video: Pain Documentation**
> *Visit mometrix.com/academy and enter Code:* **248521**

PAIN MEDICATIONS

NSAIDs

The classification, mechanism of action, side effects, and key teaching points for non-steriodal anti-inflammatory drugs (NSAIDs) are discussed below:
- Indication: relief of acute/chronic pain, inflammation
- MOA: prevent release of prostaglandins, inhibiting pain and inflammatory response
- Medications: Ibuprofen (Motrin, Advil), Naproxen (Aleve), ketoprofen, indomethacin
- Side Effects: gastric upset, stomach ulcers, increased risk of bleeding, nephrotoxicity, hypersensitivity
- Teaching:
  o Take with food or milk to decrease GI upset
  o Works well for muscle strain/spasms; works best if taken early to prevent pain.
  o Overdose: renal failure. Do not take more than daily recommended amount/amount prescribed by MD.
  o Report: dark, tarry stools, blood in vomit, gum bleeding, increased bruising, severe stomach pain, difficulty breathing, etc.
  o May be given with misoprostol, which reduces gastric acid secretion, thus preventing NSAID-related ulcers; though this medication may increase menstrual bleeding (contraindicated in pregnancy – causes miscarriage)

> ➤ **Review Video: NSAID Effects**
> *Visit mometrix.com/academy and enter Code:* **569064**

Muscle Relaxants

The classification, mechanism of action, side effects, and key teaching points of muscle relaxants are discussed below:
- Indication: acute injury, spasms caused by anxiety, inflammation, pain, trauma.
- MOA: Central acting; work in central nervous system to potentiate effects of GABA (amino acid)
- Medications: baclofen, cyclobenzaprine

- 114 -

- Dantrolene: acts directly on muscles to decrease excitability; spasticity, as well as malignant hyperthermia.
- Side Effects: drowsiness, loss of coordination, dizziness/ lightheadedness, euphoria, constipation, hepatotoxicity (dantrolene).
- Teaching:
  o Do not take with alcohol, will potentiate CNS depression
  o Increased risk of injury: monitor ambulation, do not allow to operate heavy machinery while on this mediation

Opioid Analgesics

The classification, indication, mechanism of action, side effects, and known contraindications of opioid analgesics are discussed below:
- Indication: Strong pain relief; adjunct treatment of MI (morphine)*
- MOA: Naturally derived from the opium plant, opioids attach to opioid receptors in the brain, spinal cord, and gastrointestinal tract, stopping the transmission of pain messages to the brain. They also alter how the brain perceives the incoming pain signals; common opiates are morphine, hydromorphone, oxycodone, methadone, fentanyl, and butorphanol
- Side Effects: euphoria, drowsiness, nausea/vomiting, constipation, dilated pupils and respiratory depression, CNS depression, emotional liability, risk of addiction.
- Contraindications: respiratory depression, known allergy, suspected gallbladder disease (morphine).
- Teaching:
  o Teach not to drive or operate machinery while taking these drugs.
  o Do not take with alcohol; take only as directed.
  o Patient cannot sign consent while under influence of opiates.
  o Educate on addiction, drug-sharing; other forms of pain relief.

*Morphine is often used in treating pain accompanying an MI. It decreases preload in the heart, relieving ischemia and allowing oxygen to perfuse the cells.

Reduction of Risk Potential

This domain is defined by the NCSBN as "reducing the likelihood that clients will develop complications or health problems related to existing conditions, treatments, or procedures." This section includes common diagnostic procedures and tests, laboratory values, and potential complications related to common procedures.

CT scan

The computed tomography (CT) scan offers imaging of sections of the body from various angles. CT assists in early diagnosis of disease and disease processes. The CT is approximately 100 times more sensitive than the normal x-ray. CT can be performed with or without contrast dye (media). Contrast offers enhanced views of the organs and structures being examined; an example is increased visibility of small tumors or abnormalities. The CT is used for viewing the brain, head, chest, abdomen, pelvis, spine, and bones of the body; it is used most often in determining coronary artery disease or lesions of the head, liver, and kidney. CT also assists in the diagnosis of tumors, edema, abscesses, infection, metastatic diseases, vascular disorders, stroke, and bone destruction and deformity. CT is also used to locate and identify foreign object within soft tissue. Use caution with contrast dye in patients with renal impairment. Ensure patient can lie still during test. Not an MRI – open machine. MD may order patient to be NPO before procedure. For the procedure, the patient will lie still on a table and move in and out of a hollow machine.

EEG

The electroencephalography (EEG) is a reading of the electropotentials within the brain. The electroencephalogram measures electrical impulses of brain cells, and is an assistive tool for diagnosing seizure disorders, neoplasm of the brain, cerebral vascular accident/strokes, trauma of the brain, and infectious processes of the brain and nervous system. Electroencephalogram is also used to determine brain death, and may also be useful in diagnosis of intracranial hemorrhage and intracranial abscess. The normal findings of an EEG are the same for the adult or child. Normal tracing and regular short waves are the expected findings of the EEG. Avoid sedatives, alcohol, and stimulants (caffeine) for 24-48 hours before the test ; wash the hair with normal shampoo (do not condition); use of hairspray/products/oil in hair will alter test; ***will not be painful***. Patient will simply rest quietly with electrodes placed on scalp. Can wash gel out of hair afterwards. For the procedure, electrodes with gel will be placed on different areas of the scalp, and then patient will lie in quiet room for 1-3 hours; video may be taken during test.

Babinski reflex

Babinski reflex occurs when the great toe flexes toward the top of the foot and the other toes fan out after the sole of the foot has been firmly stroked. This reflex is normal in infants, disappearing at the age of 2. In people older than 2 years, the presence of a Babinski's reflex indicates damage to the brain/nervous system. The reflex can be temporary or permanent depending on the extent of the damage. Any condition in which there is suspected neurological insult warrants testing for a Babinski reflex; if found, further testing should be done immediately to determine the cause and extent of the damage.

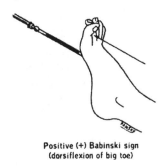

Positive (+) Babinski sign
(dorsiflexion of big toe)

Bronchoscopy

A bronchoscopy is an inspection of the interior of the tracheobronchial tree for either diagnosis, biopsy, or foreign body removal. A bronchoscopy can be used to visualize the larynx, trachea, and bronchi. With utilization of a bronchoscopy, the patient may have examinations of tissue, secretion removal, or specimen collection done. Normal findings of a bronchoscopy include normal structure and normal lining of the larynx, trachea, and bronchi. Educate the patient on the procedure, including anesthetic and relaxation techniques. Ensure consent is witnessed and on the chart; remove dentures, glasses, jewelry, and contact lenses. Monitor breathing and lung sounds post-procedure; keep NPO until they regain gag reflex/pass swallow screen. May give lozenges for sore throat after able to swallow; scant amount of blood after biopsy is normal. The nurse will obtain vital signs prior to the examination/procedure. Patient will be anesthetized, and a scope placed down trachea, and a small biopsy will be taken/ foreign object removed. Patient will not be unconscious during procedure.

Gastrointestinal series

A gastrointestinal series is an examination using x-ray. The gastrointestinal series uses fluoroscopy to visualize the esophagus, stomach, and small intestine. The patient will be asked to ingest oral contrast such as barium meal or meglumine diatrizoate. The contrast media is observed under fluoroscopy while it passes through the digestive tract. The gastrointestinal series is used to determine and diagnose inflammation, ulcerations, and tumors, and also to detect and diagnose hiatal hernias, pyloric stenosis, gastroenteritis, gastric polyps, foreign bodies, and malabsorption of the gastrointestinal system. Esophageal varices, obstructions, and strictures are also visible using a gastrointestinal series.

Bladder imaging tests

Bladder imaging tests include:
- X-ray: May show kidney stones, tumors, and size and shape of prostate.
- Intravenous pyelogram (IVP): X-rays are taken after administration of IV contrast agent to show how the dye moves through the kidneys, ureter, and bladder. Can demonstrate problems resulting from urinary retention or reflux.
- Cystoscopy: Endoscopic examination of the bladder provides direct visualization of the urethra, bladder, and ureteral orifices.
- Cystography: Contrast dye is instilled into the bladder per catheter and then x-rays are taken to outline the bladder and show any perforations.
- Voiding cystourethrography: Contrast dye is instilled into the bladder and fluoroscopy utilized while the bladder is full and during urination. Frequently used to diagnose vesicoureteral reflux.
- Ultrasound: Shows the urinary tract and abnormalities as well as tumors and urinary retention.
- CT: Can show the presence of stones, cysts, injuries, and tumors, but not adequate for diagnosis of malignancy.
- MRI: Provides detailed images of the urinary organs and shows tumors or other abnormalities.

LABORATORY VALUES

Lab levels associated with diabetes

There are two main labs that are used in diagnosis of diabetes: HbA_{1c} and fasting blood glucose. While other lab abnormalities are often seen, these two are considered diagnostic for the disease. HbA_{1c} is the major determinant for glycosylated hemoglobin; it is used to

- 117 -

determine blood sugar control over the last 90 days. This can be used to diagnose effectiveness of diabetic therapy or diagnose diabetes.
- Normal HbA$_{1c}$ is 2%-5%; anything < 7% considered controlled.
- Uncontrolled diabetes is > 8%.

Fasting Blood Glucose (sugar): Glucose is formed from carbohydrates taken in with food and stored in the liver and skeletal muscles. Glucose levels are maintained by insulin production in the pancreas. Elevated glucose (hyperglycemia) indicates not enough inadequate insulin production. Self-monitoring glucose is done with capillary blood or finger stick method.
- Blood Glucose: 70-110 mg/dL; panic level is < 40 mg/dL or > 400 mg/dL.

> **Review Video: <u>Blood Glucose Pattern Management</u>**
> *Visit **mometrix.com/academy** and enter **Code: 626814***

Thyroid function tests

Thyroid function tests include:
- Thyroid-Stimulating Hormone (TSH): TSH is a hormone secreted by the pituitary gland that stimulates the production of T4 (thyroxine) from the thyroid gland. TSH is used in the diagnosis of thyroid and pituitary gland disorders.
  - TSH: 0.35-5.5 uIU/mL
- Thyroxine (T4): T4 is the major hormone derived and secreted by the thyroid gland; used in the diagnosis of hypo- and hyperthyroidism.
  - T4: 4.5-11.5 ug/dL
- Triiodothyronine (T3): T3 is a thyroid hormone that is always present in small amounts. Serum T3 is secreted in reaction to TSH; also used to diagnose altered thyroid function.
  - T3: 80-200 ng/dL
- Calcitonin: Calcitonin is secreted by the thyroid gland and aids in the maintenance of serum calcium and phosphorus levels. Calcitonin is elevated with thyroid cancer, and hyperplasia of the adenoma.
  - Calcitonin: Male: < 40 ng/L; Female: < 25 ng/L

BMP

A basic metabolic panel (BMP) includes 14 different lab tests that are used to assess the body's metabolism. The components of the BMP and general reference ranges are listed below; note that normals may fluctuate slightly in different facilities due to calibration of laboratory machines.
- Sodium (Na): 135-145 mEq/L
- Potassium (K): 3.5-5.3 mEq/L
- Calcium (Ca): 9-11 mg/dL (total), 4.5-5.6 mg/dL (ionized)
- Chloride (Cl): 95-105 mEq/L
- Albumin: 3.9-5.0 g/dL
- Alkaline phosphatase (ALP): 44-147 IU/L
- ALT: 8-37 IU/L
- AST: 10-34 IU/L
- BUN : 7-20 mg/dL

- CO_2: 20-29 mmol/L
- Creatinine: 0.8-1.4 mg/dL
- Glucose: 70-100 mg/dL
- Total bilirubin: 0.2-1.9 mg/dL
- Total protein: 6.3-7.9 g/dL

CBC

A complete blood cell count (CBC) is a combination of red blood cells, white blood cells, erythrocyte indices, hematocrit, differential white blood cell count, and may even include the platelet count. CBCs are used as diagnostic tests to assist in determination of anemia, blood loss, blood values, and hydration status.
- RBC: Male is 4.5-6.0 µL; Female is 4.0-5.0 µL
  ↓ RBC may indicate hemorrhage, anemia, or overhydration; ↑ RBC may indicate dehydration and polycythemia vera.
- Hgb: Male is 13.5-18.0 g/dL; Female is 12.0-16.0 g/dL
  ↑ Hgb levels may indicate hemoconcentration/dehydration, and polycythemia vera. ↓ Hgb may indicate anemia, acute blood loss, and hemodilution.
- Hct: Male is 40%-54%; Female is 36%-46%
  ↓ Hct indicates anemia and folic acid deficiency. ↑ Hct may indicate dehydration and polycythemia vera.
- White Blood Cells* (WBCs) : 3.5-10 x 103/mm3
  ↑ WBC indicate infection, inflammation, tissue damage, or leukemia; ↓ WBC indicates leukopenia (caused by cancer treatments or other immune deficiencies), cancer, severe infection, or liver/spleen disease.

*The types and functions of white blood cells are as follows:
- Lymphocytes: Work closely with macrophages. Subtypes include B cells, which produce specific antibodies to destroy foreign substances; T cells, which help regulate immune response and attack virus-infected cells, foreign tissue, and cancer cells; natural killer (NK) cells, which utilize phagocytosis and destroy cancer cells and virus-infected cells.
- Monocytes: Production increases during an immune response. Mature into macrophages, which engage in phagocytosis and help activate T cells and B cells.
- Eosinophils (granulocyte): Become active in parasitic infections and allergic responses. Contain granules that are toxic to many organisms as well as tissue.
- Basophils (granulocyte): Involved in type 1 hypersensitivity (IgE-mediated) and may result in anaphylaxis.
- Neutrophils (polymorphonuclear granulocytes): Primary role is in fighting inflammation and arrive first at site of inflammation by leaving the blood and entering tissue where they act as phagocytes, ingesting and killing microorganisms.

Coagulation Studies

The following are coagulation studies:
- ApTT (Activated Partial Thromboplastin Time): ApTT will reveal clotting deficiencies, and is used to determine effectiveness of heparin management.
  - pTT: 60-70 seconds.

- PT (Prothrombin Time): Prothrombin time measures the clotting ability of factors I, II, V, VII, and X; used to monitor warfarin.
  - PT: 10-13 seconds.
- INR (International Normalized Ratio): INR is used to monitor clotting time in patients taking warfarin.
  - INR: 2.0-3.0.
- Platelet* count: The platelet count is used to determine basic elements of the blood that promote coagulation (clotting). A decreased platelet count of < 50% of the normal value will cause bleeding; this decreased platelet count places the patient at risk of hemorrhage.
  - Platelets: 150,000-400,000 μL
- Factor assay: Factor assays are ordered to detect deficiencies of blood coagulation components. There are 12 factor assays and they are equally important for blood clotting; these are generally interpreted by a hematologist.

* Platelets, also called thrombocytes, are the smallest cell-like component of human blood, originating in the bone marrow where they are fragments of a large cell, the megakaryocyte. Because platelets are fragments of a cell, they have no nucleus. In the blood, the platelets are disk-shaped but change into a globular form with pseudopodia (false feet) when activated. These pseudopodia help to form a clot in a two-step process that involves first adhesion, where the platelets bind to a wound site, and then activation, where the platelets change shape and release agents to attract other platelets. Fibrin forms from fibrinogen (a protein produced in the liver), creating a stabilizing mesh over the platelet plug to control bleeding. Normal platelet counts range from 150,000 to 400,000 per mm^3. Platelet counts may increase with infections, cirrhosis, heart disease, malignancies, pancreatitis, and polycythemia. Platelet counts may decrease with alcohol toxicity, aplastic anemia, iron-deficiency anemia, megaloblastic anemia drug toxicity, prolonged hypoxia, viral infection, and immune thrombocytopenic purpura.

Cardiac Function

The various cardiac function labs are explained below:
- Troponin: a form of globular protein found in cardiac and skeletal muscle. Troponin is released with injury or necrosis of the myocardium. There are 2 cycles of troponin release: 4-6 hours immediately post-cardiac injury, and may still rise 7 to 10 days following a cardiac injury.
  - Troponin: < 0.012 mcg/L
- CK-MB: an enzyme found in heart muscle. Elevated levels indicate acute MI/heart attack, severe angina pectoris, cardiac surgical procedures, cardiac ischemia, myocarditis, and hypokalemia.
  - CK-MB: 0-6%
- Brain natriuretic peptide (BNP): a peptide that is released into the bloodstream (circulation) of individuals with heart failure. Can be falsely elevated in severe kidney disease.
  - BNP: < 100 pg/mL

Cholesterol, HDL, LDL, and serum triglyceride levels

Lipids are fats that combine with plasma proteins to form lipoproteins (e.g., LDL, HDL), which are carried throughout the body. The primary lipids include:

- Triglycerides: This is "neutral" fat composed of glycerol and fatty acids. It is found in adipose tissue throughout the body, and its primary role is to store energy. Levels tend to elevate with obesity, alcohol use, and diabetes.
- Steroids (Cholesterol): Cholesterol is required for formation of the cell membrane and serves as a precursor for hormone synthesis of other steroids (such as estrogen, testosterone, and bile salts). Cholesterol is found in the cell membranes and the digestive and endocrine systems.
- Phospholipids: These lipids are derived from triglycerides and are important constituents of all cell membranes, forming lipid bilayers that form barriers around cells but allow passage of small molecules, such as oxygen.

Cholesterol is a blood lipid synthesized by the liver and found in red blood cells, cell membranes, and muscles. Serum cholesterol is used as an indicator of atherosclerosis and coronary artery disease. HDL is considered the friendly cholesterol and consists of 50% protein and assists with decreasing plaque deposits in blood vessels; high levels are desirable. However, LDL and triglycerides are associated with atherosclerosis and increased risk of MI; therefore, low levels are desired.

Special considerations are as follows:

- Client NPO for the 12 hours prior to the test.
- Aspirin, cortisone, and alcohol (< 24 h before test) can alter the cholesterol level, causing an increase or decrease. Ventilators, hypoxemia, and hemolysis of the specimen can cause false elevations.

The following are reference values:

- Total cholesterol: < 200 mg/dL; moderate risk: 200-240 mg/dL; high risk: > 240 mg/dL
- High-density lipoprotein (HDL): 29-77 mg/dL
- Low-density lipoprotein (LDL): 60-160 mg/dL
- Triglyceride level: 10-190 mg/dL

Rheumatoid Arthritis Labs

The following are labs associated with rheumatoid arthritis:

- ASO (antistreptolysin O): created in response to streptolysin, an agent secreted by beta-hemolytic group A *Streptococcus* that is capable of lysing red blood cells (RBCs). ASO levels that are elevated can indicate rheumatic fever, acute glomerulonephritis, and recent streptococcal infections.
  - ASO: < 100 Todd units
- ANA (antinuclear antibodies): The ANA is a diagnostic tool for screening systemic lupus erythematosus (SLE) and other collagen disorders such as rheumatoid arthritis, scleroderma, leukemia, and infectious mononucleosis.
  - ANA > 1:20 (titer).

- ESR (erythrocyte sedimentation rate): ESR is the rate in which red blood cells settle in unclotted blood in millimeters per hour. Elevated in the presence of inflammation in the body.
    - ESR: 0-20 mm/h
- CRP (C-reactive protein): appears 10 hours after the onset of an inflammatory process in which tissue destruction is involved. CRP is used to monitor acute inflammatory phases of rheumatoid arthritis and rheumatic fever; infections - *will only elevate with bacterial infections.*
    - CRP: negative.
- Rheumatoid factor (RF): Rheumatoid factor is a test utilized to measure antibodies IgM, IgG, and IgA found with rheumatoid arthritis.
    - RF: < 40-60 u/mL/1:80 titer

ABGs

Arterial blood gases (ABGs) are performed for patients with suspected blood or metabolic malfunction, as well as to evaluate the effectiveness of ventilation. The basic components and expected normal values are:
1. PO_2 75-100 mm Hg
2. PCO_2 38-42 mm Hg
3. Bicarbonate 23-26 mEq/L
4. pH 7.38-7.44
5. Oxygen saturation 95% or greater
6. Bicarbonate, serum 23-28 mEq/L

An *Allen's test* should always be performed before performing an ABG to ensure that the hand has adequate perfusion; this is done by occluding both the radial and ulnar arteries, having the patient clench fist a few times, then releasing the ulnar (pinky side) artery only and observing for the return of color to the hand. Blood drawn should be bright red; dark blood may indicate venous blood.

Liver Panel

Liver function tests:
- Alkaline Phosphatase (ALP): Alkaline phosphatase is an enzyme produced mainly in the liver and bone.
    - ALP Normal: 42-136 units/L
    - Elevated in elderly patients; bone growth
- Alanine aminotransferase (ALT): assists in the detection of liver disorders such as viral (acute) hepatitis, cancer, necrosis, alcohol abuse, and drug or chemical toxicity.
    - ALT Normal: 10-35 units/L
    - Elevated in males, infants, and elderly patients
- Aspartate aminotransferase (AST): Elevated levels assist in the determination of heart and liver muscle damage. ALT is also used in conjunction with CK and LDH in diagnosing an acute MI.
    - AST Normal: 8-38 units/L
    - Infants and elderly increased; females decreased

- Bilirubin: Byproduct of RBC destruction; increased levels cause jaundice in the patient. Indicates liver dysfunction/RBC hemolysis.
  - Bilirubin Normal: 0.2-1.3 mg/dL

Pancreatic Function Tests

Lab levels associated with pancreatic function tests are explained below:
- Amylase: an enzyme that originates within the pancreas, salivary glands, and liver that functions to change starch into sugar.
  - Amylase: 60-160 U/dL (Somogyi).
  - Elderly levels are slightly higher than that of younger adults.
  - The nurse should be aware that glucose in an IV may cause a false-negative amylase.
- Lipase: an enzyme secreted by the pancreas and digests fat. Acute pancreatitis is the most common cause of an elevated lipase level. Decreased levels may indicate late cancer, or hepatitis.
  - Lipase: 20-180 U/L

Renal Function Tests

The lab levels associated with renal function are discussed below:
- BUN (blood urea nitrogen): BUN is utilized to detect disorders of the kidney such as dehydration, liver damage, overhydration, kidney function (renal insufficiency), and sepsis.
  - BUN: 5-25 mg/dL
  - Slightly elevated in elderly patients.
- Creatinine: Creatinine is a byproduct of muscle catabolism; creatinine production is proportional to muscle mass. Creatinine is filtered by the glomeruli and is excreted in the urine. Creatinine is elevated with acute and chronic renal failure. Low magnesium and high creatinine signals renal failure.
  - Creatinine: 0.5-1.5 mg/dL
  - Females are slightly lower related to lower muscle mass.
- Albumin: Albumin levels are used to determine the amount of albumin circulating in the blood or urine. Decreased levels are associated with liver disease, burns, inflammation, shock, malnutrition, and renal disorders.
  - Albumin: 3.5-5 g/dL

Urinalysis

Urinalysis may be performed to detect problems with renal function, disease processes, urinary tract infections, diabetes, prenatal examinations, and routine examinations. The nurse should remember that drugs and foods can alter the color of urine. Normal results are as follows:
1. Color: Straw (cloudiness may be due to phosphates and urates and is considered normal)
2. Turbidity: Clear
3. Specific Gravity: 1.001-1.02 (low: sickle cell, DM, diabetes insipidus)
4. Dipstick: pH 4.5-7.5

5. Protein: Negative (positive: nephritic syndrome, renal tubular disease, pyelonephritis, and polycystic kidney disease)
6. Sugar: Negative (positive: diabetes or other endocrine disease)
7. Acetone/ketones: Negative (positive: non controlled diabetes, alcoholism, starvation)
8. Bile: Negative
9. Hemoglobin: Negative (positive: bleeding, kidney/bladder irritation)
10. Nitrite: Negative (positive: indicates bacteria)
11. Leukocyte Esterase: Negative
12. Urobilinogen: Positive

HIV and AIDS

Human immune deficiency virus (HIV) is the retrovirus that causes acquired immune deficiency syndrome (AIDS). The diagnosis of AIDS is determined by the CD4+ T-cell count (per the CDC), with AIDS currently diagnosed with a CD4+ count of < 200 cells/mm^3. HIV is transmitted in bodily fluids. The primary infection stage occurs between the times of initial infection to the development of HIV-specific antigens. Then, HIV/AIDS is staged depending on CD4+ count and conditions:

- Category A: (CD4+ count < 500). Asymptomatic or lymphadenopathy.
- Category B: (CD4+ count 200 to 499). Conditions include candidiasis, PID, bacillary angiomatosis, fever, diarrhea, herpes zoster, ITP, and peripheral neuropathy.
- Category C (AIDS): (CD4+ count < 200). Invasive diseases common. Conditions include cervical cancer, candidiasis, CMV, encephalopathy, TB, *P. jiroveci* pneumonia, Kaposi sarcoma, toxoplasmosis, wasting syndrome.

Diagnosis is based on HIV antibody tests (ELISA), Western blot assay, and viral load tests (reverse transcriptase PCR). Treatment consists of antiretroviral agents (NRTIs, NNRTIs, protease inhibitors, fusion inhibitors, integrase strand transfer inhibitors, and multiclass combination products).

Opportunistic Infections associated with AIDS
Opportunistic infections are infections that occur in AIDS patients. Due to the decreased immunity characterized by the disease, these infections now have the "opportunity" to infect the individual. Remember, AIDS patients do not die of AIDS, but of one of these diseases:

- salmonellosis, syphilis, and neurosyphilis
- tuberculosis (TB), bacillary angiomatosis ("cat-scratch disease")
- aspergillosis, candidiasis (thrush, yeast infection)
- coccidioidomycosis, cryptococcal meningitis
- histoplasmosis, Kaposi sarcoma
- lymphoma, systemic non-Hodgkin lymphoma (NHL)
- primary CNS lymphoma, cryptosporidiosis
- isosporiasis, microsporidiosis
- *Pneumocystis jiroveci* pneumonia (PCP), toxoplasmosis
- cytomegalovirus (CMV), hepatitis
- herpes simplex (HSV, genital herpes), herpes zoster (HZV, shingles)

- human papilloma virus (HPV, genital warts, cervical cancer)
- AIDS dementia complex (ADC)

> **Review Video:** <u>**AIDS Infections and Malignancies**</u>
> *Visit **mometrix.com/academy** and enter **Code: 319526***

Necrotizing enterocolitis (NEC)

Necrotizing enterocolitis (NEC) is an acute inflammatory disease of the bowel in preterm and high-risk infants. While the cause is unknown, it leads to ischemia and death of the bowel tissue, often with fatal infection if not recognized and treated promptly. Risk factors include prematurity, formula feeding, and difficult delivery. Signs and symptoms include swollen abdomen, nausea/vomiting, lethargy, refusal to eat, fever, tachycardia, and constipation/bloody stools. Diagnosis is based on x-ray, blood work, and lab studies (stool, blood, urine cultures).

Treatment includes the following:
- IV antibiotics and fluids; TPN for nutrition
- NG tube for gastric decompression
- Bowel resection if perforation occurs; temporary or permanent ostomy.
- Prevention: NPO for 24-48 h if suspected asphyxiation during birth or very low birth weight infant, breast milk is preferred food for oral feeds.

Endocarditis

Endocarditis is inflammation of the endocardium and heart valves, caused by fungi, virus, or bacteria. Factors that may contribute to infectious endocarditis include history of valvular disease, surgical procedures, immunosuppressive drug therapy such as steroids, and heroin addiction. Infectious endocarditis also may be caused by extensive indwelling catheters (PICC/central lines), and prolonged IV antibiotics. Signs and symptoms include weakness/fatigue, fever, heart murmur, dyspnea, night sweats, Janeway lesions (red spots on palms), Osler nodes (painful lesions), joint pain, and splinter hemorrhages in fingernails. Diagnosis is based on CBC, ESR, ECG, blood cultures, TEE, MRI, and physical exam.

Treatment includes:
- IV antibiotics; plasmapheresis.
- Surgery may be indicated for valve replacement.
- Monitor the patient for jaundice, arrhythmias, CHF, glomerulonephritis, emboli.
- Prevent: needle-exchange programs, *take antibiotics before dental procedures if high-risk (e.g., history of heart valve replacement)*.

Disseminated Intravascular Coagulation (DIC)

Disseminated intravascular coagulation (DIC) is a life-threatening coagulopathy that occurs secondary to other disorders that accelerate clotting, resulting in occlusions of small blood vessels and depletion of clotting factors and platelets with activation of fibrinolysis. This, in turn, results in hemorrhage. Clotting may impair functioning of the kidneys and other organs. Triggering factors may include various infections, obstetric complications, malignancies, tissue necrosis, heatstroke, toxins, fat embolism, blood transfusion reactions, cardiac arrest, and cardiopulmonary bypass. Signs and symptoms include abnormal bleeding of all types (GI, petechiae, oozing around IVs or from surgical incisions), cyanosis (especially of the extremities), impairment of renal function, nausea, vomiting, severe pain (back, abdomen, muscles), shock, and multiple organ failures. Diagnosis is based on DIC panel with prolonged prothrombin and partial prothrombin times, increased D-dimer, thrombocytopenia (below 100,000/mcL), fragmented RBCs, and decreased fibrinogen and clotting factors. Treatment consists of identifying and treating underlying cause, anticoagulants, cryoprecipitate (to increase fibrinogen), coagulation inhibitors, and replacement blood products such as FFP and platelets.

Alternate Wound-Closure Therapies

The methods and uses of alternate wound-closure therapies are discusses below:
- Whirlpool/Hydrotherapy
  - Vasodilation: blood flow brings oxygen, nutrients, white blood cells, and antibiotics to the tissues and removes metabolites.
  - Mechanical effects of whirlpool stimulate granulation tissue formation; also softens necrotic tissue/aides phagocytosis.
  - Sedation and analgesia are induced by the warm water.
  - Used for: necrotic/wounds with heavy exudate or debris; tissue that can tolerate increased circulatory perfusion.
  - Contraindications: edema, altered LOC, infection, fever, maceration, phlebitis, compromised cardiovascular/pulmonary function, renal failure, and incontinence.
- Vacuum-assisted closure/negative-pressure wound therapy
  - Special foam dressing with an attached evacuation tube is inserted into the wound and covered with an adhesive drape in order to create an airtight seal; removes excess fluid/reduces edema.
  - Increases vascularity/promotes formation of granulation tissue
  - Used for: pressure ulcers/chronic wounds; surgical wounds/large and open wounds with excess exudate or drainage.
- Hyperbaric oxygen therapy
  - Systemic therapy in which 100% oxygen is delivered in a room or chamber that is pressurized at a level greater than sea level.
  - Increases dissolved oxygen in blood = greater oxygen to wounds.
  - Used for: dry/gas gangrene, skin grafts/flaps, crush injury, wounds not responding to more conservative treatment. Also used for air/gas embolism, decompression sickness, and carbon monoxide poisoning.

Rh Incompatibility

Rh is a component of the blood, generally expressed as "positive" and "negative" blood type. Rh compatability comes into play when an Rh-negative woman is carrying the child of an Rh-positive man. Since the woman is Rh negative, her body will develop RhD antibodies if exposed to the RhD antigen. This is known as *sensitization*. Because of genetics, there is a 50% to 100% chance that the baby of an Rh-positive man will be Rh positive, depending on if he is homozygous or heterozygous Rh positive. If the baby is Rh positive, then the mother will develop anti-D antibodies when the baby's blood is mixed with hers during placental separation. The first child would remain unharmed; however, during subsequent pregnancies, the mother's anti-D antibodies can cross the placenta to the fetal blood,

- 126 -

causing agglutination and hemolysis of fetal cells to a varying degree. This could result in fetal demise, erythroblastosis fetalis, icterus gravis neonatorum, hemolytic anemia, kernicterus, or liver damage of the fetus. Screening pregnant woman for Rh status is critical to prevent Rh sensitization. If Rh negative, the woman will be required to take a medication known as RhoGAM. This is an IM injection given throughout pregnancy that prevents sensitization in the woman. RhoGAM will not work if sensitization has already occurred.

Thromboembolism

Thromboembolism includes both the formation of a thrombus (such as in the heart with A-fib and in the deep veins with immobilization) and embolism in which a clot breaks off and travels through the circulatory system. While thromboembolism may cause a heart attack or stroke, the most common presentation is a pulmonary embolism resulting from deep vein thrombosis. Signs and symptoms are as follows:
- Generally asymptomatic
- Pain at the thrombus site, which may be swollen and erythematous, typically in the lower extremity.
- When the patient develops pulmonary embolism, the usual presentation is acute onset of dyspnea.
- Some patients may have frothy sputum, cough, fever, and/or hemoptysis as well.

Diagnosis includes laboratory tests (CBC, troponins, D-dimer, ABGs, and BNP), ultrasound, spiral CT, pulmonary angiography, and ventilation/perfusion scanning. Treatment includes anticoagulants, thrombolytic therapy, oxygen, and thrombectomy. Prevention includes smoking cessation, regular exercise, discontinuation of birth control pills, early ambulation after surgery, SCDs/compression hose, control of high blood pressure, treatment for peripheral arterial disease, and avoiding prolonged sitting.

Dealing with Unexpected Responses to Therapies

While treatments and therapies often follow an expected and reliable course, there are times when a patient can have an adverse or unexpected reaction. This can be a fearful time for the patient as well as the nurse. When the patient has an unexpected response to a therapy, here are some actions that the nurse should take:
- First, immediately cease whatever therapy is causing the reaction if possible (stop the blood or IV medication, remove that patient from the area, etc.).
- Remember ABC – airway, breathing, circulation. If the patient stops breathing or loses a pulse, call for help and begin CPR immediately.
- If the patient is having an allergic reaction to a medication, notify the physician immediately and administer an antihistamine or reversal agent (often Benadryl or epinephrine for anaphylaxis).
- After resolution of the event, regardless of the outcome, be sure to thoroughly document what happened, including all the steps taken before and after the incident to ensure patient safety.

NURSING 4
The neurological exam helps determine the person's neurological health, and diagnose dementia/delerium/brain stem injury, and many other disorders. It includes:

- Level of Consciousness (LOC): most important piece of the neurological exam, and often the only level of exam completed on a regular basis during nursing assessments.
  - o Arousal/Level of Alterness: Assess as you walk into the room; may require noxious stimuli (sternal rub, nail-bed pressure).
    - ▪ Alert ⤳Lethargic ⤳Obtunded ⤳Stuporous⤳Comatose
  - o Awareness: Patient's orientation to person, place, and time.
- Advanced Neuro Screening: this is used for patients with known or suspected neurological deficit (e.g., stroke) who can respond to questions. May include NIH Stroke Scale in some facilities. Assessments may include:
  - o Orientation to time, place, person, and purpose of visit.
  - o Following commands/the use of language (fluency of spontaneous speech)
  - o Naming objects such as a pen or watch; repetition of rhymes (e.g., "Mary had a little lamb"); checking for slurred speech and dysarthria.
  - o Short-term/long-term memory (ask the patient to recall three items, such as, "rose, umbrella, truck," minutes after hearing the words).
  - o Bilateral strength and coordination testing

Assessment of the neurological system should begin by evaluation of the patient's mental status and speaking ability to determine if the patient is oriented, as well as level of consciousness (alert, lethargic, obtunded, stuporous, or comatose). The physical examination should continue with examination of the cranial nerves (I–XII), which includes assessment of smell, visual abilities, facial movement, hearing, swallowing, voice, and speech. Then the motor system is assessed, including evaluation of position of the body, involuntary movements, muscle strength, muscle tone, flexion, extension, stability, and gait. Assessment of the sensory system includes evaluation of pain, temperature, position, vibration, light touch, position, and discrimination. The reflexes are assessed and graded on a scale of 0 (no response) to 2+ (normal) to 4+ (hyperactive). Reflexes include biceps reflex (evaluates C5 and C6), triceps reflex (C6 and C7), brachioradialis reflex (C5, C6), knee reflex (L2, L3, L4), ankle reflex (S1), and plantar response (L5, S1).

The Glasgow Coma Scale (GCS) is used to measure level of consciousness (LOC) and extent of brain injury. There are 3 components:
- Eye opening: Spontaneous 4, To voice 3, To pain 2, None 1
- Verbal response: Oriented 5, Confused 4, wrong words 3, unintelligible 2, None 1
- Motor response: Obeys commands 6, Localizes pain 5, Withdraws from pain 4, Flexion (decorticate) 3, Extension (decerebrate) 2, None 1

Scoring guide (3-15): Mild, ≥13; Moderate, 9 to 12; Severe, ≤8

Reflexes are graded 0 to 4, where 0 is absent, 1 is reduced, 2 is normal, 3 is increased, and 4 is clonus. Reflexes are tested over the biceps, triceps, brachioradialis, quadriceps, and Achilles tendons.
- Reflexes graded 0 and 1 indicate lower motor neuron damage (ie, damage to anterior horn cell, anterior nerve root, peripheral nerve, or neuromuscular junction of muscle).
- Reflexes graded 3 and 4 indicate an upper motor neuron damage (ie, in the cerebrum, brain stem or spinal cord).

Posturing

Decorticate and decerebrate posturing are caused by varying levels of damage to the brain/brain stem. If either of these postures is observed, it should be considered a medical emergency and reported immediately.

Decorticate (flexion) posturing
The patient will have the following: flexion of the head and trunk, adduction and internal rotation of the arms, pronation and flexion of the forearm, flexion of the wrists and fingers, flexion of the hips, knees, ankles, and toes, internal rotation of the legs, and inversion of the feet.

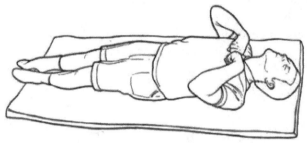

Decerebrate (extension) posturing
The patient will have the following: extension and internal rotation of all four extremities and may also show extension of the body and head (opisthotonus). Decerebrate posturing indicates a lesion of the midbrain or lower. It is also associated with a mortality rate of 70%.

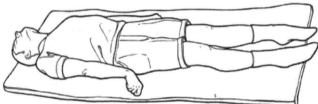

Cardiovascular System

Assessment of the cardiovascular system should begin with a health history and evaluation of any chest pain, including the location, duration, severity, and aggravating/alleviating factors. Topics to review include medications, nutrition, activities, exercise, emotional status, and sleep patterns. Physical assessment should include evaluation of the patient's general appearance and skin condition and color (noting any pallor, ecchymosis, or cyanosis). BP should be taken in supine and sitting position with 1-3 minutes between readings. Pulse rate should be evaluated both peripherally and per auscultation, noting the pulse quality on a scale of 0 (absent) to 4+ (bounding and strong), configuration, and rhythm. The heart sounds should be assessed for normal sounds (S1 and S2) and abnormal sounds (S3, S4, opening snaps, clicks, and murmurs). Jugular venous distention should be noted. The extremities should be examined with capillary refill time and any vascular changes noted, including weak or absent peripheral pulses. Edema should be evaluated by applying firm pressure for 5 seconds and then assessing on a 0 (absent) to 4+ (pitting > 8 mm) scale.

- 129 -

An understanding of the cardiovascular system includes knowing the pathophysiology of the heart. Normal blood flow through the heart is as follows:

- Deoxygenated venous blood returns to the heart per the superior vena cava, inferior vena cava, and coronary sinus (bringing blood from the coronary arteries) into the right atrium.
- When the atrium is full, it contracts and the blood flows through the tricuspid valve into the right ventricle.
- When the right ventricle is full, it contracts and blood flows through the pulmonic valve into the pulmonary artery and to the lungs.
- The oxygenated blood then flows from the lungs through the pulmonary veins and into the left atrium. When the left atrium is full, it contracts and blood flows through the mitral valve into the left ventricle.
- Once full, the left ventricle contracts and the blood flows through the aortic valve and into the aorta and the coronary arteries and general circulation.

After blood flows through the valves, the valves close to prevent backflow. Both atria and both ventricles contract simultaneously.

> **Review Video: Pulse**
> Visit **mometrix.com/academy** and enter **Code: 686534**

Pulmonary System

Assessment of the pulmonary system should begin with a health history focusing on respiratory problems, such as dyspnea, cough, sputum production, chest pain, wheezing, hemoptysis, and lifestyle choices that are risk factors, such as smoking. The upper respiratory structures (nose, sinuses, mouth, pharynx, and trachea) should be examined and palpated. The patient's chest should be exposed and the patient in supine position for examination of the anterior thorax and in sitting position if possible for examination of posterior thorax. Assessment includes observation of the rate, rhythm, depth, and effort of breathing and the patient's color. The fingers should be examined for clubbing and skin for cyanosis. Examination should include inspection, palpation, auscultation, and percussion of the lung fields. Normal breathing sounds (vesicular, bronchovesicular, bronchial, and tracheal) are assessed as well as abnormal sounds (fine or coarse crackles, wheezes, sibilant rhonchi, sonorous rhonchi, and friction rubs). Pulse oximetry is used to determine oxygen saturation.

Gastrointestinal System

Assessment of the gastrointestinal system should begin with a health history focused on GI problems, such as constipation, diarrhea, abdominal pain, nausea, flatus, and change in bowel habits. The mouth should be examined (removing dentures), including lips, gums, and tongue, using a tongue blade to depress the tongue so that the back of the mouth can be viewed. The abdomen should be examined with the patient in supine position with knees flexed. Auscultation is used to assess bowel sounds (*normal* are sounds every 5 to 20 seconds, *hypoactive* is less frequent, and *hyperactive* more frequent). Percussion is used to assess internal organs and determine the presence of masses. Light palpation is utilized to determine areas of tenderness and deeper palpation to assess masses. The patient may be placed in knee-chest, left lateral, or standing with hips flexed positions for a rectal examination. A digital rectal exam should include asking the patient to bear down so that abnormalities, such as hemorrhoids, are easier to detect.

Genitourinary System

Assessment of the genitourinary system should begin with a health history that includes sexually transmitted infections, urinary infections, incontinence, pain, dysuria, and sexual history including dysfunctions such as impotence and ejaculatory disorders. The external genitalis should be examined. The female reproductive system is usually assessed as distinct from the urinary system and requires a breast examination and pelvic examination. The genitourinary system includes the male genitals because of their proximity and dual function as part of the reproductive system and the urinary system. Physical assessment of the male should include a testicular and digital rectal examination. Assessment of the urinary system should begin with palpation of the bladder (which can usually only be felt if distended) and kidneys (although usually only part of the right kidney can be palpated in normal kidneys). Any tenderness in flank areas should be noted. If bladder percussion yields a dull sound following the patient's urination, this can indicate incomplete emptying of the bladder.

Dialysis

Dialysis is a process by which the blood is artifically filteres to get rid of waste products. It is mainly used for patients with partial or total kidney failure, using one of two processes.
- In the hemodialysis process, blood is taken from the patient via an access site, most often a fistula or graft in the arm. The blood runs through a machine called a dialyzer, which removes waste products then returns it to the patient through the same access site. Most patients that require hemodialysis go to a hospital or specialized hemodialysis center three days a week.
- During peritoneal dialysis, a cleansing solution is placed into the abdominal cavity, where it is kept for some time to absorb waste. After a catheter is sugically installed in the abdominal wall, the patient can begin cycling cleanising solution in and out of the addominal cavity, usually 3-5 times per day. When this process is done autonomously by the patient, it is known as continuous ambulatory peritoneal dialysis (CAPD). When done by a machine, it is known as continuous cyclic peritoneal dialysis (CCPD). Because there is a higher risk of infection involved with peritoneal dialysis, the patient should report bloody (if not menstruating(or cloudy dialystae, or symptoms of abdominal cramps, chills, or fever immediately.

Lithotripsy

Lithotripsy is a procedure that utilizes extracorporeal shock waves to break up stones, usually kidney stones, although it may be utilized for gallstones as well. The procedure is usually carried out with some type of anesthesia (local, general, regional) and takes 45 to 60 minutes. The patient is positioned in a tub of water or more commonly on a special cushioned table through which the shock waves pass. This procedure is more effective for small stones than large. Patients often experience some discomfort and hematuria after the procedure as the fragments of fractured stones make their way through the urinary tract and are excreted in urine. In some cases, the procedure must be repeated. Lithotripsy is used less often now in favor of ureteroscopy, which directly removes the stones. However, there are more complications, such as bleeding or perforation, which may occur with ureteroscopy.

Integumentary System

Assessment of the integumentary system should begin with health history that includes history of any allergic skin disorders, skin conditions, and skin cancer and direct observation of the entire skin area, including inspection of the inside of the mouth, the scalp, and the nails. The nurse should wear gloves if any rash or lesions are present. Skin color should be assessed, noting erythema, jaundice, cyanosis, or other discolorations. If the patient has a rash or pruritus, the area involved should be carefully examined, noting any differences in skin texture or elevations (such as may occur with a rash). Skin lesions should be carefully documented, including size, shape, and appearance. Vascular changes, such as petechia, ecchymosis, and angiomas should be noted. Both fingernails and toenails should be examined for changes, including ridging or hypertrophy, and signs of paronychia noted. The angle between the nail and its base should be assessed (normal is 160 degrees). Hair should be examined (while wearing gloves) for color, texture, distribution, and loss.

> ➤ **Review Video:** <u>Functions of the Integumentary System</u>
> *Visit **mometrix.com/academy** and enter **Code: 398674***

Physiological Adaptation

This domain is defined by the NCSBN as "managing and providing care for clients with acute, chronic, or life threatening physical health conditions." This section will discuss common diseases found in pediatric and adult patients, organized by body system.

<u>INFANT/CHILDHOOD DISEASES AND DISORDERS</u>

Cleft Lip & Palate

Cleft lip and/or cleft palate are facial malformations that occur during embryonic development in which the soft palate of the mouth does not close completely, leaving a gap. These two conditions may appear separately or together. While the cause is unknown, it is possible that heredity, maternal medications, and viruses during the first trimester may play a role in the development of cleft lip/palate. Signs and symptoms include obvious physical deformity of mouth/lips, difficulty feeding, ear infections/hearing loss, and speech difficulty. Diagnosis is based on prenatal ultrasound and physical exam. Treatment includes:

- Surgery: close lip/tubes in ears by 12 months, palate by 18 months; may protect suture with Logan bow, use Z-plasty to minimize scar retraction.
- Feeding: generally cannot breastfeed; must use special bottle that does not require high amounts of suction. Post-op: cannot put any obects in mouth; will be fed by syringe, no pacifier, wear arm restraints to prevent bringing objects to mouth

Klinefelter Syndrome

Klinefelter syndrome is a genetic disorder of males in which the child is born with an extra X chromosome (usually 47XXY), and is a common cause of hypogonadism, androgen deficiency, and infertility. Boys often appear normal but begin to have problems in school because of delayed development of language and learning disabilities, such as auditory and verbal processing problems. Children often have normal intelligence but decreased ability to access information from memory. Onset of puberty is often delayed. Boys tend to be tall and thin with extra-long extremities and wide arm span. Testicular size is abnormally small and gynecomastia is common; adolescents develop less than normal facial and body hair. Some children may also have cardiac, respiratory, and dental abnormalities. Diagnosis is based on chromosomal analysis. Testosterone replacement is started when the child is 11 to 12 years old with doses gradually increased to maintain adult levels of testosterone by age 15 to 17. This improves masculinization but does not alter infertility.

Phenylketonuria

Phenylketonuria (PKU) is an autosomal inherited recessive disorder related to the synthesis of phenylalanine, an essential amino acid required by the body. As byproducts of phenylalanine accumulate in the brain, the individual experiences developmental delays. The Guthrie test is done on all infants at birth to determine serum phenylalanine levels, as PKU was once a common yet preventable cause of intellectual disability. Signs and symptoms include urine and sweat with a musty odor, eczema, fair skin and eyes, failure to thrive, emesis, microcephaly, hyperactivity, altered behavior patterns, convulsions, and developmental delay. Diagnosis is based on blood work (Guthrie test, phenylalanine levels, etc) and genetic testing.

Treatment includes:
- Diet low in phenylalanine/protein: Lofenalac formula is given to infants, avoid sugar-free products (aspartame), milk, cheese, beef, pork, chicken, fish and beans.
- Teaching: keep food diary/track protein intake, find support groups, take special formula for protein replacement, see doctor if pregnant—uncontrolled PKU during pregnancy will harm infant.

Wilson Disease

Wilson disease is an inherited autosomal recessive condition in which high levels of copper build up in various tissues throughout the body. The key organs affected are the eyes, brain, liver, and/or kidneys. It can be difficult to differentiate between Wilson disease and other liver diseases. Signs and symptoms include gait disturbances, jaundice, tremors, abdominal pain/distention, dementia, speech problems, muscle weakness, splenomegaly, and confusion. Diagnosis is based on the following:
- Bilirubin/PT/AST increased
- Albumin/uric acid production decreased
- MRI, genetic testing, and liver biopsy
- Kayser-Fleischer rings in the eyes.

Treatment includes:
- Medications: penicillamine, trientine, zinc acetate.
- Lifestyle management: low-copper diet (avoid shellfish, nuts, chocolate, mushrooms, and liver).

- Monitor the patient for cirrhosis, muscle weakness, joint pain/stiffness, anemia, fever, hepatitis.

Legg-Calve-Perthes disease

Legg-Calve-Perthes disease is a condition in which an anatomical anomaly results in poor blood supply to the superior aspect of the femur. It is most common in boys ages 4-10, with a 5 times higher incidence rate in boys than girls. The result of this condition is the femur ball flattens out and deteriorates, leading to impaired ambulation and pain. This condition is very similar to *slipped capital femoral epiphysis*, a common hip disorder in adolescents in which the ball of the femur separates from the femur along the epiphysis. Both are diagnosed and treated similarly. Signs and symptoms include hip and knee pain, limited active and passive ROM, pain with ambulation, and unequal leg length. The child wants to cross legs and keep affected limb across the body. Diagnosis is based on x-ray, MRI, bone scan, test range-of-motion, and clinical picture. Treatment includes:
- Bracing/crutches/bed rest: keep weight off of affected hip.
- Physical therapy; strengthen affected ligaments and muscles
- Casting: keeps legs apart, allow to heal for 4-6 weeks
- Surgery: may need hip replacement/joint realignment if severe.

Cystic Fibrosis

Cystic fibrosis is an autosomal recessive disorder causing generalized malfunction of the exocrine glands, resulting in the excessive production of viscous mucus. It is caused by a genetic defect that affects sodium chloride movement in cells. People that have a family history of CF and are of Northern European descent are at an increased risk for CF. There is no cure for CF, but with early diagnosis and treatment, these patients often make it far into young adulthood. Signs and symptoms include:
- Salty-taste to skin, recurrent respiratory infections, productive cough, steatorrhea (fatty, foul-smelling stool), constipation (newborn - intestinal blockage), poor weight gain;
- Long-term – pancreatitis, infertility, and diabetes.

Diagnosis is based on sweat test, physical exam, and genetic testing. Treatment includes:
- Medications: bronchodilators, mucolytics, possible prophylactic antibiotics to prevent URIs; pancreatic enzymes, vitamin supplements (A, D, E and K especially) for digestion.
- Diet: high calories/fat, increased amounts of sodium and fluids.
- Daily pulmonary hygiene.
- Teaching: encourage activities and support groups, good nutrition is vital, avoid sick people/wash hands, report infections immediately, take enzymes *before* every meal.

Cerebral Palsy

Cerebral palsy (CP) is a non-progressive disorder of the nervous system in which the individual is unable to control voluntary muscles, present at birth or noted early in childhood (diagnosed within the first 3 years of life). CP can be acquired due to fetal injury or inherited, with males typically affected more often than females. There are 4 types of CP:
1. Spastic cerebral palsy is characterized by increased muscle tone.

- 134 -

2. Dyskinetic cerebral palsy is characterized by involuntary athetoid (constant slow) movements.
3. Ataxic cerebral palsy is characterized by poor posture and decreased muscle control and coordination.
4. Mixed: combination of any of the other three.

Signs and symptoms include poor respiration status, intellectual disability, spasticity speech and language deficits, delayed motor and sensory development, seizures, and joint contractures. Diagnosis is based on sensory/motor testing, spasticity, CT scan/MRI, and EEG. Treatment includes:

- Medications: muscle relaxers (baclofen, diazepam), anticonvulsants
- PT/OT/ST for functional deficits
- Surgery: release contractures; if severe, can cut nerves to relieve symptoms (rhizotomy)

Scoliosis

Scoliosis is an abnormal curvature of the spine to one side, defined as a deviation of greater than 10 degrees. The curvature varies from slight to severe. The spine can bend either way at any point along the spine. The chest area (thoracic scoliosis) and the lower part of the back (lumbar scoliosis) are the most common regions. Scoliosis can develop at any time during childhood and adolescence. It is more common in girls than boys, most commonly occurring at the start of adolescence, though it can occur at any time during childhood. Signs and symptoms include spinal curvature, sideways body posture, one shoulder raised higher than the other, clothes not hanging properly, local muscular aches and ligament pain. Diagnosis is based on physical exam (child stand in underwear facing away from examiner) and x-ray. Treatment includes:

- Bracing of the spine
- Surgery (if severe); if mild, may just continue to watch for further development.
- Lifestyle Modification: educate family, encourage activity for strengthening, chiropractic/physical therapy may help.

Spina Bifida

Spina bifida includes any congenital defect involving insufficient closure of the spine. Spina bifida occulta occurs when the bones of the spine do not close, but skin usually covers the defect. Myelomeningocele is the most severe form of spina bifida. In this condition, the spinal cord and meninges (the membranes covering the spinal cord) protrude out of the child's back. Signs and symptoms are as follows:

- Mild forms: asymptomatic; may have hairy patch or birth mark over lower part of spine.
- Severe: neurogenic bowel/bladder, paralysis, sepsis, scoliosis, hydrocephalus.

Diagnosis is based on x-ray, CT scan, and physical exam. It can be detected in utero with ultrasound, blood tests, and amniocentesis. Treatment for myelomeningocele includes the following:

- Cover with sterile, moist dressing to prevent infection; do not elevate to prevent increased pressure; requires surgery to fix (can be done in utero)
- May require placement of shunt to prevent/treat hydrocephalus.

- Physical and occupational therapy as child grows; be alert for learning difficulties.
- Be aware; many children with *spina bifida* have latex allergy (avoid balloons, bananas, latex catheters)

Kawasaki Disease

Kawasaki disease is a short-lived childhood autoimmune disease of unknown origin that attacks the heart, blood vessels, and lymph nodes, causing widespread inflammation and damage. Generally, the child will make a full recovery with no long-term effects. However, these patients should be monitored for coronary aneurysm and heart attack/stroke during the acute phase of the disease, and should also have follow-up appointments to ensure there is no coronary damage. Signs and symptoms include fever lasting longer than 5 days; joint pain; swollen lymph nodes; peripheral edema; rashes, papillae (small bumps) on the tongue; and chapped and peeling red lips, hands, and feet. Diagnosis is primarily based on S&S; may also do blood work and echocardiogram. Treatment includes:
- Immune globulin (human) infusion: prevents long-term complications
- High-dose aspirin: decreases inflammation, pain, and fever
- Education: early diagnosis and treatment is vital!

RSV

Respiratory syncytial virus (RSV) is a virus that attacks the respiratory system, usually of infants and young children; however, it can affect all age groups. It is highly contagious, and can spread throughout nurseries and day cares. It is a family of viruses, so there is no active immunity against the disease. Signs and symptoms include fever, SOB, cyanosis, wheezing, nasal congestion, and croupy cough. Diagnosis is based on chest x-ray, ABGs, and physical exam. Treatment includes:
- Medications: ribavirin, bronchodilators.
- IV fluids for rehydration, thin secretions.
- May require ventilator in severe cases.
- Symptom management: Infants – sleep with head propped up (blocks under crib legs), frequent small feedings, suction nose and mouth (mouth first to prevent aspiration) with bulb suction, monitor for wheezing/respiratory distress (accessory muscle use, retractions, and cyanosis).
- Monitor the patient for pneumonia, respiratory failure, and otitis media.

Tonsillitis

Tonsillitis is infection of the palatine tonsils, masses of soft tissue on each side of the throat. Tonsillitis may be a viral or bacterial. Strep throat, caused by *Streptococcus pyogenes*, may result in rheumatic fever if untreated. Signs and symptoms include severe sore throat with red swollen tonsils, sometimes with purulent drainage, rhinitis, difficulty swallowing, fever, headache, nausea, earache (from referred pain), and rash. Diagnosis is based on clinical examination and culture and sensitivities (if bacterial infection suspected). Treatment includes:
- Viral tonsillitis usually clears within a few days without treatment.
- Bacterial tonsillitis, especially strep throat, may require antibiotic therapy.
- Other treatments are supportive and include gargling with salt water and NSAIDs and/or acetaminophen for fever and discomfort.

- Tonsillectomy may be indicated for repeated tonsillitis or enlarged tonsils that interfere with breathing or sleeping. Postoperatively, the patient should be given cool liquids, acetaminophen, and an ice pack to relieve swelling and pain. An oral viscous lidocaine solution may be used to relieve pain as well.

NOTE: Frequent swallowing is warning sign of hemorrhage!

Epiglottitis

Epiglottitis is an infection of the epiglottis (the flap of tissue that closes off the larynx during swallowing) and the area around the voice box (larynx) caused by *Haemophilus influenzae* type B (HIB). HIB is an aggressive bacterium that used to be responsible for many serious infections in children younger than 5. However, since vaccinations are routinely given, epiglottitis is much more rare, sometimes caused by burns in the throat, trauma, or other organisms. Signs and symptoms include drooling/difficulty swallowing, sore throat, difficulty breathing, stridor (noisy breathing, "crowing" sound when inhaling), hoarseness, chills, shaking, fever, and cyanosis. Diagnosis is based on x-ray of throat/chest ("thumb" sign), blood/throat cultures, and physical exam.

Treatment includes the following:
- Fluids, antibiotics, steroids for swelling
- Surgery: possible tracheotomy if severe respiratory distress
- Teaching – vaccinate children according to schedule, teach S&S of respiratory distress; wash hands frequently, do not share food/personal objects
- NEVER stick anything into the mouth of a child who has suspected epiglottitis, or try to start IV/do anything distressing; could cause acute throat closure. Must ensure patent airway first.

Otitis Media

Otitis media is a common bacterial infection of the inner (middle) ear or tympanum causing fluid buildup and inflammation, often occurring in young children related to their short, wide eustachian tubes. Otitis media is often associated or accompanied by upper respiratory infections. Children in day care, bottle-fed babies, and those exposed to second-hand smoke are at an increased risk. Signs and symptoms include ear pain, tugging/pulling at ears and irritability in infants, fever, altered or decreased hearing, vertigo, and/or loss of balance. Diagnosis is based on physical exam (pneumatic otoscope), hearing exam, and tympanometry. Treatment includes:
- Medications: Tylenol for pain, antibiotics if bacterial or systemic symptoms, often "wait and see" approach taken first.
- May place tubes in ears if recurrent: tubes drain fluid, preventing ear infections; fall out on their own in ~6 months.
- Prevention: wash hands/avoid respiratory infections, breastfeed/feed child in upright position, avoid second-hand smoke, vaccinate appropriately.

> **Review Video: Otitis Media**
*Visit **mometrix.com/academy** and enter **Code: 328778***

Wilms' Tumor

Wilms' tumor is traditionally a malignant tumor of the kidney characteristically diagnosed in childhood prior to the fifth year of life, and has traits of an inherited autosomal dominant disorder. Those with a family history of Wilms', of African-American descent, and born with other abnormalities such as hypospadius, anridia, and undescended testicles have an increased risk of Wilms' tumor. While it is rare, it often has a very good prognosis. Signs and symptoms are as follows:

- Often asymptomatic
- Palpable abdominal mass, fever, anemia, blood in urine, abdominal ascites, well-defined abdominal wall veins, and metastases to the gonadal area

Diagnosis is based on blood work, CT/MRI, and physical exam. Treatment includes:

- Surgery to remove tumor and possibly kidney, followed by chemotherapy and radiation depending on staging of disease.
- Teaching: ensure family has adequate support, use language understandable to child and parents, frequent rest during chemo.
- NEVER palpate the stomach of a child with diagnosed/suspected Wilms' tumor—it could cause metastasis!

Childhood Cancers

Childhood cancers usually originate in non-epithelial or embryonic cells, especially in preadolescent cancers. These cancers tend to be fast growing with the child rapidly deteriorating over a period of weeks or months. Childhood cancers may result from:

- Congenital genetic abnormalities (such as retinoblastoma and Wilms tumor)
- Impaired immune system, such as from AIDS or immunosuppression (increased risk of non-Hodgkin lymphoma, Hodgkin disease, leiomyosarcoma, Kaposi sarcoma)
- Chromosomal abnormalities, such as Down syndrome (trisomy 21) (markedly higher risk of leukemia)
- External/Environmental carcinogens resulting in genetic mutations (diethylstilbestrol, anabolic androgens, immunosuppressants, radiation exposure, and toxic chemicals) (may result in primary or secondary cancers)

While signs and symptoms vary according to the type of cancer, common findings include pain, palpable mass, cachexia, bruising, recurrent infections, anemia, and neurological impairment. Diagnostic tests include bone marrow biopsy, CBC, LP, and ANC, as well as CT, MRI, and ultrasound and surgical biopsy. Incidence of childhood cancers varies according to the age of the child:

- Infancy to younger than 5 years: Acute leukemia is most common, followed by brain and CNS tumors, sympathetic nervous system tumors, and kidney tumors. Less common are soft tissue, eye, and other tumors, as well as lymphomas.
- Ages 5 to 9 years: Acute leukemia remains most common followed by brain and CNS tumors, lymphoma, and soft tissue cancers. Less common are bone, kidney, eye, and other tumors, as well as sympathetic nervous system tumors.
- Ages 10 to 14 years: Incidence of acute leukemia, lymphoma, and brain and nervous system tumors are relatively equal followed by bone cancer, carcinoma, soft tissue cancer, germ cell cancer, and others.

- 138 -

- Ages 15 to 19 years: Incidence shifts with lymphoma as the most common cancer, followed by carcinoma, germ cell cancer, and then acute leukemia. Less common cancers include sarcoma, bone cancer, and other.

NEUROLOGICAL DISORDERS

Anatomy of the Brain

The brain comprises three primary areas: cerebrum, cerebellum, and brain stem. The cerebrum is divided into two hemispheres (joined by the corpus callosum), thalamus, hypothalamus, and basal ganglia. The outer layer of the hemispheres is called the cerebral cortex and is comprised of gray matter while the innermost layer is comprised of white matter (myelinated nerve fibers and neuroglia cells). The cerebral hemispheres are further divided into pairs (right and left) of lobes:
- Frontal: controls information storage, memory, personality, problem solving, motor functions of speech, and judgment.
- Parietal: interprets sensory input, such as temperature, touch, pressure, and pain, as well as aids in understanding speech and using words to express ideas.
- Temporal: Responsible for hearing, remembering visual scenes, learning, music, and interprets sensory experiences.
- Occipital: Responsible for vision and associates visual images with other sensory experiences.

The sympathetic nervous system is composted of adrenergic receptor sites, activated by epinephrine or norepinephrine. These sites are also where adrenergic drugs bind and produce their effect. They are divided into alpha-adrenergic and beta-adrenergic receptors, depending on whether they respond to norepinephrine or epinephrine. Both alpha- and beta-adrenergic receptors have subtypes designated 1 and 2. Medications classified as alpha-blockers and beta-blockers bind to the receptor sites for norepinephrine and epinephrine, blocking the stimulation of the sympathetic nervous system. The locations of receptors are as follows:
- $Alpha_1$: muscles of veins and arteries.
- $Alpha_2$: central nervous system.
- $Beta_1$: primarily located in the heart
- $Beta_2$: smooth muscle of bronchioles, arterioles, and visceral organs

There are two different glands in the brain that secrete hormones which control the functions of the body. They include the anterior and posterior pituitary glands. The anterior pituitary gland (adenohypophysis) hormones include:
- Growth hormone (somatotropin): Protein that stimulates cells to enlarge and divide, increases rate of protein synthesis, decreases rate cells utilize carbohydrates, increases rate cells utilize fats, and stimulates elongation of bones. Peak secretion is during the night.
- Prolactin: Protein that promotes production of milk after labor and delivery. May help maintain sperm production in males.
- Thyroid-stimulating hormone (thyrotropin): Glycoprotein that controls secretions of thyroid hormones and may stimulate excess growth (goiter) if levels are high.
- Adrenocorticotropic hormone: Peptide that controls the manufacture and secretion of adrenal hormones.

- Follicle-stimulating hormone: Glycoprotein that controls growth and development of follicles that contain eggs in the female ovaries. Stimulates the follicles to secrete estrogens. In males, stimulates production of sperm cells in testes.
- Luteinizing hormone: Glycoprotein that stimulates secretion of sex hormones in both males and females and controls release of egg cells from ovaries.

The posterior pituitary gland is responsible for the secretion of the hormones vasopressin/ADH and oxytocin. These hormones are synthesized in the hypothalamus, stored in the posterior pituitary, and secreted into the blood.
- Vasopressin/ADH
  o Works in the kidneys to retain more water in the blood; decreases urination and increases blood pressure.
  o Synthetic drugs: vasopressin, desmopressin, and lypressin (intranasal)
  o Uses: diabetes insipidus, hypotension, chronic ADH deficiency
- Oxytocin
  o Stimulates contractions of the uterus to initiate and sustain labor; also causes "let-down" reflex, releasing milk in response to infant's sucking on breast
  o Synthetic: oxytocic drugs such as oxytocin
  o Uses: induce labor, treat atonic uterus/postpartum hemorrhage, stimulate lactation

Dementia And Delirium

Dementia and delirium are both alterations in mentation that result from some sort of physiological origin. Dementia is a chronic condition in which mentation becomes progressively altered, and cognizant and or orderly thought processes begin to cease. Dementia is a syndrome that encompasses any disorder characterized by multiple cognitive deficits that include memory impairment. This includes Alzheimer disease, end-stage HIV, permanent brain damage, Parkinson disease, and vascular compromise. An essential feature of a dementia is the development of cognitive deficits that include memory impairment and at least one of the following problems: aphasia, apraxia, agnosia, or a disturbance in executive functioning. Delirium is an acute alteration in consciousness that cannot be explained by a preexisting or evolving dementia. It tends to fluctuate over the course of the day and attention span is impaired. Delirium is often accompanied by a disturbance in the sleep-wake cycle and psychomotor behavior. Delirium is considered a medical emergency because it can indicate many underlying pathological processes (such as a UTI, MI, severe pain, or pneumonia). It also can be superimposed upon an existing dementia; any sudden change in cognition in a person with dementia has to be evaluated for an underlying physiological cause.

Coma, persistent vegetative state, and brain death

Coma is a state of unconsciousness in which both wakefulness and awareness are absent. The patient cannot be aroused and does not display any purposeful reactions to noxious stimuli. The coma state is a continuum from light to deep and patients can fall anywhere on the continuum regarding their level of reactions. In a persistent vegetative state, wakefulness is present but awareness is absent. Sleep wake cycles and hypothalamic and brain stem functions are present but they are not aware of self or environment due to lack of cerebral function. Brain death, is complete, irreversible cessation of function of the entire brain and brain stem. Spinal reflexes may or may not be present. When brain death occurs, the patient is considered dead regardless of the presence of a heartbeat, or mechanical ventilator-assisted respirations.

Generalized seizures

Generalized seizures are neurologic events of unknown origin that cause loss of musculoskeletal control and cognitive awareness in an individual. Seizures can be caused by numerous conditions; patients with repeated seizures of unknown origin are diagnosed with epilepsy. Absence seizures (petit mal) have abrupt onset characterized by episodes of staring, cessation of activities lasting approximately 30 seconds. Myoclonic seizures have a brief shock-like contraction of muscles. This may be limited to a certain limb or area or include the entire body. Tonic-clonic (grand mal) seizures involve loss of consciousness and sustained muscle contraction of entire body, with occasional jerking; may last 1-2 minutes. Diagnosis is based on exam, EEG, PET scan, blood work, and lumbar puncture. Treatment includes the following:
- Medications: lorazepam IV for emergency; long-term therapy:
  o Absence: valproate, and ethosuximide
  o Myoclonic seizures: valproate
  o Tonic-clonic seizures: carbamazepine, phenobarbital, phenytoin, primidone, and/or valproate
- Instruct patients to NEVER stop taking medications.
- Avoid known "triggers": get rest, avoid flashing lights, etc.

Educate on first aid: lower to floor, never restrict/ put anything in mouth, place on side with pillow under head.

Meningitis

Epidemic meningitis, seen most frequently in college dormitories and military barracks, is an inflammation of the meninges of the brain and spinal cord. *Neisseria* and *Streptococcus* bacterium are often the cause, transmitted by airborne droplets. However, there are also viral and fungal forms of meningitis. Signs and symptoms include:
- Headache, photosensitivity, nausea/vomiting, nuchal rigidity, fever, lethargy.
- Brudzinski sign: When the neck is flexed, flexion of the knees also occurs. Flexion of the neck is passive.
- Kernig sign: Flexion of the knee with the lower extremity in a "raised position" that causes pain.

Diagnosis is based on blood culture, x-ray/CT scan, and lumbar puncture. Treatment includes:
- Medications: antibiotics (bacterial meningitis), steroids for brain swelling, pain medication.
- Supportive care: bed rest, fluids, seizure precautions.
- Prevention: stay on schedule with vaccines, wash hands/practice good hygiene; if pregnant, avoid unpasteurized products such as raw cheeses, diary, etc. Cook deli meat and hot dogs thoroughly.

MS

Multiple sclerosis (MS) can range from relatively benign to devastating, as communication between the brain and other parts of the body is disrupted. In the case of MS, it is the nerve-insulating myelin that comes under assault. Such assaults may be linked to an unknown environmental trigger, perhaps a virus. Most people experience their first symptoms of MS between the ages of 20 and 40; often symptoms come and go in a relapsing/remitting pattern. Signs and symptoms include vision abnormalities, paresthesia, generalized pain, difficulty with speech, tremors, dizziness, cognitive impairments, and depression. Diagnosis is based on blood levels, MRI, lumbar puncture. Treatment includes:

- No cure; symptom management.
- Medications, including corticosteroids for acute attacks, and beta-interferons and immunosuppressant drugs to prevent relapse.
- Lifestyle modification: avoid extreme heat (may precipitate relapse), take frequent rest periods, join support groups to prevent feelings of depression/isolation.

Myasthenia gravis

Myasthenia gravis is an autoimmune disorder that results in sporadic, progressive weakness of striated (skeletal) muscles because of impaired transmission of nerve impulses. Myasthenia gravis usually affects muscles controlled by the cranial nerves, although any muscle group may be affected. Many patients also have thymomas. Signs and symptoms include increasing weakness and fatigue that worsens throughout the day. Patients often exhibit ptosis and diplopia. They may have trouble chewing and swallowing and often appear to have masklike facies. If respiratory muscles are involved, patients may exhibit signs of respiratory failure. Myasthenic crisis occurs when patients can no longer breathe independently. Tests include electromyography and the Tensilon test (IV injection of edrophonium or neostigmine, which improves function if patient has myasthenia gravis). Additionally, CT or MRI to diagnose thymoma. Anticholinesterase drugs (neostigmine, pyridostigmine) relieve some muscle weakness but lose effectiveness as the disease progresses. Corticosteroids may be used. Thymectomy is performed if thymoma present. Tracheotomy and mechanical ventilation may be needed for myasthenic crisis. Instruct patients to take medications at the same time every day, first thing in the morning.

> ➤ **Review Video:** <u>Myasthenia Gravis</u>
> *Visit **mometrix.com/academy** and enter **Code: 715123***

Bell's palsy

Bell's palsy occurs when nerve impulses of the seventh cranial nerve (facial) are blocked because of an inflammatory reaction of the nerve, usually at the internal auditory meatus. Onset is rapid, but symptoms usually subside within 2 months, although the condition may recur on the same or opposite side. The causes may include infection, tumor, trauma, or hemorrhage, but the cause is often not clear. Signs and symptoms include sudden onset of unilateral facial weakness with mouth drooping, distorted taste perception, difficulty chewing and swallowing, facial pain, and incomplete eye closure on affected side. Diagnosis is made per assessment of signs and symptoms. Electromyography may help to confirm diagnosis and determine likely recovery time. Prednisone is usually administered to relieve inflammation for 2 weeks. Moist heat to affected area may relieve discomfort, and electrotherapy and massage may help to maintain muscle tone. The patient may need to wear an eye patch to protect the eye, especially if outside. Patients may need a modified soft diet, avoiding hot foods because of lack of sensation.

Cerebrovascular Vascular Accident

Cerebrovascular accident (CVA; stroke) is sudden impairment of circulation in one or more of the blood vessels supplying the brain because of thrombosis (most common), embolism, or hemorrhage, with strokes classified as ischemic or hemorrhagic. The lack of oxygen to the brain tissue can result in permanent brain damage. Risk factors include history of transient ischemic episodes (TIEs), atherosclerosis, hypertension, rheumatic heart disease, diabetes, gout, cardiomyopathy, oral contraceptives, cigarette smoking, and dysrhythmias. Signs and symptoms vary depending on the site of the occlusion. If the stroke occurs on the left side, then right-sided paresis/paralysis occurs and *vice versa*, although damage to facial nerves results in nerve dysfunction on the same side. Diagnosis may be based on CT, MRI, EEG, and/or angiography. Treatment includes:

- Ischemic strokes are treated with aspirin and tissue plasminogen activator (tPA) (within 4.5 hours) as well as supportive treatment.
- Hemorrhagic strokes may require supportive care and surgical repair (coil, clip, AVM repair, radiosurgery, intracranial bypass)
- Short-term or long-term physical and rehabilitative therapy

Parkinson's disease

Parkinson's disease is a neurological disorder characterized by a lack of dopamine (a neurotransmitter) in the brain. The deficiency of dopamine may occur related to degeneration, vascular disorders, or inflammatory changes. It most often occurs in men older than 60, but rarely occurs in younger people as well. Signs and symptoms include rhythmic muscle tremors ("cogwheeling"), rigidity with movement, shuffling gait in which the trunk, legs, knees, and hips are flexed, but remain stiff, festination- quickened gait, droopy posture, tremors of the hands ("pill rolling"), mask-like facial expression, weight loss, difficulty with enunciation, and small hand-writing (micrographia). Diagnosis is based on physical exam, neurological exam – no specific tests. Treatment includes:

- Medications: levodopa/carbidopa, antidepressants.
- PT/OT/ST for functional deficits
- Teaching: small frequent meals, increased amounts of liquid in the diet and increased fiber in the diet, ensure family has adequate support system.

> ➤ **Review Video: Parkinson's Disease**
> Visit *mometrix.com/academy* and enter *Code:* **110876**

Conjunctivitis

Conjunctivitis (also known as "pink eye") is the inflammation of the conjunctiva caused by viruses or bacteria. If it is viral, it is highly contagious. Conjunctivitis can also be caused by chemicals or allergic reactions. Recurring conjunctivitis can indicate a larger underlying disease process. Signs and symptoms include inflamed, pink-colored eyes; purulent discharge from eyes; crusts; itching/burning eyes; and blurred vision. Diagnosis is based on physical exam and clinical picture. Treatment includes:

- Antibiotic eye drops: place drops into eye without touching lashes, do not share bottle to avoid spread, do not use same wash cloth/eye drops between infected/non-infected eyes.
- Symptom management; warm cloths to the eye are helpful, as well as OTC "artificial tears" for irritation/burning, throw away contact lenses/eye makeup used during infection, wear glasses.
- Prevention: wash hands frequently, do not share eye makeup/contact lenses, avoid touching eyes.

Glaucoma

Glaucoma is a condition in which the pressure inside of the eye is increased due to poor drainage of aqueous humor inside the eye, leading to damage to the optic nerve. The exact cause is often unknown, but a family history of glaucoma, diabetes, impaired vision, and increased age are all recognized risk factors. Signs and symptoms are as follows:
- Often asymptomatic
- Loss of peripheral vision, halos around lights, eye pain, headaches, hazy-looking eyes (infants).

Diagnosis is based on complete eye exam, including tonometry and vision test. Treatment includes the following:
- Eye drops: Ensure pressure is held on the inner canthus of the eye for a minimum of 30 seconds to prevent systemic effects.
  - Prostaglandins: latanoprost (common)
  - Beta-blocker: timolol
  - Carbonic anhydrase inhibitors: end in –amide; also given as oral medications: acetazolamide
  - Adrenergic: brimonidine
  - Miotics: pilocarpine and carbachol
- Surgery: increases drainage out of the eye
- Teach: Vision loss is irreversible, but early intervention and treatment can prevent further loss of vision.

> **Review Video: Biggest Differences between Glaucoma and Cataracts**
> Visit **mometrix.com/academy** and enter **Code: 937483**

CARDIOVASCULAR DISORDERS

Hypertension

Hypertension is a condition in which the blood pressure of the body is elevated, generally about 120/80 mm Hg. It can be transient, such as in disease states, or prolonged. Prolonged hypertension is a leading cause of heart attack and stroke, and is associated with stenosis, peripheral vascular disease, and increased vascular resistance.
Blood Pressure (BP) = cardiac output (CO) x systemic vascular resistance (SVR)
Hypertension is often known as the "silent killer." Patients with HTN are generally asymptomatic. However, with severe hypertension (SBP > 170), the patient may experience a headache at the base of the skull, flushing, and blurred vision, sensation of pounding in

head, neck, or chest. Diagnosis is based on physical exam and blood pressure monitoring. Treatment includes the following:

- Medications: antihypertensives, diuretics such as hydrochlorothiazide.
- Lifestyle modification: low-sodium diet, regular low-impact exercise, stress management, and weight loss are all known to lower blood pressure.

> ➢ **Review Video:** <u>Hypertension</u>
> *Visit **mometrix.com/academy** and enter **Code: 458989***

Atrial Arrhythmias

The following are types of atrial arrhythmias:
- Atrial tachycardia: AT is a supraventricular (arising above the ventricles) tachycardia with an atrial rate ranging from 150 to 250 bpm. AT may be transient and is sometimes associated with excess caffeine use, marijuana use, electrolyte imbalance, or physical or emotional stress. AT may also occur with cardiac disorders, such as MI or cardiomyopathy.
- Atrial fibrillation: results from chaotic electrical stimulation of the atria, resulting in an unpredictable irregular rhythm. The atrial rate may exceed 300 bpm but the AV node blocks some impulses so the ventricular rate is usually between 100 and 150 bpm.
- Atrial flutter: AF is a supraventricular tachycardia with an atrial rate of about 300 bpm in a rapid but regular rhythm with a ventricular rate that is commonly 60 to 100 but may be 125 to 150. A common finding is a 2:1 conduction rate, which is an atrial rate of 300 bpm with a ventricular rate of 150 bpm.

Heart Block

The following are different types of heart block:
- Atrioventricular (AV) block, first degree: Conduction of impulses from the atria to the ventricles is delayed with block usually at AV node or bundle of His. Atrial and ventricular rhythms are regular.
- AV block, second degree, type I (Mobitz I): Some impulses are conducted and some are blocked, with each successive impulse from SA node delayed longer than previous until an impulse fails to be conducted, after which the pattern repeats. This block is usually secondary to drug effects or conditions (such as CAD or MI) and is usually transient.
- AV block second degree, type II (Mobitz II): Impulses from the SA node sometimes fail to conduct to the ventricles. Blocks, which may be consecutive, are below the AV node at the bundle of His or bundle branches.
- AV block, type III: This life-threatening complete heart block allows no impulses to reach the ventricle with block at the level of the AV node, the bundle of His, or the bundle branches.

Ventricular arrhythmias

Ventricular arrhythmias originate from the ventricles, often detected by the lack of a discernible P wave. Three main types of ventricle arrhythmias include:

1. Premature Ventricular Contraction (PVC) - A wide and bizarre, premature QRS complex, followed by compensatory pause.
2. Ventricular Tachycardia - Presence of 3 or more PVCs, rate of 150-200 bpm, possible abrupt onset. Possibly due to an ischemic ventricle or electrolyte imbalance.
3. Ventricular Fibrillation - Completely abnormal ventricular rhythm with no discernible QRS complex; ventricles are literally quivering. Requires emergency intervention.

Diagnosis is based on ECG, physical exam, and blood work (BMP). Treatment is as follows:
- **CHECK FOR PULSE;** if no pulse, activate code and begin CPR
- PVCs: occasional PVCs are common, especially with caffeine or stress. However, check electrolytes if frequent (> 6/minute), as this increases risk of V-tach/V-fib.
- V-Tach: Use <u>LAMB</u> to remember treatment:
  o <u>L</u>idocaine
  o <u>A</u>miodarone
  o <u>M</u>agnesium/Mexiletine
  o <u>B</u>eta-Blocker

Acute Coronary Syndromes

Acute coronary syndrome (ACS) is a condition in which there is a sudden decrease of blood flow/oxygen supply to the cardiac tissue. The most common forms of ACS are unstable angina and myocardial infarction. Acute coronary syndromes develop when atherosclerotic plaque buildup lines the walls of the vessels, causing occlusion of the vessel. ACS can also be caused by an embolus or arterial vasospasm. Unstable angina that occurs as a result of occlusion is reversible ischemia. Irreversible ischemia causes myocardial infarction and muscle death and damage. Signs and symptoms include chest pain/pressure, may radiate to left arm, jaw and shoulder; nausea/vomiting; diaphoresis; and SOB/dyspnea on exertion. Diagnosis is based on EKG, blood work (troponin and CK-MB), and physical exam.

Treatment includes the following:
- Medications: nitroglycerin (angina), morphine for pain and decreases cardiac workload, aspirin, may use thrombolytic such as TPA if clot is suspected and cath lab not readily available
- Place on oxygen, and bedrest.
- Cardiac Catheterization - to open vessels/ablate clot; may require open heart surgery (CABG) if disease is severe.
- Teaching: Angina – Causes (4 E's): **E**xertion, **E**ating, **E**motional Distress, **E**xtreme Temperature; weight management, low-cholesterol/low-sodium diet, monitor for S&S of heart failure/cardiogenic show
- **MONA** for chest pain: **M**orphine, **O**xygen, **N**itroglycerin, **A**spirin.

*See Coronary Artery Disease teaching card for more information.

Valvular Diseases

The following are common valvular diseases:
- Mitral stenosis: A thickening and contracture of the mitral valve cusps of the heart. This thickening and constriction causes narrowing of the mitral valve and produces

a resistance to diastolic filling of the left ventricle. The most common cause of mitral stenosis is rheumatic fever.

- Mitral insufficiency: An incompetent deformity of the mitral valve. Also termed valvular regurgitation and is characterized by valves that do not close completely, resulting in retrograde blood flow back up into the atrium from the ventricles.
- Aortic valve stenosis: A narrowing of the opening between the left ventricle and the aorta. It is the most commonly caused by a genetic disorder, rheumatic fever, or atherosclerosis.
- Aortic insufficiency: Characterized by deformed flaps of the heart valves that prevent proper closure. Without proper closure, the blood flows back from the aorta into the left ventricle.
- Tricuspid stenosis: A restriction of the tricuspid valve.
- Tricuspid insufficiency: A regurgitation of the blood from the right ventricle to the right atrium that occurs during ventricular systole.

Heart Failure

Heart failure is a condition in which the heart becomes unable to adequately pump blood throughout the body. It encompasses ventricular dysfunction, ischemic cardiomyopathies, and systolic and diastolic dysfunction. Heart failure generally starts as left-sided, and proceeds to the right side as the condition worsens. There is no known cure for chronic heart failure, so treatments focus on symptom management and palliative care. Signs and symptoms are as follows:

- Right-sided: generalized edema, jugular vein distention, and hepatomegaly.
- Left-sided: dyspnea on exertion, cough with blood-tinged or frothy sputum, orthopnea (difficulty breathing while laying down)

Diagnosis is based on blood work (BNAP > 100), echocardiogram, and ECG. Treatment includes the following:

- Furosemide/bumetanide: Loop diuretics to decrease fluid overload; thiazide diuretics may also be used.
- Blood pressure management: often use ACE inhibitor—relaxes blood vessels, decreasing workload of the heart; ends in "–pril"
- May also include beta-blockers, and digoxin for increased cardiac strength
- Lifestyle modification: low-sodium and fluid-restricted diet, low level exercise, may require oxygen during end stages, weigh self-daily, same time, report > 1-2 lb in a day/> 3-5 in a week.

Cardiac tamponade

Cardiac tamponade occurs when fluid, usually blood, accumulates in the pericardial sac. If the fluid accumulates rapidly, the walls of the pericardial sac do not have time to stretch to accommodate the fluid, so the patient may quickly develop pulseless electrical activity (PEA) with fluid accumulation of 50 to 250 mL. If fluid accumulates slowly, such as with pericardial effusions associated with cancer, patients may tolerate up to 2L of fluid before symptoms become acute. Cardiac tamponade compresses the heart and limits the venous return to the heart and blood flow into the ventricles, thereby reducing cardiac output. Beck's triad of symptoms typical to acute cardiac tamponade include decreased arterial blood pressure, increased jugular venous distention, and muffled heart sounds. Diagnosis is per symptoms, ECG, chest x-ray, and/or echocardiography. Treatment is pericardiocentesis to relieve pressure. In some cases, a drain may be placed in the pericardial sac or a window cut to allow drainage into the pleural cavity if there is a large effusion.

Buerger Disease

Thromboangiitis obliterans (Buerger disease) is an inflammatory process of the arteries and veins. Thromboangiitis obliterans occurs most often in young and middle-aged men, especially those who smoke. Thromboangiitis obliterans is characterized by occlusions of the extremities (both upper and lower) that are caused by inflammation and thrombus formations that occlude the vessels. Signs and symptoms include ulcerations of the extremities, coolness and pallor in the hands and feet, increased sensitivity to cold, paresthesia, intermittent claudication in legs, and cyanotic hands and feet. Diagnosis is based on blood work, Allen test, angiogram, and clinical picture. Treatment includes:
- Smoking cessation is cornerstone of treatment to halt progress of disease; medications to dilate vessels; compression stockings.
- Monitor patient for infection and gangrene.
- **Note:** Do not confuse with *Raynaud disease*, a condition that most commonly occurs in young/middle-aged woman, caused by arterial vasospasm of hands and feet; similar symptoms, and often related to psychological illness.

HEMATOLOGICAL DISORDERS

Anatomy and Physiology of the Immune System

The body's first line of defense against microorganisms is the innate (primary) immune response, which is a *nonspecific* form of defense against infection. This includes the skin, mucous membranes, body fluids, and bacterial flora of the intestines:
- The skin provides a barrier to entry of bacteria. Fatty acids and lactic acids of sweat and sebaceous secretions also contribute to the first line of defense.
- The mucous lining of the respiratory and GI tracts traps bacteria and the trapped particles are removed by coughing and sneezing, aided by ciliated epithelial cells.
- Tears, saliva, and urine contain enzymes and acids that kill bacteria.
- Normal bacterial flora in humans defends against infectious bacteria by competitive inhibition—competing for nutrients, space to grow, etc.

Innate immunity is also called natural immunity. Innate immunity consists of all the immune defenses that lack immunologic memory. Innate immunity is acquired at birth and all humans have a resistance to certain types of organisms. Acquired immunity includes active acquired immunity and passive acquired immunity. Acquired immunity is gained after birth as a result of an immune response. Active or passive immunity is related to the stimulation process and whether the response is activated by a donor or by the host. It can also be further classified as natural vs. artificial.
- Active acquired immunity: Active acquired immunity is produced by a host after exposure from an antigen or immunization.
  - o Active natural: immunity after sick from disease
  - o Active artificial: immunity after receiving immunization
- Passive acquired immunity: Passive acquired immunity is when antibodies are given to the host.

- 148 -

o Passive natural: breast-fed infants receive antigens from milk
o Passive artificial: infusion of antigens to combat disease

Immunoglobulins are antibodies that are produced from serum glycoprotein in plasma cells in response to pathogens. Immunoglobulins are receptors on the surfaces of mature B cells. Immunoglobulins have specific sensitivity to antigens. There are five molecular classes of immunoglobulin. The five classes of immunoglobulin are IgG, IgA, IgM, IgE, and IgD.

- IgG is responsible for most antibody functions, and can be found in all the fluids of the body. They fight most bacteria and viruses, and are responsible for activities such as precipitation, agglutination, and complement activation. IgG is also the only antibody that can pass from mother to baby through placenta.
- IgA is found in body secretions, such as those in the ear, nose, throat, digestive tract, vagina, etc. The IgA antibodies protect the body from infectious enzymes and secretions.
- IgM is the largest immunoglobulin and is the first antibody produced during the initial primary response to an antigen.
- IgD is found in low concentrations in the blood and peritoneal lining, and the function is unknown.
- IgE is the least concentrated immunoglobulin in circulation, primarily found in the respiratory system. IgE is the primary antibody with allergic reactions, and also responds to parasitic infections.

Antigens are molecules or molecular complexes that react with preformed components of the immune system such as lymphocytes and antibodies. Antigenicity is the molecules' innate capacity to react with those preformed components. Self-antigens are produced within the body and nonself antigens are foreign to the body or not formed by the body. Immunogens are antigens that have the capacity to initiate an immune response. Immunogens and antigens result in stimulation of an immune response by the body. The body responds with antibodies or immune cells when activated to protect the body from invasion of bacteria, viruses, and/or any other inflammatory process, illness, or injury.

Humoral immunity is associated with circulating antibodies, and B cells are the primary source of humoral immunity. The primary immunocyte of the immune response is the lymphocyte. The process of humoral immunity involves the lymphocyte migration through lymphatic system and blood vessels. As lymphocytes make their way through the lymph, they become B cells. B cells that encounter antigens are stimulated to mature into plasma cells that produce antibodies.

Cancer

Cancers (neoplasms) are the uncontrolled or uncontrollable proliferations of abnormal cells. Cancer cells typically are immature, abnormal, and encapsulated, allowing for easy metastasis and invasion of surrounding cells. Causative factors associated with cancers include viruses, chronic irritation of skin or other tissues (e.g., sunburns), chemical exposure, high-fat /low-fiber diets, and/or genetics. **CAUTION UP** is a helpful mnemonic to assist you to remember the early warning signs of cancer.
Change in bowel or bladder
A lesion that does not heal
Unusual bleeding or discharge
Thickening or lump in breast or elsewhere

Indigestion or difficulty swallowing
Obvious changes in wart or mole
Nagging cough or persistent hoarseness
Unexplained weight loss
Pernicious anemia

Diagnosis is based on blood work, CT, MRI, PET scan, and biopsy. Treatment includes:
- Chemotherapy; systemic agents that destroy cancer in the body
- Radiation: using radioactive particles to destroy cancer; local.

Prognosis depends on cancer type and progression at diagnosis.

Neoplasms

The four different classifications of neoplasms are:
1. Carcinoma: Originates from the epithelial tissue of the skin, lung, gastrointestinal tract, breast and uterine lining. Carcinomas traditionally begin to spread via the lymph system, followed by the bloodstream. The two major types of carcinoma are the glandular (adenocarcinoma) and squamous cell carcinoma. Squamous cell carcinoma is the most frequently diagnosed type of cancer.
2. Sarcoma: A neoplasm of the connective tissue. Sarcomas have an increased risk of malignancy, and originate from an excessive proliferation of mesodermal cells. Sarcomas are common in bone and muscle, and are generally characterized by large masses that may or may not metastasize to other areas of the body.
3. Lymphoma: Neoplasms of the lymph or reticuloendothelial tissue. Lymphomas are typically solid tumors that traditionally appear in the lymph nodes, spleen, or any other organ tissue. Hodgkin disease is an example of lymphoma. Lymphomas are categorized according to cell involvement (B or T cells).
4. Leukemia: Both acute and chronic and encompasses the blood-producing organs. Leukemia is a progressive proliferation of abnormal leukocytes. Categorized by cell type and duration from initial onset to time of demise.

> ➢ **Review Video: Leukemia**
> *Visit **mometrix.com/academy** and enter **Code: 940024***

Iron Deficiency Anemia

Iron deficiency anemia is a lack of circulating hemoglobin resulting from a lack of iron in the blood. There are several causes for this disease:
- Inadequate supply: rapid growth (prematurity, adolescence, pregnancy), poor eating habits.
- Impaired absorption: malabsorption disorders
- Blood loss: hemorrhage, parasitic infections
- Hemodilution of pregnancy: increased blood volume results in a relative deficiency of circulating hemoglobin and other components of the blood.

Signs and symptoms include pallor, poor physical/cognitive development (infants), infections, edema, irritability, tachycardia, fatigue, glossitis, spoon-shaped fingernails (termed koilonychia), and PICA (eating non-food substances, such as ice chips or soap).

Diagnosis is based on complete blood cell count with differential and fecal occult blood. Treatment includes the following:

- Increase dietary iron: dark, leafy vegetables, red meat, do not use cow milk for infants ≤ 1 year of age.
- Iron supplementation:
  - Oral - can cause darkening of stools and stomach irritation. Take with a meal.
  - IV – Do not give with other medications. Watch for extravasation, which will cause irritation of tissues.
- Blood Transfusion (severe cases)

Aplastic Anemia

Aplastic anemia is characterized by a decreased production of red blood cells within the bone marrow, causing a decreased amount of circulating erythrocytes, leukocytes, or platelets in the blood. Causes of aplastic anemia include, but are not limited to, exposure to drugs and/or chemicals, anti-tumor agents, 6-mercaptopurine, antimicrobials, heavy metals, radiation, and pregnancy (rare). Signs and symptoms include dyspnea, ecchymoses, petechiae, fatigue, fever, hemorrhage, menorrhagia, occult blood, epistaxis, pallor, palpitations, weakness, retinal hemorrhage, and weight loss. Diagnosis is based on blood work (CBC), bone marrow biopsy, and physical exam.

Treatment includes:

- Blood transfusion, stem cells
- Medications: immunosuppressants, bone marrow stimulants (epoetin alfa, sargramostim, filgrastim), antibiotics for infection
- Lifestyle modification: wash hands frequently/avoid sick people, rest frequently, avoid contact sports/other things that increase risk of injury and subsequent bleeding

Hemophilia

Hemophilia is an inherited x-linked chromosomal disorder that results in impaired clotting of the blood. Because it is x-linked, hemophilia most often occurs in males, and is inherited from their mothers. Types of hemophilia are:

- Hemophilia A: "Classic hemophilia," deficiency of factor VII.
- Hemophilia B: "Christmas disease," deficiency of factor IX.
- Hemophilia C: mild form, occurs equally in males and females.

Signs and symptoms include mild to severe bleeding from minor wounds, joint pain, bruising, and nosebleeds. Diagnosis is based on blood work (pTT/INR/blood clotting factors) and physical exam. Treatment includes:

- Medications: desmopressin, antifibrinolytics, replacement of missing factor, blood transfusions; cannot take NSAIDs or blood thinners.
- PT/OT for joint damage from bleeding; may require surgery if joint bleeding severe.
- Teaching: treat wounds immediatley, report excessive bleeding, exercise regulary to strengthen muscles/must avoid contact sports; practice good oral hygeine to prevent gum bleeds, wear medical alert bracelet/educate caregivers

Sickle Cell Anemia

Sickle cell anemia is an autosomal recessive disorder that occurs primarily in African Americans. Patients have sickle cell crises, during which there is partial or complete replacement of normal Hgb with abnormal hemoglobin S (Hgb S). This results in elongated, "sickle"-shaped red blood cells that are rigid and obstruct capillary blood flow. These microscopic clots cause damage to organs of the body, especially the spleen. Patients are at increased risk of heart attack and stroke due to clots. Precipitating factors for a crisis are most commonly anything that causes hypoxia in the tissues, including trauma, infection, fever, physical and emotional stress, dehydration, increased altitude (even poorly pressurized airplanes), hypoventilation, and hypothermia.

Signs and symptoms are as follows:
- Extreme pain, especially in joints/chest, shortness of breath
- Long-term effects include infections, delayed growth, swollen hands/feet.

Diagnosis is based on blood smear, sickle turbidity test, serum electrophoresis, and newborn screening. Treatment includes the following:
- *Treat underlying cause of crisis!
- Medications: antibiotics, analgesics* (will require high amounts due to tolerance).
- Oxygen, IV fluids, moist heat for discomfort, possible routine blood transfusions.
- Surgery: splenectomy if recurrent splenic sequestration.
- Bed rest to maximize energy and improve oxygenation.
- Teach: stay hydrated, get adequate nutrition, and report S&S of infection immediately.

*Sickle cell pain is considered real pain on the NCLEX; priority to treat.

> ➤ **Review Video: <u>Sickle Cell Disease</u>**
> *Visit **mometrix.com/academy** and enter **Code: 603869***

Thalassemia

Thalassemia is an autosomal inherited recessive trait characterized by the abnormal formation and decreased life span of red blood cells that occurs primarily in the Asian, Middle Eastern, and Mediterranean populations. The decreased lifespan of RBCs leads to increased serum iron/increased bilirubin. There are two types of thalassemia, alpha and beta. Signs and symptoms include pallor, jaundice, bronzed/freckled appearance, anorexia, hepatomegaly, splenomegaly, fatigue, decreased appetite and poor diet, altered growth patterns/delayed sexual maturation, dyspnea, gallstones (cholelithiasis), and pathologic (unexplained) fractures. Thalassemia may cause mongoloid faces in older children. Diagnosis is based on blood work (CBC, BMP), family history, and clinical picture. Treatment includes the following:
- Blood transfusions: desired hemoglobin will be 9.3 g/dL at minimum.
- Folate may be given and iron chelation therapy (a mechanism of treatment to remove specific particles from the blood) may be utilized.
- Daily penicillin may be used as a prophylactic mechanism.
- The nurse should counsel the patient to avoid strenuous exercise, and also to avoid iron rich foods.

Note: Cooley anemia is beta-thalassemia major.

HUS vs. TTP

Hemolytic uremic syndrome (HUS) and thrombotic thrombocytopenic purpura (TTP) are characterized by microangiopathic hemolytic anemia (platelet-rich clots forming in capillaries and arterioles) and thrombocytopenia. The hemolytic anemia occurs when red blood cells pass through areas with thrombi and become fragmented by the turbulence.

There are, however, some differences between HUS and TTP:

HUS	TTP
Affects primarily children younger than 5 or older adults Commonly results in renal impairment Cause is usually severe diarrhea from Shiga-toxin producing E. coli S&S: Fever, dehydration, abdominal tenderness, acute renal failure, neurological impairment. Diagnosis: CBC, coagulation tests, stool cultures, kidney function tests. Treatment is supportive care and dialysis. Plasma exchange has not been as effective with HUS. Eculizumab for treatment of atypical HUS. Blood/platelet transfusions may be indicated.	Primarily affects adults Commonly results in neurological impairment Cause is genetic, autoimmune, or drug-induced S&S: altered mental status, fatigue, petechiae, fever, and hemoglobinuria. Diagnosis: CBC, coagulation tests, assessment of von Willebrand factor–cleaving protease (ADAMTS13) activity Treatment is total plasma exchange with FFP. Platelet transfusions are usually avoided. Corticosteroids may also be administered. Refractory cases may respond to vincristine.

RA

Rheumatoid arthritis (RA) is a chronic autoimmune disease characterized by cartilage damage that results in inflammation, cartilage and bone deformities, and decreased mobility. Phagocytes (neutrophils and macrophages) form enzymes that cause inflammation and degrade synovial tissue and articular cartilage. This inflammatory process can result in hemorrhage, coagulation, and fibrin deposits within the synovial fluid. Signs and symptoms include fever, fatigue, joint pain and swelling, decreased ROM, hand/feet deformities, numbness, skin color changes. Diagnosis is based on evaluating rheumatoid factor tests, C-reactive protein, ESR, synovial fluid exam, and x-rays of involved joints. Treatment includes:

- Symptom management; no cure.
- Medications: corticosteroids, anti-malarial drugs, COX-2 inhibitors, NSAIDs
- Physical therapy, moist heat, splinting for symptom relief.

SLE

Systemic lupus erythematosus (SLE) is an autoimmune disorder that causes widespread inflammation in the joints, skin, and various organ systems. Exacerbations and remissions are part of the disease process of SLE. Possible contributing factors include immunology, environmental factors, hormone abnormalities, and genetics. It is 9 times more common in females. Signs and symptoms include "butterfly" rash - a red or pink rash spread across the nose and cheeks, weight loss, fever, hair loss, abdominal pain, mouth sores, fatigue, seizures, arthritis, nausea, joint pain, and psychosis. Diagnosis is based on CBC, chest x-ray, ANA test, Coombs' test, urine analysis, and testing for various antibodies. Treatment includes the following:

- Medications: NSAIDs, cytotoxic drugs, hydroxychloroquine.
- Monitor the patient for seizures, anemia, myocarditis, infection, renal failure.
- Teaching: avoid sunlight, wear sunscreen and a hat while outside, contact health care provider if ill or suspect infection; conserve energy, and avoid stress as much as possible.

Lymphomas

Lymphomas are cancers of the lymphocite cells that make up the immune system. Lymphoma is further classified as Hodgkin or non-Hodgkin lymphoma:

- Hodgkin lymphoma:
    - Identified by the prescence of Reed-Sternberg cells
    - More prevalent in 15-19 years of age; also in men > 50.
    - May be sub-staged as "A" or "B," indicating prescence of symptoms
- Non-Hodgkin lymphomas (NHL)
    - More prevalent in children < 14 years
    - Approximately 60% of pediatric lymphomas are NHL

Signs and symptoms are as follows:

- Stage A - asymptomatic.
- Stage B - persistent fever, night sweats, unexplained weight loss; enlarged, firm, nontender lymph nodes; itching, difficulty breathing, malaise

Diagnosis is based on blood tests, bone marrow biopsy, PET scan, and chest x-ray. Therapeutic management consistst of :

- Radiation/ Chemotherapy (alone or with radiation)
- Prognosis depends on severity/progression of the disease

> ➢ **Review Video: Lymphoma**
> *Visit **mometrix.com/academy** and enter **Code: 513277***

PULMONARY DISORDERS

Respiratory terminology

Tympanic percussion — lung is hyper expanded with air as in asthma, emphysema, chronic bronchitis, and cystic fibrosis.

Dull percussion — lung filled with fluid, pus (pleural effusion).

Decreased breath sounds — over obstructed areas (cancer), or decreased lung tissues (emphysema), atelectasis.

Crackles — sounds like small, cracking/popping noises – indicates fluid in lungs, like that found in fluid overload or pneumonia.

Rhonchi — Rough, "course" lung sounds – indicates congestion.

Wheezes — high, musical sounds resulting when bronchi are narrowed (asthma, chronic bronchitis, cystic fibrosis, localized tumor).

Alterations In Respirations

The following are alterations in respirations, including signs and symptoms of respiratory distress:
- Tachypnea: respiratory rate > 20 breaths per minute
- Hypopnea: respiratory rate < 12 breaths per minute
- Dyspnea: shortness of breath, often accompanied by anxiety, gasping, and sitting upright
- Ataxic respirations: completely irregular pattern of respirations with increasing periods of apnea, often associated with brain damage (stroke, TBI) and poor outcome.
- Cheyne-Stokes: The patient breathes shallowly at first and then progressively deeper and finally progressively more shallowly until breathing stops for periods of apnea that vary from 30 seconds to 2 minutes before the cycle repeats, associated with dying patients.
- Biot's breathing: pattern includes periods of regular but rapid respirations followed by periods of apnea, associated with damage to the medulla in the brain from stroke or tentorial herniation. May also be associated with long-term opioid use.
- Kussmaul's respirations: pattern of hyperventilation with the patient increasingly gasping for air, associated with metabolic acidosis/diabetic ketoacidosis.
- Apneustic respirations: Prolonged inspiration followed by markedly prolonged expiration, which may be apneic. Associated with damage to respiratory center of the brain.

Pulmonary Hypertension

Pulmonary hypertension (PH) is a condition in which the pulmonary arteries that carry blood from the right atrium to the lungs become constricted so that the pressure inside rises, causing the right atrium to apply increasing pressure in order to facilitate blood flow. This causes the right atrium to expand and weaken to the point it is unable to adequately pump blood to the lungs. PH may be primary or secondary (causes include sarcoidosis, metastases, vascular obstruction, COPD, and scleroderma). Primary hypertension is most common in females (20-40 years) and is usually fatal within 3-4 years. Signs and symptoms include increasing dyspnea, weakness, syncope, and right heart failure (peripheral edema, jugular venous distention, hepatomegaly, and ascites). Diagnosis is based on ABGs, ECG, cardiac catheterization, pulmonary angiography, echocardiogram, 6-minute walk test, V/Q scan, and pulmonary function tests. Treatment includes diuretics (furosemide), anticoagulants (warfarin), inotropic agents (digoxin), oxygen therapy, monitoring of blood gases, daily weight, intake and output, bosentan (blocks endothelin, which constricts arteries), epoprostenol or treprostinil sodium (dilates pulmonary arteries), and sildenafil (relaxes smooth muscles). Definitive treatment is lung or heart/lung transplantation.

- 155 -

Pleural Effusion & Empyema

Pleural effusion is the accumulation of fluid in the pleural space, usually secondary to other disease processes, such as heart failure, TB, neoplasms, nephrotic syndrome, and viral respiratory infections. The fluid may be serous, bloody, or purulent (empyema), and transudative or exudative. Signs and symptoms depend on underlying condition but include dyspnea, from mild to severe. Tracheal deviation away from affected side may be evident. Diagnosis is based on chest x-ray, lateral decubitus x-ray, CT, thoracentesis, and pleural biopsy. Treatment includes treating underlying cause, thoracentesis to remove fluid, insertion of chest tube, pleurodesis, and pleurectomy or pleuroperitoneal shunt (primarily with malignancy). Empyema is a pleural effusion in which the collection of pleural fluid is thick and purulent, usually as a result of bacterial pneumonia or penetrating chest trauma. Empyema may also occur as a complication of thoracentesis or thoracic surgery. Signs and symptoms includes acute illness with fever, chills, pain, cough, and dyspnea. Diagnosis is based on chest CT and thoracentesis with culture and sensitivity. Treatment includes antibiotics and drainage of pleural space per needle aspiration, tube thoracostomy, or open chest drainage with thoracotomy

Pneumonia

Pneumonia is an infection caused by fluid in the lungs. There are several types of pneumonia, including viral pneumonia, "walking pneumonia," *Legionella* pneumonia, CMV pneumonia (AIDS), aspiration pneumonia, and atypical pneumonia. Pneumonia is a leading cause of death in hospitals, and requires rigorous attention to prevent and treat to avoid complications. Regardless of the cause, pneumonias are all treated similarly. Signs and symptoms include fever, headache, difficulty breathing, feeling short of breath, cough, and inspiratory chest pain. Diagnosis is based on chest x-ray, CT scan, pulmonary perfusion scan, CBC, sputum culture, and auscultation of crackles. Treatment includes the following:

- Antibiotics if caused by a bacterial infection.
- Respiratory treatments to open airways.
- Steroids: decrease swelling in lungs.
- IV fluids; thin secretions to cough up, rehydrate.
- Supplemental oxygen and pain medication for discomfort.
- Prevention: pneumococcal vaccine for high-risk individuals/those older than 65, incentive spirometry/teaching hospitalized patient's to cough/deep breathe, early ambulation.

ARDS

Acute respiratory distress syndrome (ARDS) is inflammation of the lungs. In ARDS, the pulmonary neutrophils gather in excessive amounts at the site of inflammation, along with fibrin and platelets. Injury to capillaries from inflammation leads to edema. The fluid contains plasma proteins that can inactivate the surfactant of the alveoli, causing alveolar collapse. Fibrin clotting then causes obstructed airspaces. The result is decreased respiratory compliance, decreased function, decreased residual volumes, and dead airspace. The end result for the patient is ventilation perfusion mismatching, intrapulmonary shunting, and hypoxemia, and subsequent death. ARDS can be caused by trauma, chemical inhalation, pneumonia, or septic shock. Signs and symptoms include respiratory distress, hypoxemia, cyanosis, hypotension, tachycardia progressing to bradycardia. Diagnosis is based on arterial blood gases, chest x-ray, CBC, blood cultures, and physical exam. Treatment is as follows:

- Mechanical ventilation/intubation with high tidal volumes and PEEP.
- Treat the underlying condition; IV antibiotics, etc.
- Monitor the patient for pulmonary fibrosis, MODS, ventilator-associated pneumonia, and acidosis.

Asthma

Asthma is a chronic obstructive pulmonary disease of the airways that causes them to tighten. During acute attacks, the air supply to the lungs may be shut off completely. Status Asthmaticus is when the respiratory distress continues despite vigorous therapeutic measures. Signs and symptoms include chest tightness, shortness of breath, wheezing, cough, and wheezing followed by sudden silence (ominous sign). Diagnosis is based on physical exam and pulmonary function tests (PFTs). Treatment includes:

- Emergency Medications: epinephrine IV (status asthmaticus) albuterol, ipratropium, oral/IV steroids.
- Long-term medications: corticosteroids, sympathomimetics (e.g., terbutaline), bronchodilators (e.g., salmeterol), theophylline (monitor serum levels), leukotriene modifiers (e.g., montelukast).
- Chest physiotherapy (CPT)
- Hyposensitization - allergy shots.
- Avoid exacerbation/allergens.
- Monitor function with peak flow meter.
- Regular exercise to promote pulmonary health.

> **Review Video: Asthma and Allergens**
> Visit **mometrix.com/academy** and enter **Code: 799141**

COPD

Chronic obstructive pulmonary disease (COPD) is an umbrella term for diseases of the bronchi that cause irreversible narrowing of the airways, and forced expiration is decreased. COPD includes chronic bronchitis and emphysema most often, but also includes asthma, cystic fibrosis, and bronchiectasis.

- Chronic bronchitis: productive cough for at least 3 months over the span of 2 years; copious sputum production and cough, morning headache; "blue blowers" – cannot get enough oxygen in.
- Emphysema: overfilling/dilation of alveolar sacs, leading to decreased expiratory effort; minimal cough, wheezing and decreased lung sounds; "pink-puffers" – retain CO_2.

Signs and symptoms include difficulty breathing, dyspnea on exertion, wheezing/tight lung sounds, increased posterior-anterior chest diameter ("barrell chest"), and weight loss. Diagnosis is based on ABGs, pulmonary function tests (PFTs), and clinical picture.

Treatment includes the following:

- Supplemental O_2; however, do not give more than 2-3 liters, as these patients have hypoxic drive to breath.
- Nutrition: hypermetabolic state (increased work of breathing) requires increased calories; however, may limit carbohydrates to limit hypercarbia
- Teaching: frequent rest/ energy conservation, and pursed lip breathing to increase alveolar resistance, smoking cessation, and avoidance of respiratory irritants (aerosols, allergens, etc)

* See COPD teaching card for more information

GASTROENTEROLOGICAL DISORDERS

Digestion terms

Ingestion — Ingestion is the initial step of placing food in the oral cavity (mouth).

Digestion — Digestion is further classified as mechanical or chemical digestion. Mechanical digestion takes place after ingestion in the form of chewing. Chemical digestion is the process of digestive enzymes mixing with foods to form altered compounds that facilitate absorption as well as passage through the digestive tract.

Motility — Motility is the way foods are transported through the digestive system; terms associated with motility include peristalsis and segmentation; these refer to the musculature of the digestive tract.

Secretion — Secretion occurs when digestive liquids are excreted during the digestive process.

Absorption — Absorption occurs when nutrients are broken down into particles small enough to move through the intestinal mucosa and into the bloodstream.

Elimination — Elimination is the formation of feces in the rectum, and defecation of stool via the anal canal and anus.

Anatomy and Physiology of the Digestive System

The digestive system is a sequence of organs that function together to breakdown ingested nutrients for digestion and absorption. Digestion is a method of altering foods into smaller and smaller particles until the nutrients are absorbed into the body. The digestive system is also considered a protective mechanism for the body as it relates to absorption of microorganisms and/or noxious substances. The process of digestion takes place as follows: first, the oral cavity (mouth) facilitates chewing to break down ingested materials. The salivary glands are located in the oral cavity, which produce saliva rich in amylase that lubricates the ingested materials and begins the initial phase of carbohydrate breakdown. Swallowing is facilitated by the pharynx. Food is moved from the oral cavity into the stomach via the esophagus. The stomach secretes acid and maintains motion to break down foods. The liver produces digestive bile, which the gallbladder concentrates and stores. Bile is then secreted into the small intestine to break down fats. The pancreas produces bicarbonate (a base) that assists in the regulation of stomach acid and the production of insulin (a hormone) to regulate blood glucose levels. The small intestine is responsible for

- 158 -

the absorption nutrients once food has been broken into particles small enough to cross the cell membrane of the digestive mucosa. The large intestine is responsible to absorb mostly water; by the time food reaches the large intestine, it is a mass that is known as feces. The rectum is the distal portion of the large intestine and stores feces. The anus serves as the outlet for fecal material.

Absorption is the body's process of assimilating the nutrients from digested food. Absorption takes place when microscopic digested food particles diffuse through the walls of the mucosa of the small intestine into the bloodstream or lymph fluid. There are several types of diffusion that must occur depending on which nutrient the body is absorbing. Passive diffusion is the simplest type, where molecules travel from an area of high concentration to low concentration. Facilitated diffusion is used when nutrient molecules being transported through the cell membrane must use transporter proteins to get inside, though still moving from high to low conentration. Finally, active transport takes place when cellular energy is used to transfer molecules into areas of high pressure via transporter proteins.

Metabolism occurs when absorbed nutrients are utilized by the body to maintain proper function, energy levels, and maintenance. Metabolism occurs in two forms: catabolism and anabolism. Catabolism is when food particles are broken down into molecular particles. The body mainly uses catabolism to produce chemical and heat energy. Anabolism, however, is the formation of new substances using the catabolized nutrients to build larger molecules. Anabolism is responsible for the production of new tissue. To maintain proper metabolic function, the patient's nutritional intake must be in balance with their body's requirements for daily functional needs. Maintaining this balance is critical in preventing and treating obesity, cachexia, and other forms of malnourishment.

When the body is deprived of adequate nutrients, the functioning of the immune system is altered, leaving the body vunerable to disease. The immune system activates a response to infectious organisms as a measure of protection for the body. If the immune system is compromised, its defense mechanisms will become altered. With malnutrition, the skin becomes less elastic and healing is delayed, giving a point of entry for bacteria. Under-nourishment causes the microvilli of the mucous membranes in the intestines to flatten, further decreasing the amount of nutrient absorption and antibody excretion. At the cellular level, the different white blood cells and antibodies may be slow to respond and/or may not have enough energy to mount a cell-mediated immune response if not properly supplied with nutrients to create adenosine triphosphate (ATP). This could allow the invasion of harmful viruses/bacteria and the growth of organisms.

The term "iatrogenic" means "related to health care/health treatment." Iatrogenic malnutrition is malnutrition that occurs with prolonged hospitalization, surgical procedures, and/or prescribed treatments. Monitoring diet, hydration status, level of consciousness, fatigue, and overall health are some ways nurses can prevent iatrogenic malnutrition in hospitalized patients. Some populations at an increased risk of iatrogenic malnutrition include patients with cancer, pulmonary disorders, or Alzheimer disease, and elderly patients with fractures.

GERD

Gastroesophageal reflux disease (GERD) is esophagitis caused by reflux of stomach acid back up into the esophagus. There is an increased risk of GERD with decreased sphincter tone with smoking, alcohol, and fatty meals. Reflux is also worsened with obesity, pregnancy, impaired gastric emptying, prone positioning, and peristaltic dysfunction. Signs and symptoms include heartburn after meals and less commonly, morning cough or hoarseness (irritation of larynx). It is often asymptomatic. Diagnosis is based on physical exam/clinical picture, EGD, and pH monitoring.

Treatment includes:
- Medication: PPIs (esomeprazole, etc.)/H2 blockers (cimetidine, etc.), antacids (TUMS, etc.).
- Lifestyle modification: decrease irritating foods in diet (coffee, alcohol, carbonated beverages, fatty foods, citrus, tomatoes/tomato products, chocolate, etc.); stay upright an hour after meals, and raise head of bed when sleeping.
- Teach risk of prolonged exposure (especially nocturnal): mucosal damage, including ulceration, erosion, and Barrett esophagus (intestinal metaplasia; higher risk of cancer of esophagus) - may require surgery.

> **Review Video: What is GERD?**
> *Visit mometrix.com/academy and enter Code:* **806648**

Peptic Ulcer Disease

Peptic ulcer disease refers to gastric or duodenal ulcers (erosions of mucosa), which may be associated with NSAID use, aspirin use, Helicobacter pylori infection, or chronic alcohol use. Peptic ulcers may be acute or chronic. Gastric ulcers tend to be superficial and associated with normal to decreased gastric secretions while duodenal ulcers are more likely to be penetrating and associated with increased gastric secretions. Both types may result in perforation, hemorrhage, or obstruction. Signs and symptoms are as follows:
- Gastric ulcers—pain or burning in high epigastrium 1 to 2 hours after meals
- Duodenal ulcers—pain, cramping, burning in mid-epigastrium, upper abdomen, and back; 2-4 hours after meals as well as between meals and middle of the night.

Diagnosis is based on endoscopy and laboratory tests, including CBC and stools for blood. Barium studies if patient is unable to tolerate endoscopy. *H. pylori* test. Treatment consists of antibiotics if positive for *H. pylori*, H2-receptor blockers, cytoprotective drugs, and antacids. Some patients may benefit from TCAs to reduce stress.

> **Review Video: Peptic Ulcers and GERD**
> *Visit mometrix.com/academy and enter Code:* **775788**

Dumping Syndrome

Dumping syndrome is a rapid cycle of gastric emptying. When large volumes of food are placed into the small intestine too quickly, fluid is pulled from within the cells to accommodate digestion and hypovolemia occurs, causing the symptoms associated with dumping syndrome. Dumping syndrome is generally the result of gastric surgery, such as gastric bypass or surgery to remove stomach cancer. Signs and symptoms take place 30-60 minutes after a meal: flushing, diaphoresis, weakness, dizziness, nausea, abdominal cramping, diarrhea, and potential vasomotor failure (tachycardia, orthostatic or positional hypotension). Diagnosis is based on clinical symptoms, gastric emptying test, and serum glucose. Treatment is as follows:

- Avoid carbohydrates and simple sugars; eat high-fiber foods and protein.
- Do not drink water with meals; eat multiple small meals throughout the day.
- Lie down after eating to ease dizziness and slow gastric emptying.

Gastroparesis

Gastroparesis is a condition in which the muscles that cause peristalsis slow down or stop working all together, resulting in delayed gastric emptying and abdominal discomfort. Patients who have been diagnosed with diabetes have an increased risk of gastroparesis related to diabetic neuropathy of the vagal nerve that innervates the stomach area. Other high-risk patients include those with nervous system diseases, recent surgery, hypothyroidism, and certain cancer and other medications. Signs and symptoms include bloating, feelings of fullness and/or nausea, vomiting, gastric pain, and heartburn. Diagnosis is based on Esophagogastroduodenoscopy (EGD)/upper GI exam/barium swallow, gastric-emptying exam, breath test. Treatment includes:

- Medications: metoclopramide for motility, ondansetron/ antiemetics for nausea/vomiting.
- Surgery: place feeding tube/gastric vent; generally temporary.
- Lifestyle modification: low carbohydrate diet, small, frequent meals are helpful; some patients find that low-fat/fiber, soft or liquid diets assist with food toleration, low-level exercise after eating.

IBS

Inflammatory bowel disease (IBS) is a chronic disorder of the large or small intestine with an unknown cause. Chronic ulcerative colitis (CUC) and Crohn disease are designated as inflammatory bowel diseases. Crohn disease occurs most often between 15 and 35 years, and CUC most often between the ages of 15 and 30 years or between 50 and 70 years. Patients will often experience remissions/exacerbations. Signs and symptoms of include constipation/diarrhea, weight loss, abdominal pain, fever, joint pain, GI bleeding, fistula formations, fat-malabsorption, enlarged colon (megacolon), and obstruction of the bowel. Symptoms of ulcerative colitis are massive bleeding with stools; mostly in lower colon. Symptoms of Crohn disease are skipping, "cobble-stone" lesions from mouth to anus. Diagnosis is based on barium enema, ESR, CRP, and colonoscopy. Treatment includes:

- Corticosteroids, mesalamine, azathioprine, folate supplements.
- Surgery: drain abscesses, fistula repair, and ostomy (severe).
- Monitor the patient for ankylosing spondylitis, liver disease, carcinoma, infection, hemorrhage, perforated colon.
- Teaching: NSAIDs, stress, and certain dietary choices will aggravate IBS; report floating stools/limit fat, sitz baths and careful peri-care for comfort. Increase insoluble fiber in diet with diarrhea stools.

Celiac Disease

Celiac disease occurs when the microvilli of the small intestine are damaged by gliadin, a protein of gluten found in wheat, rye, oats, and barley. Celiac disease is generally diagnosed in children, but can occur in adulthood. Atrophy and inflammatory processes in the small intestine are the result of celiac disease, leading to the impaired absorption of vitamins and minerals, causing malnutrition, anemia, and clotting disorders. Signs and symptoms are loose stools, often diarrhea, fatty stools (steatorrhea), flatus, bloating, weakness, vitamin and nutrient deficiencies, anemia, failure to thrive, changes in personality such as lethargy or irritability. Diagnosis is based on clinical symptoms, blood tests for antigens, and scope of intestines. Treatment is as follows:

- No cure: must remove products that contain gluten from the diet including wheat, rye, oat, and barley. Patients cannot digest even a small amount of these foods, nor can they eat food prepared in the same kitchen as foods with gluten.
- Monitor weight on a routine basis, document diet consumption, monitor growth patterns.

Diverticulitis

Diverticulitis is inflammation of diverticula, which are bulging herniations in the intestinal wall, most commonly found in the sigmoid colon, although they can occur anywhere within the GI tract from pharynx to anus. Diverticulitis may result in bowel obstruction, infection, perforation, or hemorrhage as undigested food and bacteria accumulate in diverticula, forming a fecalith (hard mass) that can impair circulation. Signs and symptoms include acute pain (usually LLQ), abdominal distention, nausea, flatus, fever, constipation, irregular bowel habits, and leukocytosis. Diagnosis is based on upper GI, barium enema, and CBC. Colonoscopy is often avoided during acute diverticulitis because of the bowel prep needed. Mild to moderate cases are treated with bedrest, stool softeners, and liquid or bland diet followed by high residue diet and bulk-forming laxatives once symptoms subside. With severe diverticulitis, surgical resection of the bowel may be required, sometimes with a temporary colostomy.

Hiatal hernia

Hiatal hernia is an area of the stomach that has protruded upward into the chest via the esophageal hiatus. Hiatal hernias may occur due to weakness in the diaphragm, eructation (belching) on a routine basis, pregnancy, reduced motility of the esophagus (scleroderma), and gastric emptying delays. Disease processes such as Zollinger-Ellison syndrome, and Heller's myotomy are also known causes of hiatal hernia. Signs and symptoms include heartburn, belching, chest/abdominal pain, and GI bleeding. Diagnosis is based on blood work, x-ray/barium swallow, and endoscopy (EGD). Treatment includes the following:

- Medications: H2 antagonists, such as ranitidine, famotidine, or cimetidine. Proton pump inhibitors (PPIs), such as esomeprazole or lansoprazole, are also used.
- Lifestyle modification: refraining from lying flat in bed/going to bed directly after consuming a meal, avoiding restrictive clothing, weight loss, avoiding caffeine and spicy foods.
- Clinical note: the H2 receptor agonists all have the suffix -ine, and PPIs all end in -azole.

Intussusception

Intussusception is the inversion of one portion of the intestine into another resulting in intestinal obstruction, often called *telescoping* of the bowel. It is often found in infants and toddlers, but can occur in older adults as well. The cause is often unknown in children, but can be caused by tumors or adhesions in adults. Signs and symptoms include severe intermittent or constant abdominal pain with drawing up of the lower extremities, abdominal distention, emesis with bile, diarrhea, or jelly-type stools (presence of blood and/or mucus), lethargy, palpable abdominal mass, fever and pallor. Diagnosis is based on EGD, MRI with contrast, x-ray (shows "bullseye"), and air/barium enema. Treatment includes the following:

- NG tube and IV fluids for rehydration and gastric decompression.
- A barium/ air enema will diagnose as well as fix the problem for most children. Adults generally require surgical repair.
- Monitor for signs of peritonitis and dehydration.

Appendicitis

Appendicitis is an acute inflammation of the vermiform appendix. More commonly found in males than females, appendicitis can be deadly if not diagnosed and treated promptly. Signs and symptoms include McBurney sign (rebound tenderness), Psoas sign (pain with right thigh extension), abdominal pain that starts near the umbilicus and moves to the right lower quadrant, guarding of the area, anorexia, nausea and vomiting, constipation or mild diarrhea, elevated temperature, and rapid heart rate. Diagnosis is based on blood work, rectal exam, CT scan, and ultrasound. Treatment includes the following:

- Fluids for correction of any fluid or electrolyte imbalances
- Broad-spectrum antibiotics
- Surgical procedures to remove the appendix or drain any abscess that may have occurred.
- Teaching: full activity should return within 6 weeks post-op, resume diet as bowel function resumes (typically 24 to 48 hours post-op).
- Monitor for nausea, vomiting, pain, fever and chills; could be peritonitis

Acute pancreatitis

Acute pancreatitis is an inflammatory process of the pancreas caused by autodigestion of trypsin. Causes of pancreatitis include gallstones (microlithiasis), alcohol, and trauma, treatment for AIDS, antibiotics, diuretics, and treatments for inflammatory bowel disorders. Signs and symptoms include:

- Epigastric pain that radiates to the back, nausea and vomiting, fever, shock, hypotension, jaundice
- Grey Turner Sign is flank discoloration (bluish)
- Cullen sign - umbilical discoloration.

Diagnosis is based on blood work (amylase/lipase), C-reactive protein, CT/MRI, endoscopic ultrasound, and stool studies. Be aware that insulin and steroids have the potential to alter lab results in these patients.

Treatment: **PANCREAS**
P: pain control: generally narcotics, pain is severe.
A: arrest and shock will require intravenous (IV) fluids.
N: nasogastric tube; clear liquids or NPO; possibly TPN.
C: calcium monitoring.
R: renal function evaluation (BUN/creatinine).

$\underline{E}$: ensure adequate pulmonary function (risk of acidosis).
$\underline{A}$: antimicrobial therapy.
$\underline{S}$: surgical or other procedures to assist with treatment.

Treatment also includes the following:
- Teaching: bedrest, position with pillows for comfort.
- Smoking and drinking cessation.
- Increase fluids, low-fat/high-protein diet; may take supplemental enzymes to aid digestion.

Hepatitis cirrhosis/portal hypertension

Portal hypertension or hepatitis cirrhosis is a disruption in the normal configuration of hepatic lobules or obstruction of the portal vein leading to increased portal venous pressure and subsequemt cell death. Portal hypertension occurs predominantly in older adult males. Risk factors for portal hypertension include cirrhosis, alcohol abuse, viral hepatitis B, hepatitis C, and hemochromatosis. Signs and symptoms include hepatosplenomegaly, caput medusa (varicose veins that radiate from the umbilicus), umbilical bruit, hemorrhoids, spider angiomata, gynecomastia, testicular atrophy, and digital clubbing. <u>Diagnosis is based on</u> blood work (AST/ALT), EGD, and x-ray. Treatment is as follows:
- Treat underlying cause: antivirals, drinking cessation, etc.
- Nutritional and metabolic support.
- Monitor for changes in level of consciousness (LOC) as this is the first sign of hepatic encephalopathy (buildup of ammonia causing damage to brain).

RENAL / GENITOURINARY DISORDERS

UTIs

Urinary tract infections (UTIs) are bacterial infections that cause inflammation in one or more areas of the urinary tract. *Escherichia coli* is the most common causative organism with urinary tract infections, often transmitted from the GI tract. "Urinary tract infection" is an umbrella term used to discuss cystitis (bladder infection), pyelonephritis (kidney infection), and urethritis. Types of UTIs are:
- Recurrent—repeated episodes.
- Persistent—bacteriuria despite antibiotics.
- Febrile—typically indicates pyelonephritis.
- Urosepsis—bacterial illness; urinary pathogens in blood.

Signs and symptoms include:
- Fever, polyuria, and urgency with urination
- Dysuria, urinary retention, and enuresis (episodes of incontinence).
- Pain in low back, flank area, and lower abdominal area.
- Elderly: only sign may be change in mental status
- Pediatric - asymptomatic until septic.

Diagnosis is based on urinalysis, blood tests, and physical exam. Treatment includes the following:
- Antibiotic therapy; may culture urine to use most effective medicine.

- Fluids: hydrate and flush out bacteria; cranberry juice may help.
- Teach: stay hydrated, avoid hot tubs and baths, Woman – urinate after sex, wipe front-to-back.

Acute Glomerulonephritis

Acute glomerulonephritis is characterized by inflammation of the glomeruli in the kidneys, most often caused by an antigen-antibody response to group A beta-hemolytic *Streptococcus*. Signs and symptoms include cola-colored urine (hematuria), foamy urine, oliguria/anuria, edema, hypertension, protein, nitrates, cells, epithelial cells, and casts in urine. Diagnosis is based on blood work (creatinine, BUN, ESR), urinalysis, x-ray/CT, and renal biopsy. Ask if patient has had a sore throat in the past 2 weeks, or history of heart valve replacement. Treatment includes the following:
- Controlling blood pressure is priority: ACE inhibitors/angiotensin II blockers, diuretics.
- Usually will resolve on own without specific treatment.
- Teach: report and treat sore throat promptly to prevent systemic spread of strep infections.

BPH

Benign prostatic hypertrophy (BPH) is the enlargement of the prostate to the point that it begins to compress the urethra and cause some degree of urinary obstruction. BPH commences with changes in the periurethral glandular tissue. The enlarged tissue may obstruct the urethra or create a pouch within the bladder that results in urinary retention. BPH may result from hormonal changes, inflammation, or metabolic changes. Early indications include reduced urinary stream in both volume and force, difficulty initiating urination, urinary retention, and urgency. Later symptoms include frequent urination, nocturia, incontinence, and urinary obstruction. Diagnosis is based on urinalysis and culture positive for hematuria and/or pyuria, elevated BUN and creatinine (with impaired renal function), IVP, and cystourethroscopy. The prostate may be palpable on rectal exam. Conservative treatment includes sitz baths and prostatic massage. Definitive treatment is surgical prostatectomy. Transurethral resection of the prostate (TURP) is usually done if the prostate weighs less than 2 ounces. If patients are poor candidates for surgery, an indwelling Foley catheter (usually suprapubic) may be inserted.

Gout

Gout is a disorder of altered purine metabolism characterized by elevated uric acid levels that cause inflammation. This results in a sudden onset of crystal deposits and sodium urate in the connective tissues and articular cartilage, usually affecting the joint of the big toe. Risk factors for gout include severe arthritis, family history, male sex, obesity, recent surgery/trauma, and alcohol abuse. Signs and symptoms include acute onset of swelling, severe pain (even weight of sheet will seem unbearable), erythema in 1 or more joints, and soft tissue redness and warmth. Diagnosis is based on blood work (uric acid, creatinine), joint fluid biopsy, physical exam, and ultrasound. Treatment includes:
- Medications: colchicine, NSAIDs, steroids for acute flareup.
- Fluids and rest; keep pressure off of affected area.

- Prevention: allopurinol or febuxostat lowers uric acid in blood, and probenecid increases excretion of uric acid from the body.
- Teaching: Take medications as directed to prevent flareups: gout is a recurring disorder; diet restrictions: low fat, low or no alcohol, decrease red meat/seafood, no sardines, anchovies, liver, or sweetbreads.

ENDOCRINE DISORDERS

Cushing syndrome

Cushing syndrome is an abnormal production of ACTH, which causes elevated cortisol levels. It can be caused by prolonged use of corticosteroids or tumor on adrenal cortex. Signs and symptoms include muscle weakness, central obesity distribution, hyperglycemia, hyperkalemia, bone and joint pain, hypertension, mood changes, headaches, frequent urination, moon-shaped facies, weight gain, acne, hirsutism, and immunosuppression. Diagnosis is based on dexamethasone suppression test, cortisol level check, and MRI-check for tumors. Treatment includes the following:
- Surgery to remove tumor.
- Monitor corticosteroid levels; avoid prolonged use of steroids.
- Symptom management; wash hands frequently to avoid infection, low-carb diet to manage blood sugar/weight gain, etc.
- Monitor the patient for kidney stones, HTN, diabetes, fractures.

Thyroid Disorders

The thyroid is an important organ of the body that secretes hormones that stimulate growth and metabolism. The thyroid hormones are thyroxine (T4) and triiodothyronine (T3). Thyroid hormones contain iodine compounds that are crucial to normal development. Patients can either have hyperactive thyroid (Graves' disease) or hypothyroidism. Patients must be placed on life-long treatment to avoid ill effects. Signs and symptoms include:
- Hyperthyroidism: hyperactive, hot, weight loss, fatigue
- Hypothyroidism: depression, cold, weight gain, fatigue, constipation, goiter, myxedema, coma
- Congenital Hypothyroidism: jaundice (> 24 h), difficulty feeding, inactivity, constipation, umbilical hernia, wide-set eyes, broad, flat noses, tongue protrusion, and coarse, brittle hair, delayed dentition, anemia, developmental delays.

Diagnosis is based on blood work (TSH/T4 levels) and physical exam. Treatment includes:
- Medication: will get regular blood work to assess efficacy
  - Hyperthyroidism: propylthiouracil (PTU), methimazole
  - Hypothyroidism: levothyroxine
- Surgical removal of thyroid (hyper); must then replace hormones with levothyroxine.

> **Review Video: Graves' Disease**
> Visit **mometrix.com/academy** and enter **Code: 543173**

Classifications of Diabetes

The National Institutes of Health (NIH) recognizes the following as classifications of diabetes:

- Diabetes Mellitus (DM): an umbrella term that includes type I diabetes (insulin-dependent diabetes) and type II (non-insulin dependent diabetes). Type II divides into nonobese non-insulin dependent or obese non-insulin dependent diabetes.
- Impaired Glucose Tolerance (IGT): Impaired glucose tolerance occurs when there is an increased amount of circulating blood glucose after consuming an increased amount of carbohydrates.
- Gestational Diabetes Mellitus (GD): Gestational diabetes is a form of diabetes mellitus that occurs during pregnancy, characterized by the pregnant woman's intolerance of carbohydrates.

Type I Diabetes Mellitus

Type I Diabetes Mellitus or insulin dependent diabetes mellitus (IDDM) was formerly called childhood-onset diabetes because it typically surfaces early in life, before the age of 30. In these individuals, the beta cells of the islets of Langerhans have suffered damage, usually due to autoimmunity, childhood disease, exposure to toxins, or congenital damage. This results in the inability of the pancrease to produce insulin, and results in inability of the body to use glucose. Signs and symptoms include polyuria, polydipsia, polyphagia, weight loss, weakness, fatigue, increased rates of infection, and increased healing time. Diagnosis is based on fasting blood glucose and glucose tolerance test. Treatment includes the following:

- Insulin replacement: use of short-acting and long-acting insulins to replace function of pancreas.
- Teaching: S&S of hypo/hyperglycemia, lifestyle modification (diabetic diet, sick-day rules, when and how to check blood sugar, etc)
- Ketoacidosis from fat metabolism when insulin is under-administered; teach S&S as this complication can be life-threatening if not treated properly.

People with type I diabetes produce no insulin of their own, so all insulin must be supplemented. Therefore, stabilization of blood glucose levels is the priority of care with the type I diabetic patient. Insulin therapy is the only course of medications that can be used with the type I diabetic patient; insulin injections serve to replace what is not being produced by the body. Clinical diabetic patients are educated on food exchanges to maintain the proper carbohydrate, protein, and fat ratios that promote normal blood glucose levels. Carbohydrates represent 50% of the diabetic diet, protein represents 20%, and fat represents the remaining 30% of the diabetic diet

*See Diabetic Teaching card for more information.

*Clinical note: Oral antidiabetic agents stimulate insulin production in the pancreas; in a patient with the type I diabetes, the pancreas is not capable of producing insulin. Therefore, oral antidiabetic agents are not effective for these individuals.

> **Review Video: Diabetes and Insulin**
> *Visit **mometrix.com/academy** and enter **Code: 666371***

> **Review Video: Diabetes Type I**

Type II Diabetes Mellitus

Type II Diabetes or non-insulin dependent diabetes mellitus (NIDDM) is characterized by insulin resistance in the peripheral tissues along with a decreased production of insulin by the beta cells of the pancreas. Obesity and increased age increase the risk of developing NIDDM. Diabetes mellitus type II causes the same systemic effects as type I diabetes, neuropathy, retinopathy, and increased rates of atherosclerosis leading to cardiovascular disease. Signs and symptoms include polyuria, polydipsia, polyphagia, weight loss, weakness, fatigue, increased rates of infection, and increased healing time. Diagnosis is based on fasting blood sugar and glucose tolerance test.

Treatment includes:
- Oral hypoglycemics: desired glucose range is 70-110 mg/dL.
- Home glucose monitoring should be done before every meal and at bedtime and PRN.
- Diet education: Diet that consists of 10%-20% protein; < 10% fats, rest carbohydrates. Limit sugar.
- Lifestyle modification: regular exercise, weight loss can actually reverse disease process.

*See Diabetic Teaching card for more information.

DKA

Diabetic ketoacidosis (DKA) is a condition that occurs in diabetic patients in which the body metabolizes fat instead of carbohydrates in the absence of insulin. As the body is utilizing fatty acids for energy, it begins producing an abnormal amount of ketones (ketosis). With ketoacidosis, the glucose level is elevated and the patient is suffering life-threatening hyperglycemia. Extreme physiological stress, illness, and poor blood glucose management are all potential causes of DKA. Signs and symptoms include Kussmaul respirations, fruity odor to the breath, dehydration, anorexia or polyphagia, polydipsia, hypotension, hypothermia, confusion, tachycardia, tachypnea, hypothermia, weakness, malaise, lethargy, nausea, and/or vomiting. Diagnosis is based on blood work (BMP/CBC), urinalysis (ketones), ABGs, chest x-ray, clinical picture, and ECG.

Treatment includes the following:
- Fluid resuscitation -1000 mL the first hour is standard.
- Intravenous insulin.
- Monitor blood glucose and serum potassium closely, as both will drop dramatically with movement of glucose into cells.
- Prevention: follow diabetes management plan, check sugar more often in times of illness and stress, report ketones in urine right away.

SKIN/ORTHOPEDIC DISORDERS

Acne

Acne is a disease that involves the sebaceous glands and hair follicles of the skin. Excessive sebum production causes the overgrowth of *Propionibacterium acnes* bacteria, causing the formation of pustules on the skin of the face, back, and chest. Acne is more common in boys than girls, and peak age is 16-17 years old for young women and 17-18 years for young men. A combined approach to treatment is most effective:

- General - well-balanced diet, rest, decrease stress
- Cleansing - acne not caused by dirt or oil on the skin; however, gentle cleansing daily/ twice a day prevents spread of bacteria
- Medication
    - Topical: Retinoid and Benzoyl Peroxide: use 30 minutes after cleansing. Can cause photosensitivity; wear sunscreen outdoors.
    - Oral: Accutane (isotretinoin [13-cis-retinoic acid]); only in severe cases; contraindicated in pregnancy (causes severe birth defects).
- Female only: Oral birth control is sometimes prescribed as it is found helpful in treating hormonal forms of acne.

Contusions and hematomas

A contusion (bruise) is characterized by bleeding into the skin when it is crushed or squeezed and not broken. The progressive color changes of bruises or contusions reflect the time or duration of the bruise; initial contusions begin as red or deep purple, fade to blue or black, then yellow and/or green before fading back to normal skin tone. The discoloration relates to the extent of vascular injury. A hematoma is characterized by blood that has collected or pooled into the soft tissue of an enclosed space. Hematomas may cause problems when they exert pressure on adjacent structures.

- Subdural Hematoma: A subdural hematoma is a pooling or collection of blood between the dura mater and the surface of the brain. Subdural hematomas result from shearing of small veins that connect the subdural space.
- Epidermal Hematoma: An epidermal hematoma is a collection or pooling of blood between the inner surface of the skull and the dura. Epidermal hematomas are the result of arterial tears.

Document placement, size, and coloration—do not diagnose.
Note: multiple bruises in different stages of healing/on the torso could indicate abuse.

Phases of Wound Healing

The four phases of wound healing are as follows:
- Phase 1: Inflammation
  Edema of the tissues as injured cells leak contents; angiogenesis - growth of new blood vessels in damaged tissue; phagocytosis – white blood cells destroy invading pathogens.
- Phase 2: Granulation/Proliferation
  Lasts 5-30 days; formation of granulation tissue, which helps rebuild lost cells in the base of the wound.
- Phase 3: Contraction
  Fibroblasts bring wound edges closer together to aid in closing the wound.
- Phase 4: Maturation

Scab forms over wound, which eventually falls off and leaves scar tissue in some cases

The following are factors that influence healing:
- Moist, crust-free environment enhances wound healing
- Poor nutrition, stress, infection, diseases, and decreased circulation can all increase healing time

Atopic Dermatitis

Atopic dermatitis is an inflammatory reaction that is traditionally caused by allergens that come in contact with the skin. The nurse will need to assess for secondary infection related to scratching. Signs and symptoms include erythema, papules, vesicles, and macules that may or may not produce exudates. The individual will experience itching (pruritus) and erythema to the affected areas. Lesions may appear on the face, trunk, limbs, or head. At the time of initial exam, the nurse should assess for exposure to chemicals, history of skin infections, climate exposure that includes excessive heat and cold, as well as determination of any changes taking place within the household. Instruct patient to limit or avoid stress as possible, minimize over exposure to heat or cold, take tepid baths, use oatmeal in the bath to help with pruritus, decrease or limit the use of perfumed soaps, decrease sun exposure, and avoid lotions that contain alcohol. Stress the use of emollient creams for symptom relief.

Fractures

A fracture is a full or partial break in a bone, and classified as open (compound) vs. closed (simple) fractures. Open (compound) fractures are fractures in which the bone protrudes out of the skin. Types include:
1. Pathological fractures: Breaks at the site of an abnormality/existing weakness (tumors, osteoporosis, infection, and metabolic disorders)
2. Stress fractures: result from repeated stress placed on the bone
3. Oblique fractures: occur at a curve or slope.
4. Greenstick: incomplete fracture caused by excessive bend (pediatric)
5. Transverse: broken bone at right angle to axis
6. Comminuted: fractured into several pieces
7. Buckled/impacted : ends of bone are driven into each other (pediatric arm fractures)

Signs and symptoms include swelling/bruising, obvious deformity, pain with movement, and loss of ROM. Diagnosis is based on x-ray and physical exam. Treatment includes the following:
- Casting/immobilize bone
- Surgery: may require pins/rods to help reconstruct bone
- Teaching: do not stick anything into cast, cover during shower, may have to do PT/OT to regain strength in limb.

Note: *If casted, watch for compartment syndrome (#1 symptom = pain unrelieved by narcotics).*

Neurovascular compromise, Compartment Syndrome, and Arterial Occlusion

Compartment syndrome is excessively high pressure in a compartment of the body (most often the legs, arm, or abdomen) that usually results from blood or edema filling the area. This commonly happens after cast application or circumferential burns. Acute arterial occlusions happen when blood flow to an extremity (most often the leg) is suddenly stopped. It occurs most often in patients with a history of peripheral artery disease or in the postoperative period after many cardiovascular surgeries.

These are both considered medical emergencies; if left untreated, they will result in tissue necrosis and death. The following are the key signs and symptoms of neurovascular compromise (6 P's):
- **P**araesthesia
- **P**ain out of proportion to injury; not relieved by narcotics (key)
- **P**aralysis
- **P**allor
- **P**ulselessness
- **P**oikilothermia (temperature difference between injured and uninjured limbs)

Scleroderma

Scleroderma is a diffuse connective tissue disorder in which insoluble collagen forms and accumulates in the tissues, leading to fibrotic changes, loss of elasticity, and impaired movement. The disorder starts in the hands and spreads systemically to the heart, lungs, and digestive system. Scleroderma usually starts with Raynaud phenomenon in the hands. Symptoms are referred to as CREST syndrome:
- **(C)**alcium deposits in the skin,
- **(R)**aynaud's phenomenon (spasm of blood vessel due to cold or emotional stress)
- **(E)**sophageal hardening (acid reflux),
- **(S)**clerodactyly (thickening of skin on fingers/hands),
- **(T)**elangiectasia (capillary dilation that forms vascular lesions).

Diagnosis is based on symptoms, skin biopsy, pulmonary studies, esophageal studies, echocardiography, and ANA (positive ANA indicates connective tissue disorder). There is no specific treatment for the disease but counseling and support should be offered to patients. Calcium channel blockers and antihypertensive may help alleviate Raynaud phenomenon, and NSAIDs may help relieve inflammation and pain. Careful skin care is indicated to prevent skin breakdown. Patient teaching must include protective measures to avoid cold, which will worsen Raynaud.

MULTISYSTEM DISORDERS

Hypothermia

Hypothermia is a condition that results when more heat is lost than the body can generate, and is defined as an internal body temperature less than 95°F. Symptoms usually develop slowly; someone with hypothermia typically experiences gradual loss of mental acuity and physical ability; may be unaware of the need for emergency medical treatment. Older adults, infants, young children, and people who are underweight are at particular risk. Signs and symptoms include shivering, bradycardia, slurred speech, abnormally slow breathing, cold/pale skin, loss of coordination, fatigue, lethargy, and coma. Diagnosis is based on vital signs and clinical picture.

Treatment includes the following:
- Emergency management: infusion of warmed IV fluids, Bair-Hugger (circulates continuously warmed air around patient), warm blankets, give warm fluids; use rectal temperature
- Prevention: community education about shelters during cold weather, avoid prolonged exposure to cold, layered clothing.

Note: Severe hypothermia can hide pulse and blood pressure: *"They're not dead until they're warm and dead."*

Heat cramps, Heat Exhaustion, and Heat Stroke

Heat-related illnesses are a consequence of prolonged or intense exposure to elevated temperatures. There are three main types of heat-related illnesses:
1. Heat cramps are painful muscle spasms in the abdomen, arms, or legs following strenuous activity. The skin is usually moist and cool and the pulse is normal or slightly raised.
2. Heat exhaustion means the body is becoming overheated. The person may be thirsty, giddy, weak, uncoordinated, nauseous, and *sweating profusely*; the pulse is slowed and weak. The skin feels cold and clammy to the touch.
3. Heat stroke can be ***life threatening***! Immediate medical attention is essential. Body temperature above 104°F: may exhibit confusion/combativeness, lethargy/faintness, staggering, strong rapid or extremly slowed pulse, *dry flushed skin,* lack of sweating, possible delirium or coma.

If a person is exhibiting signs of heat-related illness, immediately move him/her into a cool and shaded area. Remove any excess clothing, and offer fluids, preferably something with electrolytes. If symptoms do not immediatley begin to improve, get immediate medical help. Stay hydrated when outdoors during hot weather, wear light-colored clothes, and avoid hours of peak heat (2-5 PM).

Dehydration

Dehydration occurs when fluid intake is not adequate for fluid loss. Dehydration may occur as the result of polyuria, diarrhea, high fever, vomiting, heat exposure, and excessive exercise, especially if coupled with high heat. Symptoms vary according to the severity of the dehydration, and young children and older adults may not exhibit typical thirst, making dehydration more difficult to diagnose. Signs and symptoms are as follows:
- Mild/Moderate—dry mouth, thirst, decreased urination, headache, constipation, dizziness, and lethargy.
- Severe—severe thirst, dry mucous membranes, irritability, confusion, decreased or absent urination, concentrated urine, sunken fontanels (infants), tearless crying, fever, poor skin turgor, tachycardia, tachypnea.

Diagnosis is based on CBC, electrolytes, urinalysis, and urine osmolality. Treatment depends on severity:

- Mild/Moderate—increased fluid intake, including oral rehydration solutions for children and water or other liquids for adults (although carbonated beverages should be avoided). Salt pills are not recommended as they may result in hypernatremia.
- Severe—may require electrolyte replacement and intravenous fluids.

> ➤ **Review Video: <u>Dehydration</u>**
> Visit ***mometrix.com/academy*** *and enter* ***Code: 972181***

SIRS

Systemic inflammatory response syndrome (SIRS) is a generalized systemic inflammation in organs remote from the initial insult. The many causes of SIRS include infection (especially of heart and lungs), pancreatitis, trauma with massive tissue injury/ischemia, shock, massive transfusion, and autoimmune diseases. Signs and symptoms are as follows:

- Temperature < 36°C or > 38°C
- Heart rate > 90 beats/min
- Respiratory rate > 20 breaths/min or $PaCO_2$ < 32 mm Hg;
- WBC > 12,000/mm³ or < 4000/mm³, or ≥ 10% immature (bands) forms

Diagnosis is based on blood work (CBC/BMP) and physical exam/clinical picture. Treat the underlying cause (IV antibiotics, fluids, parenteral nutrition, supportive treatment). Be alert for progression to multiple organ dysfunction syndrome (MODS)!

MODS

Multiple Organ Dysfunction Syndrome (MODS) results from a systemic inflammatory response syndrome (SIRS), and is progressive physiologic failure of two or more separate organ systems. MODS is the major cause of death of patients in the critical care units. Outcome is directly related to the number of organs that fail. The failure of three or more organs is associated with a 90% to 95% mortality rate. Organ failure may occur in a progressive pattern or organs may fail simultaneously. The lungs are generally the first organ and the most common organ to be affected. Signs and symptoms include lethargy, altered level of consciousness, an elevated body temperature, lower than normal lymphocyte counts, lack of energy, ascites, and possibly an alteration in bowel pattern or decreased peristalsis. Cardiovascular instability and central nervous system dysfunction may be present. Diagnosis is based on blood work, clinical symptoms/examination, and various testing. Treatment includes the following:

- Intensive antibiotic therapy to treat underlying infection.
- Hypermetabolic states: requires increased calories; often placed on TPN or another alternate form of nutrition.
- Monitor in intensive care unit; anticipate need for intubation if respiratory system collapses.

Shock

Shock is characterized by inadequate cellular metabolism due to poor tissue perfusion. There are four main types of shock:
1. Hypovolemic shock: Decreased blood volume.
    - Causes: massive hemorrhage, dehydration.
2. Cardiogenic shock: Heart cannot circulate blood adequately.
    - Causes: heart attack, heart failure, and arrhythmias.
3. Neurogenic shock: Mass vasodilation, resulting in decreased venous return/cardiac output.
    - Causes include general anesthesia (deep sedation), injuries to the central nervous system, barbiturate intoxication, spinal anesthesia, and fainting.
4. Septic shock: Toxic substances/infectious organisms cause inflammation and dilation blood vessels.
    - Causes of septic shock include gram-positive organisms such as pneumococci, staphylococci, and streptococci.

Signs and symptoms include tachycardia, hypotension, tachypnea, weak pulse, cool, clammy skin, altered LOC, and decreased urine output. Diagnosis is based on vital signs, clinical picture, and blood work. Treatment is as follows:
- Treat underlying cause; generally fluid resuscitation and vasopressors required.
- Can progress to uncompensated shock: fatal at this point.

Burn Injuries

Burns occur when intense or prolonged heat causes injury to the cells. The types of burn injury are as follows:
- Thermal burns - (common) flames, hot objects/water
    o Complications: massive skin loss – skin grafts.
- Chemical burns - acids or alkaline; internal or external.
    o Complications: tissue destruction may continue for 72 h
- Electrical burns - electrical current (coagulation necrosis)
    o Complications: fractures, cardiac arrest/arrhythmias (24-48 h), metabolic acidosis, renal failure (myoglobinuria)
- Smoke & inhalation injury -hot air or noxious chemicals
    o Complications: airway obstruction – look for singed nasal hairs/eyebrows, hoarse voice/cough, darkened membranes; obstruction can occur 24 h post burn.
    o Severity = Time of Exposure + Intensity of Heat

The degree and extent of burns are ways to determine the severity of the injury. These are determined by the depth of the injury, as well as the total body surface area (TBSA) affected:
- Depth of injury
    o 1st degree—superficial: reddened skin, but intact
    o 2nd degree—partial thickness; loss of skin, into dermis (most painful)
    o 3rd degree—full thickness; all skin is lost, can see fat/muscle
    o 4th degree—full thickness + underlying tissue; can see to bone

- o Both 3rd and 4th degree are not painful as nerves are lost; however, will not heal without skin grafting.
- TBSA - Rule of Nines
  - o Adults:
    - Head and neck - 9%
    - Anterior torso - 18%
    - Posterior torso - 18%
    - Each leg - 18%
    - Each arm - 9%
    - Genitalia/perineum - 1%
  - o Children:
    - Head/Neck increased to 18%
    - Legs only 13.5% each.
    - Note: 10% of total surface area burned in school-aged child or younger may be fatal.

The following are the three phases of burn management:
1. The Emergent Phase (Resuscitative Phase)
   - o 24-48 h; begins with fluid loss/edema formation and continues until fluid motorization and diuresis begins.
   - o Complications: hypovolemic shock and obstructed airway (often delayed 24 h), pneumonia, arrhythmias, compartment syndrome (circumferential burns), acute tubular necrosis/ renal failure.
   - o Interventions: fluid resuscitation, vasopressors, artificial airway, escharotomy (restores circulation).
2. The Acute Phase:
   - o Weeks/months: diuresis to complete wound healing.
   - o Complications: infection/sepsis (usually gram-negative); gastroparesis/intestinal ileus, ulcers, stress-induced diabetes mellitus, contractures.
   - o Interventions: IV antibiotics – culture wounds/IV/Foley/etc. for bacteria/sensitivity, pain management, skin grafts, NG tube, PPIs for ulcer, wound care/debridement, passive/active ROM.
3. The Rehabilitative Phase:
   - o Weeks to months: from wound covered to optimal functioning.
   - o Complications: joint/skin contractures and scarring, permanent disability, regression/depression.
   - o Interventions: physical/occupational therapy, splints/pressure garments. May need psychiatric counseling for body image alterations and self-esteem issues, encourage support groups and counseling, protect grafts from sunlight for 1 year.

> **Review Video: Rule of Nines**
*Visit **mometrix.com/academy** and enter **Code: 988486***

Treatment for burns is as follows:

BURNS:
Breathing/**B**ody Image: watch for distress, counseling
Urine output: 30 mL/hr minimum (0.5mL/kg/hr most accurate)

<u>R</u>esuscitation (Fluid): first 24-48 h
<u>N</u>utrition: increase protein and calories
<u>S</u>hock/<u>S</u>ilvadene: Keep CVP ~12 cm water pressure, monitor U/O
- Tetanus if not up to date on vaccinations.

Burn patients are at exceptional risk of infection because the barrier of protective skin is breached, and eschar provides a medium for microorganisms, along with the immunosuppression which occurs. There are a number of reservoirs of infection for organisms to grow, and many of these reservoirs can serve as sources for transmission on the hands of health care workers:
- Burn wounds are colonized within the first few hours by gram-positive organisms from sweat glands and hair follicles and within days by gram-negative organisms, so collectively the burn wounds of all patients on the unit may harbor organisms that can spread from one patient to another.
- Gastrointestinal tract flora can contaminate burn wounds directly if wounds are in proximity to fecal material or indirectly through cross-contamination.
- Normal flora, especially gram-positive cocci, on the skin are the cause of early burn infections, and an increasingly important reservoir, with nasal colonization often implicated in burn infections.
- Environment can harbor organisms on many inanimate surfaces. Hydrotherapy equipment has been a frequent cause of wound infection because contaminated equipment spreads the infection to subsequent patients being treated.

Infection Control: Transplant Patients

Infections pose a serious threat to transplant patients, especially during the first year. While opportunistic infections have decreased, nosocomial infections have increased, most related to bacterial infections. Transplant patients consistently show higher rates of infection than other patients. There are numerous potential sources:
- Donor-infected organs can transmit HBV, HBC, herpesvirus, HIV, and human T-cell leukemia virus type I. Additionally, donors who are immunocompromised prior to harvesting of the organs may have nosocomial bacterial or fungal infections that can be transmitted. Organs can also become infected during harvesting.
- Health care workers may transmit pathogens through droplets, airborne particles, or contact, frequently transmitting pathogens on their hands or clothing.
- Blood and blood products can transmit CMV, but transmission is rare. HCV transmission has been reduced to < 1%.
- Environmental reservoir sources can include the water system, demolition activities, equipment, and surfaces. Some pathogens, such as MRSA and VRE, may be endemic to the hospital environment.

Several viral infections are more likely to occur in transplant patients due to their immunocompromised state:
1. Cytomegalovirus (CMV): the most common pathogen related to transplant infections, affecting 40%-90% of recipients
2. Herpes simplex virus: reactivated/new - may disseminate to liver
3. Human herpesvirus-6 – mostly reactivation, newer strain
4. Varicella-zoster virus: new – may disseminate to viscera
5. Hepatitis B and C viruses: causes liver failure; also affects kidney transplant patients

6. BK virus (BKV): causes renal dysfunction; transmission unknown
7. Adenoviruses (AdV): bone marrow transplant; can become systemic

Prevention consists of the following:
- Serologic matching can prevent primary transmission but the limited supply of organs may make this impractical.
- Early diagnosis with serum assay for targeted treatment.
- Antiviral prophylaxis in high-risk patients can be effective.
- Immunization has proven to be safe and highly effective, reducing the incidence of infection and the severity.
- Immunoglobulin is given to susceptible transplant patients exposed to certain viruses.
- Reduction in immunosuppressive medications if possible.
- High-dose acyclovir for some viruses may reduce severity of infection.
- Targeting patients at the highest risk of disease through surveillance and using proper transmission-based precautions are the most practical methods of infection control.

The following are common bacterial infections after transplant surgery:
- Staphylococcus aureus is the most common cause of bacterial infection in liver, heart, kidney, and pancreas transplant patients. Intravascular cannulas cause about 54% of MRSA infections, but nosocomial transmission occurs.
- Vancomycin-resistant enterococci (VRE) causes 10%-15% of liver failures, according to recent studies. Nosocomial transmission occurs frequently, especially with prolonged hospitalization and ICU stay. VRE colonization puts patients at continued risk of infection and poses a reservoir for nosocomial infections.
- Nocardia is found in the soil and decaying vegetation, and transmission is through inhalation. Lung, heart, and intestinal transplants have the highest rates of infection. Mortality rates are high for those who are infected. Risk factors include high-dose cortisone, high levels of immunosuppressants, and CMV infection within 6 months.

Infection control strategies include:
- Handwashing and basic clean technique are still the best methods of infection control in these patients.
- Environmental monitoring
- Antibiotic prophylaxis is effective.

Aspergillus infections primarily involve pneumonia and sinusitis, but 25%-35% disseminate systemically, and *Aspergillus* pneumonia infections have mortality rates up to 85%. *Aspergillus* is a serious fungal infection in immunocompromised transplant patients, especially lung transplant patients with 8% infection rates within 9 months of surgery. Liver transplant patients have infection rates of 1%-4% but disease occurs earlier, within 2-4 weeks. Heart transplant infection rates are 1%-6% with disease within 1-2 months. Aspergillus affects renal transplants the least with < 1% infection rates. Prophylaxis with antifungals has not proven to be effective. Infection control strategies include:
- Monitoring environment and improving air filtration with HEPA filtration or use of laminar air flow rooms for patients at high risk.
- Construction precautions to prevent dust and debris from circulating in patient care areas.

- Standard precautions
- High-resolution CT scans should be used for early diagnosis rather than chest x-rays so treatment with voriconazole (drug of choice) can begin.

Infection Control: Spinal Cord Injuries/Patients with Impaired Mobilization

Infection control strategies for neurology/spinal cord injuries target the most common types of infection:

- Urinary tract infection: Patients should be monitored for fever and/or changes in spasms or voiding habits that may indicate infection. When possible, intermittent catheterization (sterile rather than clean while in the hospital) should be used rather than continuous. Antibiotic prophylaxis has not proven to be effective but bacterial interference, colonizing of the urinary tract with nonpathogenic E. coli 83972, has shown promising results.
- Decubital ulcers: Procedures for regular monitoring of skin condition, turning patients, and avoiding friction to prevent pressure from developing are critical. Both staff and patients must be educated about prevention, skin care, and cleanliness. Nutrition and hydration must be adequate to maintain integrity of the skin.
- Respiratory infections: Proper use of ventilation equipment must be monitored. Assisted coughing, such as through respiratory therapy and postural drainage, can reduce infections. Prophylactic antibiotics are not recommended, but patients should receive immunizations for pneumonia.

ELECTROLYTE IMBALANCES

Magnesium Imbalances

Magnesium is a crucial extracellular ion that is vital to muscle and bone health. When imbalance occurs, it is crucial to identify and correct it quickly to prevent adverse effects:

- Hypomagnesia
  - Causes:
    - Prolonged suction, vomiting, diarrhea, malnutrition
    - Diuretic therapy, diabetic acidosis, alcoholism,
    - High serum levels of calcium, aldosterone, ADH, T4/TSH
  - Symptoms:
    - N/V
    - Irritability
    - Muscle cramps
    - Hallucinations
    - Seizures
- Hypermagnesemia
  - Causes:
    - Magnesium overdose
    - Renal failure
    - Overdose of certain magnesium-containing medications (antacids, laxatives, etc)
  - Symptoms:
    - Diarrhea
    - Lethargy

- Diminished reflexes
- Muscle atony
- Bradycardia
- Hypotension
- Coma.

Treatment for magnesium imbalance includes the following:
- Correct imbalance: magnesium replacement OR furosemide, IV calcium gluconate, or dialysis.
- Treat underlying cause (vomiting, alcoholism, etc)

Potassium Imbalances

Potassium is a critical intracellular ion important for muscle function, cellular health, and especially cardiac conduction. Potassium imbalances are:
- Hypokalemia:
  - Causes:
    - Excessive diarrhea, malnutrition, diuretic use
    - Alcoholism, hyperaldosteronism.
  - Symptoms:
    - Weakness
    - CNS depression
    - Disorientation
    - Muscle weakness
    - Cardiac arrhythmias.
- Hyperkalemia:
  - Causes:
    - Traumatic injury
    - Burns
    - Acidosis
    - Renal failure
    - Addison's disease
    - ESRD
    - Potassium-sparing diuretics
    - Excessive intake of salt-substitutes or foods high in potassium
  - Symptoms
    - Muscle cramps
    - Arrhythmias
    - Neuropathies
    - Respiratory distress

Treatment of potassium imbalances includes the following:
- Correct imbalance: potassium PO/IV OR sodium polystyrene, IV insulin with dextrose, dialysis.
- Correct underlying cause: kidney failure, medications, etc.

Sodium Imbalances

Sodium (Na) is a critical extracellular ion important for nerve and brain function, as well as the regulation of the fluid balance in the body. The following are sodium imbalances:

- Hyponatremia:
  - Causes:
    - Diarrhea
    - Excessive water intake/infusion of hypotonic fluids
    - Burn patients (eschar, hydrotherapy, silver nitrate)
    - SIADH
    - Pneumonia
    - Heart failure – edema/fluid overload.
  - Symptoms:
    - Weakness
    - Dizziness
    - Confusion
    - Headache
    - Muscle cramps
    - Tachycardia.
- Hypernatremia:
  - Causes:
    - Dehydration
    - Excessive intake
    - Diarrhea/vomiting
    - Rigorous exercise or fever (profuse sweating)
    - Diabetes Insipidus
    - Hypertonic infusions
    - Diuretics - excessive fluid loss
  - Symptoms:
    - Ascitics
    - Edema
    - Dry mouth
    - Decreased urine output
    - Irritability/confusion
    - Hypertension
    - Low-grade fever.

Treatment of sodium imbalances includes the following:
- Correct Imbalance: infusion of hypertonic/hypotonic solution, sodium supplements/diuretics, diet/lifestyle modification.
- Correct underlying cause

For additional review help, please check out our NCLEX video tutorials, which can be found on the Mometrix Academy:
http://www.mometrix.com/academy/nclex-exam/

NCLEX Test Question Strategies

Sometimes when you are testing, you may know an answer immediately on reading the choices. Other times, you may need to choose an answer without being certain. In those situations, here are some tips to help you eliminate the answer choices most likely to be incorrect. Use these strategies to dissect complex nursing questions and improve your NCLEX test taking skills.

Do NOT select an answer choice that:
- Asks "**Why**?"
- Requires you to **speculate** or read extra information into the question that isn't there.
- Is based on a scenario you may have seen at **work** or in **clinicals**; instead focus only on the information you are given.
- **Degrades** the patient, a nurse, or a colleague.
- Involves bringing up potentially **controversial** material.
- Goes against a **general rule**.
- Involves **leaving** the patient, unless absolutely necessary.
- Tries to **persuade** the patient to make a choice or agree with something; instead look for answers that are associated with **caring** about the client's feelings.
- Tells the patient not to **worry**; this minimizes the patient's concerns and feelings.
- Tries to avoid **responsibility** or passes it to someone else.
- Is **unreasonable** or under normal circumstances could/should not be done.
- Involves "**doing nothing**" or "waiting" for an unspecified period of time unless you are absolutely certain it is the best option.
- Makes **absolute** statements involving words like always, never, or must.
- Only cites a **hospital rule** for its rationale. If the hospital has a rule about something, there will be an **underlying reason**, usually patient **safety** or hospital **liability**, which you should be aware of.
- You have never heard of or are **unfamiliar** with.

Additionally, if 2 answers are exact **opposites** of each other, one of them is likely correct. If 2 or more answers are **similar**, likely none of them is correct.

If you are asked to pick which nursing action to take next, remember that every answer choice listed could be a correct action to take, but the question is asking for the **highest priority action**.

Practice Tests

Practice Test #1

1. A client is to receive 1,000 mL of potassium chloride in 5% dextrose injection (D5W) intravenously over 3 hours and 20 minutes using a drop factor of 15 drops/mL. What is the required flow rate (drops) per minute? Record your answer using a whole number.

2. A client develops mastitis in the postpartum period. Which of the following instructions does the nurse anticipate when notifying the physician? *Select all that apply.*
   a. Antibiotics for 7 to 10 days.
   b. Opioid analgesia.
   c. Alternating hot and cold compresses to relieve the pain.
   d. Discontinuation of breastfeeding.
   e. Continuation of breastfeeding.

3. The nurse is teaching a new parent about the use of car seats for infants. Which of the following information should the nurse include? *Select all that apply.*
   a. The shoulder straps should be fed through slots at or below the infant's shoulders.
   b. Infants should always be in rear-facing car seats.
   c. The mother should place padding on the car seat underneath the infant.
   d. The harness clip should be positioned at the infant's abdomen.
   e. The car seat should be positioned so that the infant's head does not fall forward.

4. A client is to wear a Holter monitor for continuous cardiac monitoring for 48 hours. The nurse should advise the client to avoid which of the following activities during the monitoring period? *Select all that apply.*
   a. Watching television.
   b. Using a remote control.
   c. Using an iPad or other wireless device.
   d. Showering and bathing.
   e. Drinking caffeinated beverages.
   f. Exercising.

5. A client requires insertion of a nasogastric tube. When preparing the client for the procedure, the nurse should place the client in which of the following positions?
   a. High Fowler's position with the head tilted forward.
   b. High Fowler's position with the head tilted backward.
   c. Semi-Fowler's position with the head in a neutral position.
   d. Semi-Fowler's position with the head tilted backward.

6. A client returns to his room after a liver biopsy. The nurse should place the client in which of the following positions?
   a. Left side-lying with a folded towel under the biopsy site.
   b. Right side-lying with a folded towel under the biopsy site.
   c. Supine with a pressure dressing over the biopsy site.
   d. Prone with a small pillow under the biopsy site.

7. Following insertion of a nasogastric (NG) tube, the nurse aspirates the gastric contents to check the pH to determine if the NG tube is correctly placed. Which of the following pH values is consistent with gastric secretions?
    a. 8.
    b. 6.
    c. 5.
    d. 4.

8. A client with a tracheostomy is exhibiting difficulty breathing, and respirations are increasingly noisy. Secretions are very thick. Which of the following initial interventions is most indicated?
    a. Increase humidification, and suction the tracheostomy tube.
    b. Notify the physician.
    c. Sit the client upright, and encourage the client to breathe deeply and cough.
    d. Gently irrigate and suction the tracheostomy tube.

9. A client has a chest tube in place with a three-chamber chest drainage system. The nurse notes continuous bubbling in the water seal chamber. This indicates which of the following?
    a. Pneumothorax.
    b. Suction is adequate.
    c. System air leak.
    d. The tube is positioned incorrectly.

10. An elderly client with moderate Alzheimer's disease lives with her daughter and appears dirty and disheveled and has lost five pounds over the previous month. Which of the following does the nurse suspect?
    a. Physical abuse.
    b. Caregiver neglect.
    c. Self-neglect.
    d. Psychological abuse.

11. The nurse is reviewing medications with a client who is to be scheduled for outpatient rotator cuff repair. Which of the following medications does the nurse anticipate the client will be advised to avoid on the morning of the surgery?
    a. Metoprolol.
    b. Synthroid.
    c. Aspirin.
    d. Prozac.

12. A patient with hypothyroidism states that she takes Synthroid® 0.112 mg daily, but the pharmacy has issued the drug labeled in micrograms. How many micrograms of Synthroid® is equivalent to 0.112 mg? *Record your answer using a whole number.*

13. The nurse is caring for an unvaccinated child who developed complications related to German measles (rubella). Which of the following infection control protocols is appropriate?
    a. Standard only.
    b. Standard and contact.
    c. Standard and droplet.
    d. Standard and airborne.

14. A client is scheduled for knee replacement surgery, and the nurse is reviewing preoperative laboratory results. The nurse should notify the physician about which of the following abnormal laboratory results?

a. Platelets 119,000.
b. Glucose 83.
c. Hemoglobin 13.7.
d. Sodium 141.

15. The nurse is caring for a client with diabetes mellitus, type 1. Which of the following signs and symptoms are indicative of diabetic ketoacidosis? *Select all that apply.*

a. Increased appetite.
b. Polyuria.
c. Hyperventilation.
d. Polydipsia.
e. Hypertension.
f. Abdominal pain.

16. A 15-year-old client was involved in an auto accident and requires emergency surgery to control bleeding, but both parents are out of town and unable to sign the consent form. Which of the following is the most appropriate action?

a. The client signs the consent form.
b. The parents give telephone consent with two witnesses listening.
c. The parents give email consent.
d. The physician operates without consent because of the emergency situation.

17. The nurse is administering an intermittent tube feeding to a client through a nasogastric tube. Which of the following positions is optimal for tube feedings?

a. The head of the bed is elevated to 45°.
b. The head of the bed is elevated to 90°.
c. The head of the bed is elevated to 30°.
d. The head of the bed is flat with the client supine.

18. When considering fluid balance, if 60% of an adult's body is composed of water, approximately what percentage of this is found in intracellular fluid?

a. 33%.
b. 25%.
c. 67%.
d. 8%.

19. Whole blood is primarily indicated for which of the following purposes?

a. To treat extreme loss of blood volume.
b. To increase clotting factors.
c. To increase oxygen-carrying capacity for those with anemia.
d. To control acute bleeding.

20. A client who has undergone a thyroidectomy complains of numbness, tingling, and stiffness in her hands, feet, and face as well as muscle tremors, spasmodic muscle contractions, and anxiety during the postoperative period. Which laboratory tests does the nurse anticipate that the physician will request?

    a. Hemoglobin.
    b. Sodium.
    c. Thyroid-stimulating hormone (TSH).
    d. Calcium.

21. A client receiving chemotherapy and opioids for renal cancer has had no bowel movement for five days and no results from two doses of laxatives in the past 48 hours. The client is passing no flatus and complains of increasing abdominal pain and nausea. Which of the following does the nurse anticipate?

    a. Abdominal examination and abdominal x-ray.
    b. Oil retention enema and manual removal of impaction.
    c. Oil retention enema followed by a soapsuds enema.
    d. Another dose of laxative followed by a soapsuds enema if there are no results in 24 hours.

22. An 82-year-old female complains of generalized fatigue and has new onset of urinary incontinence as well as anorexia, hyperventilation, and low-grade fever. The nurse anticipates that the client will be evaluated for which of the following?

    a. Diabetes mellitus.
    b. Bladder cancer.
    c. Urinary tract infection.
    d. Influenza.

23. The nurse administers a dose of acetaminophen to the wrong client. Which of the following actions is the most appropriate after notifying the physician?

    a. Notify her supervisor and complete an incident report.
    b. Ask the physician for an order of acetaminophen to cover the inadvertent administration.
    c. Take no further action because acetaminophen is relatively benign.
    d. Document in the client's record that an error in drug administration occurred.

24. The nurse is aware that African-Americans are at higher risk than Caucasians for which of the following conditions? *Select all that apply.*

    a. Hypertension.
    b. Diabetes mellitus.
    c. Asthma.
    d. Skin cancer.
    e. Osteoporosis.

25. The nurse is instructing a client who has had an eye removed in the proper procedure for inserting a prosthetic eye. Place the following steps of prosthetic-eye insertion (in Roman numerals) in the correct sequence from the first to the last.
    I.   Raise the upper eyelid.
    II.   Pull the lower eyelid down.
    III.   Slide the prosthesis under and behind the upper eyelid.
    IV.   Identify landmarks on the prosthetic eye for the inner and outer areas and the superior and inferior aspects.
    V.   Check the positioning.
    VI.   Cleanse the prosthetic eye according to the manufacturer's directions.
    a. (First)
    b. (Second)
    c. (Third)
    d. (Fourth)
    e. (Fifth)
    f. (Sixth)

26. A client's wife states that her elderly husband has begun to slightly slur his words and drop word endings, he has become increasing withdrawn socially, and he is irritable, accusing her of talking behind his back and whispering at him. The nurse suspects that the client should be initially evaluated for which of the following?
    a. Depression.
    b. Alzheimer's disease.
    c. Hearing loss.
    d. Stroke.

27. Which of the following tasks are appropriate for the nurse to delegate to unlicensed assistive personnel? *Select all that apply.*
    a. Checking temperature and vital signs for a client acutely ill with sepsis.
    b. Checking routine temperature and vital signs for clients at the beginning of the shift.
    c. Emptying catheter bags and measuring the urinary output from Foley catheters.
    d. Monitoring the transfusion of red blood cells.
    e. Assisting an ambulatory client to walk to the bathroom.

28. Two days' postpartum, a nursing mother develops swollen, taut, and very painful breasts. Which of the following is the most likely cause?
    a. Engorgement.
    b. Insufficient milk.
    c. Blocked milk ducts.
    d. Mastitis.

29. Following surgical repair of a fractured femur, a client's hemoglobin falls to 7.4 and the physician orders one unit of packed red blood cells (250 mL) to be administered over two hours with a drop factor of 10 drops/mL. What flow rate (drops per minute) is needed? *Record by rounding to the nearest whole number.*

30. Place the following metric capacity measures (in Roman numerals) in the correct position in the table below.
   I.   Deciliter
   II.   Milliliter
   III.   Dekaliter
   IV.   Kiloliter.
   V.   Hectoliter.

(A)		Centiliter	(B)		Liter	(C)		(D)		(E)

   a.
   b.
   c.
   d.
   e.

31. A client with recurrent episodes of gout has been advised to eat a low-purine diet. Which of the following foods should the nurse advise him to limit or avoid? *Select all that apply.*
   a. Liver.
   b. Sardines.
   c. Wine.
   d. Low-fat yogurt.
   e. Beef broth.
   f. Potatoes.

32. A client develops anaphylaxis syndrome and loses consciousness after eating fruit salad containing kiwi fruit, to which the client is severely allergic. The nurse is aware that the initial concern is which of the following?
   a. Establish a patent airway.
   b. Administer intravenous fluids.
   c. Administer oxygen at 100% high flow.
   d. Administer epinephrine.

33. An infant is to receive 250 mL of 5% dextrose/0.45 normal saline (D5/0.45 NS) in five hours. The pediatric IV system has a drop factor of 60 drops per mL. What is the flow rate (in drops per minute)? *Record your answer using a whole number.*

34. A client states that he takes five grains of aspirin daily, but the hospital issues aspirin in milligrams. How many milligrams are approximately equivalent to five grains of aspirin?
   a. 81 mg.
   b. 120 mg.
   c. 325 mg.
   d. 500 mg.

35. A child who weighs 40 kg is prescribed clarithromycin 15 mg/kg per day for 10 days in two divided doses for acute strep throat. If the medication is provided in suspension with 250 mg/5 mL, how many total milliliters of medication are required to complete the treatment? *Record your answer using a whole number.*

36. The physician had prescribed 10 mL of oral suspension twice daily for a child, but the mother is confused about the metric system and wants to know how many teaspoons of medication to give the child. How many teaspoons are equivalent to 10 mL of oral suspension? *Record your answer using a whole number.*

37. An electrical fire occurs in a client's room shortly after the client returns from the recovery room after repair of a hip fracture with insertion of a prosthesis. What is the best method of removing the client from the room?
    a. Place the client in a wheelchair.
    b. Transfer the client to a gurney.
    c. Move the bed with the client on it.
    d. Do a two-person carry.

38. A client is confused after receiving morphine for analgesia and repeatedly tries to pull out the intravenous (IV) line in her left arm. Which of the following actions is the best initial solution?
    a. Attempt to camouflage the IV and tie a piece of tubing to the bedrail so the client can pull on that safely.
    b. Apply wrist restraints.
    c. Apply wrist and vest restraints.
    d. Discontinue the IV line and reinsert at a more distant site.

39. A nurse must teach a client how to do wound care and dressing changes prior to discharge. Which of the following are barriers to learning? *Select all that apply.*
    a. The client is 55 years old.
    b. The client is fearful.
    c. The client is illiterate.
    d. The client is weak and frail.
    e. The client has many questions about the procedures.
    f. The client is hard of hearing.

40. A client is prescribed 0.25 mg terbutaline subcutaneously, but the medication is provided as 1 mg/mL. How much medication is needed to provide the correct dosage? *Record your answer using a decimal to two places.*

41. A client has returned from surgery after removal of a tumor of the colon and creation of a temporary colostomy. She refuses to take a deep breath and cough then refuses to turn. Which of the following should the nurse assess first in trying to understand her lack of cooperation?
    a. Delirium status.
    b. Vital signs.
    c. Oxygen saturation.
    d. Level of pain.

42. When assisting a client with range-of-motion exercises, which movements should be carried out on the client's elbows? *Select all that apply.*
   a. Supination.
   b. Flexion.
   c. Circumduction
   d. Pronation
   e. Extension.
   f. Hyperextension.

43. A client has had a long leg cast removed after eight weeks. Which of the following actions is the correct method of cleansing the skin after cast removal?
   a. Advise the client to use a bath brush on his skin during a shower.
   b. Advise the client to soak in a tub of water and wash his leg with a washcloth.
   c. Apply a cold-water enzyme wash to the client's skin, leave it in place for 20 minutes, and then rinse it off with warm water.
   d. Wash the skin with hot, soapy water and then rinse with warm water.

44. The nurse has documented a treatment on the wrong client's record. Which of the following methods of indicating the error is correct?
   a. The nurse draws a straight line through the incorrect entry and writes "error" above it and initials the correction.
   b. The nurse uses correction fluid to cover the incorrect entry.
   c. The nurse draws multiple lines through the incorrect entry so it is unreadable, writes "error" above it, and initials the correction.
   d. The nurse leaves the incorrect entry in place, writes "error" in the margin, and initials and dates the notation.

45. A client in Dunlop traction experiences numbness of the thumb and index finger and cannot move the thumb to touch the tips of the other fingers. The capillary refill time is four seconds. Which of the following actions is indicated?
   a. Remove and reapply the forearm elastic bandage more loosely.
   b. Decrease the weights on the traction.
   c. Release the countertraction.
   d. Increase the weights on the traction.

46. For which of the following reasons would the nurse use the Braden Scale to assess a client?
   a. To determine if the client is suffering from delirium.
   b. To determine if the client is at risk for developing pressure sores.
   c. To determine if the client is at risk for falls.
   d. To determine if the client is at risk for substance abuse.

47. Following a disaster with multiple victims and danger to those present, which group should have priority for protection from injury?
   a. The clients/victims.
   b. The firefighters and police officers.
   c. The bystanders and news reporters.
   d. The healthcare providers.

48. Which of the following statements by the client suggests that the client has not made informed consent for a craniotomy?
    a. "I know that surgery could cause a stroke, and I'm scared."
    b. "I told the doctor I didn't want to know anything about the surgery, and she agreed."
    c. "I have one more question before I sign the consent form."
    d. "This is a really complicated procedure. So many things could go wrong."

49. The computers for documenting client care and treatment are located at the nursing station. Which of the following is the most important consideration regarding the computers?
    a. Height of the computer stations.
    b. Ratio of computers to staff.
    c. Positioning of the computer screens away from the line of sight of unauthorized persons.
    d. Brand of computer and operating system.

50. The physician has ordered that a serum trough level be drawn for a medication. Which of the following is the correct time to draw blood for a trough level?
    a. At the midpoint in time between two scheduled doses of the drug.
    b. At the time the drug peaks.
    c. Immediately after a scheduled dose is administered.
    d. Immediately before a scheduled dose is due.

51. A client tells the nurse that she is on a high-protein diet and averages 75 g of protein daily, 120 g of carbohydrates, and 40 g of fat. If fat is equal to 9 calories per gram and protein and carbohydrates are equal to 4 calories per gram, how many total calories is the client averaging each day? *Record your answer using a whole number.*

52. An elderly preoperative client seems very anxious but denies concerns when the nurse asks; however, the client's son confides that the client is very superstitious and believes it is bad luck that he is in room 113. Which of the following actions is the best response?
    a. Reassure the client that the room number will not affect his surgery outcome.
    b. Contact the admissions department and request that the client be reassigned to a different room.
    c. Ask the physician for medication to relax the client.
    d. Ask the son to stay with the client to reassure him.

53. A transient homeless client with a history of mental illness and substance abuse is to be discharged. Which of the following support systems are most likely to provide social support for the client? *Select all that apply.*
    a. Self-help programs.
    b. Internet-based programs.
    c. Community agencies.
    d. Governmental agencies.
    e. Friends.
    f. Family.

54. A client is receiving oxygen therapy at 3 L/min per nasal cannula. Which of the following fraction of inspired oxygen (FiO_2) measurements does the nurse expect that the client is receiving?
    a. 24%.
    b. 60%.
    c. 32%.
    d. 100%.

55. A 43-year-old client has developed progressive frontotemporal dementia and is exhibiting inappropriate and compulsive behaviors, difficulty with language, and impaired judgment. Which statement by the client's wife suggests that she has not accepted a permanent role change in their relationship?
    a. "I need my husband to take care of financial matters."
    b. "It's so frustrating that my husband refuses to bathe."
    c. "My husband doesn't pay attention to anything I try to tell him."
    d. "I want my husband to do the things that he can still manage independently."

56. A client undergoing "cold-turkey" withdrawal from years of substance abuse is most at risk of serious life-threatening complications with which of the following substances?
    a. Heroin.
    b. Cocaine.
    c. Alcohol.
    d. Marijuana.

57. The nurse finds a client smoking marijuana in the hospital and tells her that no smoking or use of drugs is allowed in the facility. The client responds by shouting, "What business is it of yours? Leave me alone!" Which of the following initial responses is the best for the nurse to use to defuse the situation?
    a. "It's my business because I'm your nurse."
    b. "If you don't put that out immediately, I will call security."
    c. "You are violating the facility policies and the law!"
    d. "I'm sorry, but I have to ask you again to put out your marijuana cigarette."

58. A client who served three tours of duty in Afghanistan has been diagnosed with posttraumatic stress disorder (PTSD). Which of the following signs and symptoms does the nurse expect the client to exhibit? *Select all that apply.*
    a. Recurring flashbacks.
    b. Detachment from others.
    c. Anger.
    d. Hyperacute memory regarding the events associated with the trauma.
    e. Nightmares.
    f. Excessive sleeping.

59. A diabetic client self-administers insulin four times daily. Which of the following statements by the client indicates the need for further education?
    a. "I flush the used needles down the toilet."
    b. "I carry glucose tablets with me at all times."
    c. "I eat a little dessert occasionally."
    d. "I avoid wearing sandals."

60. A hospice client is to receive 4 mg of morphine sulfate (MS) subcutaneously from a vial that contains 10 mg/mL. How many milliliters of MS should the patient receive to equal a dose of 4 mg? *Record your answer using one decimal place.*

61. Which of the following findings are indicative of peripheral arterial insufficiency? *Select all that apply.*
    a. Throbbing, cramping pain that increases with exercise.
    b. Aching pain that increases with dependency.
    c. Capillary refill time of less than two seconds.
    d. Shiny skin with decreased hair.
    e. Brown pigment about the ankles and lower legs.
    f. Pale color on elevation and redness on dependency.

62. The nurse is assisting a client with a colostomy irrigation. The client is positioned on the toilet and has removed the colostomy pouch, and the irrigation bag is filled with 1000 mL of warm water. Place the following actions (in Roman numerals) in the correct order from first to last.
    I.   Allow 15 to 20 minutes for evacuation and then fold the sleeve, secure it, and leave it in place for 30 to 45 minutes before removing it.
    II.   Allow the solution to flow in for 5 to 10 minutes and then clamp the tubing and close the top of the irrigation sleeve.
    III.   Apply gloves, lubricate the cone tip, and insert it into the stoma, holding it securely.
    IV.   Apply the irrigation sleeve over the stoma.
    V.   Hang the irrigation solution with the bottom of the bag being 20 inches above the stoma.
       a. (First)
       b. (Second)
       c. (Third)
       d. (Fourth)
       e. (Fifth).

63. A client complains of sleeping poorly, arousing many times during the night, awakening with a headache, and feeling tired and sluggish in the morning and throughout the day. For which of the following tests does the nurse anticipate that the client will be scheduled?
    a. Electroencephalogram.
    b. Electrocardiogram.
    c. Nocturnal polysomnogram.
    d. Magnetic resonance imaging (MRI) of the brain.

64. A pregnant woman undergoes a 40-minute nonstress test for evaluation of the fetal heart rate (FHR) and accelerations. Which of the following test results is normal (reactive)?
    a. One acceleration of the FHR of 10 beats per minute (bpm) above the baseline for 10 seconds.
    b. Two accelerations of the FHR of 10 bpm above the baseline for 15 seconds.
    c. No accelerations of the FHR.
    d. Three accelerations of the FHR of 15 bpm above the baseline for 20 seconds.

65. The nurse is conducting an aphasia assessment of a client who has suffered a stroke. Which of the following observations should the nurse include in the assessment? *Select all that apply.*
    a. Spontaneous speech.
    b. Comprehension of the spoken and written word.
    c. Ability to name objects.
    d. Ability to describe objects.
    e. Ability to write.
    f. Ability to recall four named items after five minutes.

66. The nurse must obtain wound cultures for anaerobic and aerobic bacteria from the traumatic leg wound of a three-year-old child, but the wound is quite painful even with analgesia. Which is the best approach?
    a. Do the cultures in the child's room with the child in bed and the mother assisting.
    b. Do the cultures in the child's room with the child in bed with a nurse assisting and the mother comforting the child.
    c. Do the cultures in a separate treatment room with the mother holding the child and a nurse assisting.
    d. Do the cultures in a separate treatment room with a nurse assisting and the mother comforting the child.

67. A nurse is at a local swimming pool, and a man collapses with a cardiac arrest after exiting the pool. The man is still wet when the nurse begins cardiopulmonary resuscitation (CPR), and another person brings the automated external defibrillator (AED). Which of the following should the nurse do next?
    a. Apply the AED pads and deliver a shock.
    b. Wipe the chest dry with an available cloth or towel.
    c. Continue CPR because a client who is wet cannot receive a shock.
    d. Wipe the chest with an alcohol hand wipe to speed the evaporation of the water.

68. The client's intravenous (IV) line has a gauze pad wrapped around the IV catheter at the insertion site and a transparent dressing over the gauze dressing. How long after application should the nurse change the dressing?
    a. At the normal rotation time for the IV.
    b. When the transparent dressing loosens.
    c. In 48 hours.
    d. In 24 hours.

69. Which of the following groups of neonates should be screened for hearing loss?
    a. Premature neonates.
    b. Neonates with risk factors for hearing loss.
    c. Neonates with abnormal Apgar scores.
    d. All neonates.

70. A child weighing 20 kg is to receive 45 mg/kg of amoxicillin per day in a divided dose every 12 hours. The oral suspension contains 250 mg/5 mL. How many milliliters should the child receive in each dose? *Record your answer using a whole number.*

71. A client has a rate-responsive permanent pacemaker in his upper chest. The nurse understands rate-responsive to mean which of the following?
    a. A pacemaker function prevents excessive changes in the pacing rate.
    b. The pacing rate increases above the normal pacing rate with sudden bradycardia.
    c. The pacemaker switches from atrial tracking mode to nontracking mode with atrial fibrillation.
    d. The pacing rate increases when the sensors note increased activity.

72. The "5 A's" of smoking cessation intervention begin with which of the following?
    a. Advise all clients who smoke to stop smoking.
    b. Ask all clients about tobacco use at every visit.
    c. Assess clients' willingness to stop smoking.
    d. Assist the client to stop smoking.

73. The nurse is educating a client about lifestyle modifications to manage hypertension. Which of the following modifications should the nurse recommend? *Select all that apply.*
    a. Limit fluid intake to 2000 mL daily.
    b. Engage in regular aerobic exercise (30 minutes most days).
    c. Adopt the dietary approaches to stop hypertension (DASH) eating plan.
    d. Lose weight.
    e. Eliminate all alcoholic beverages.
    f. Stop smoking.

74. The nurse is caring for a Muslim client who is recovering from an automobile accident and is unable to cleanse herself after a bowel movement. Which of the following should the nurse do to show respect for the woman's cultural and religious beliefs?
    a. Use the left hand to cleanse the client's rectal area.
    b. Ask a female family member to assist the client.
    c. Wear gloves when cleansing the client's rectal area.
    d. Ask the client's husband to assist the client.

75. A client with multiple sclerosis tires easily, so the nurse is instructing the client in energy-conservation techniques. Which of the following techniques may help the client conserve energy? *Select all that apply.*
    a. Sit down to perform activities instead of standing.
    b. Keep frequently used items close at hand on the floor or on a high shelf.
    c. Rest 10 minutes out of every hour.
    d. Plan ahead to avoid extra movements.
    e. Watch for stress signals, such as dyspnea or fatigue.
    f. Pull objects instead of pushing them.

76. The mother of a 24-month-old child tells the nurse that she is concerned that her child's language abilities are delayed. Which of the following language milestones does the nurse expect the child to exhibit?
    a. Understands 300 words and uses two- and three-word sentences.
    b. Says and understands a few words, such as "Mama" and "Dada," and can imitate animal sounds, such as "moo" and "woof."
    c. Says and understands four to six words but understands more and can point to items he wants.
    d. Says and understands up to 20 words and can point to his body parts.

77. A client who experienced a cardiac arrest and resuscitation is exhibiting characteristics of mild anoxic brain injury. Which of the following characteristics does the nurse expect her to exhibit? *Select all that apply.*
    a. Decreased ability to concentrate.
    b. Seizures.
    c. Memory impairment.
    d. Semicomatose state.
    e. Decreased balance.
    f. Restlessness.

78. A client has developed osteomyelitis of the bones of the left foot following the infection of a diabetic ulcer. The nurse anticipates which of the following treatments to be the primary focus?
    a. Warm wet soaks.
    b. Analgesia.
    c. Surgical debridement.
    d. Intravenous (IV) antibiotic therapy.

79. During the second stage of labor, the baby's head becomes compressed because the mother has a narrow, bony pelvis. Which of the following is the most common result for the infant from this type of compression?
    a. Cerebral palsy.
    b. Intellectual disability.
    c. Cranial molding.
    d. Epilepsy.

80. A client with rheumatoid arthritis tells the nurse that she is having increasing difficulty cooking, cleaning, and attending to activities of daily living. Which of the following referrals is the most appropriate?
    a. Occupational therapist.
    b. Physical therapist.
    c. Home health agency.
    d. Assisted-living facility.

81. If the nurse is teaching a group of clients about risk factors for diabetes mellitus, type 2, the nurse should include which of the following? *Select all that apply.*
    a. Obesity
    b. Hypertension and/or heart disease
    c. 45 years or older
    d. Caucasian race
    e. Family history of diabetes mellitus, type 2

82. The nurse is assessing an older adult. The client does not appear to always understand the questions, sometimes answering incorrectly, and stares at the nurse's mouth rather than the nurse's eyes when the nurse is speaking. The client answers in an unusually loud voice. Which of the following impairments should the nurse suspect?
    a. Hearing impairment
    b. Cognitive impairment
    c. Vision impairment
    d. Anxiety

83. A client is to be discharged 48 hours after a normal vaginal delivery of an infant with no laceration or episiotomy. Which of the following danger signs should the client be advised to report to her physician? *Select all that apply.*
    a. Temperature higher than 38°C/100.4°F
    b. Difficulty urinating
    c. Swelling, redness, or pain in one or both legs
    d. Fatigue
    e. Foul-smelling vaginal discharge

84. When assessing a client's skin, the nurse notes a scattered red rash on the trunk. The individual lesions are about 0.5 cm in diameter and are flat, nonpalpable, and circumscribed. How would this type of lesion be classified?
    a. Papule
    b. Nodule
    c. Macule
    d. Patch

85. An older client says that she frequently experiences stress incontinence and may have to stop playing golf because swinging the golf club often results in small amounts of urinary incontinence. Which of the following suggestions may be **most** effective?
    a. Take a deep breath while swinging the golf club.
    b. Utilize the "knack" (precisely timed muscle contractions).
    c. Wear incontinence pads.
    d. Urinate immediately before playing golf.

86. A client has had a recent below-knee (BK) amputation of the right leg because of a traumatic injury. After removing the elastic wrap, which the client had applied, the nurse notes an unusual pattern of swelling. Which of the following is the **most** likely reason for this observation?
    a. Wound infection
    b. Impaired circulation to the stump
    c. Incorrect wrap technique
    d. Bleeding into the tissues

87. A client has recurrent episodes of constipation and fecal impaction. The nurse is assisting the client with a bowel-training regimen. Which of the following interventions should be included? *Select all that apply.*
    a. Scheduled toileting
    b. Stool softeners
    c. High-fiber diet
    d. Daily laxatives
    e. Periodic enemas
    f. Routine exercise

88. Which of the following descriptions is typical of a Parkinsonian gait?
    a. Uncoordinated and unsteady, wide-based, staggering, high stepping, flat footed step
    b. Short, slow, stiff steps with thighs crossing while moving forward
    c. Decreased speed and balance, slight flexion of hips and knees, stooped posture, and short or shuffling steps
    d. Slight flexion of hips and knees, short shuffling steps, trunk leaning forward, and no arm swing

89. A client has increasing pain in both hands. On examination, the nurse notes that the metacarpophalangeal and proximal interphalangeal joints are enlarged and swollen, swan-neck deformity is evident, and the fingers on both hands show ulnar deviation. These findings are consistent with which of the following disorders?
    a. Osteoarthritis
    b. Rheumatoid arthritis
    c. Gouty arthritis
    d. Psoriatic arthritis

90. A client with pelvic skin traction for low back pain is at risk of which of the following problems associated with decreased mobility? *Select all that apply.*
    a. Orthostatic hypotension
    b. Muscle weakness
    c. Venous stasis
    d. Dysuria
    e. Confusion

91. If a client weighs 132 lb and has a caloric requirement of 28 calories per kg of body weight per day, what is the number of calories that the client needs each day to maintain body weight? *Record your answer using a whole number.*
    _____calories

92. If a client has had repair of a right fractured hip and has an overhead trapeze on the bed to assist with movement, which of the following instructions should the client receive about use of the assistive device? *Select all that apply.*
    a. The client should always grasp the bar with both hands before moving.
    b. The client should grasp the bar with the left hand and place the right hand flat on the bed to assist movement.
    c. The client should flex the left hip and knee and place the foot flat on the bed before moving.
    d. The client should keep the left hip and knee extended when moving.

93. If a 6-year-old child has influenza with a fever and cough, which statements by the child's caregiver suggest a need for education? *Select all that apply.*
   a. "If his fever gets too high, I'll give him a bath in cold water."
   b. "I try to offer him plenty of liquids."
   c. "Sipping hot lemonade seems to help relieve his cough."
   d. "I've been giving him baby aspirin to lower his fever."
   e. "I alternate giving him acetaminophen and ibuprofen for this fever."

94. Nutrients per serving:

Nutrients	Lunch meat	Peanuts	Cheese	Apple
Fat	6 grams	14 grams	9 grams	0.3 grams
Carbs	1 gram	5 grams	1 gram	25 grams
Insol. Fiber	0	1 gram	0	5 grams
Protein	7 grams	7 grams	7 grams	0.5 grams

Which of the snacks—lunch meat, peanuts, cheese, or apple—has the lowest number of calories per serving?
   a. Lunch meat
   b. Peanuts
   c. Cheese
   d. Apple

95. The nurse must administer in one syringe a combined dose of two different insulins from two vials. The procedure includes:
   I.   Cleanse tops of vials.
   II.   Inject air into vial 1.
   III.   Withdraw medication from vial 1.
   IV.   Change needles.
   V.   Withdraw medication from vial 2.
   VI.   Inject air into vial 2.

Place the steps (Roman numerals) in the correct order in the chart below.

Step	Procedure
1	(A)
2	(B)
3	(C)
4	(D)
5	(E)
6	(F)

96. If teaching a client to use a metered-dose inhaler (MDI) without a spacer, how far away from the mouth should the nurse advise the client that the inhaler be positioned when administering a dose of inhaled medication?
   a. The inhaler should be enclosed within the client's lips.
   b. The inhaler should be immediately outside of the client's lips.
   c. The inhaler should be 1 to 2 inches away from the client's lips.
   d. The inhaler should be 3 to 4 inches away from the client's lips.

97. A client is receiving an opioid per patient-controlled analgesia (PCA) pump to control postoperative pain; however, when the nurse assesses the client, she finds the client is pale and hypotensive, and has a respiratory rate of 6 breaths per minute. The PCA pump record shows that the limit for maximum dosage was set far too high, resulting in an overdose. The client is very somnolent and barely responsive. What interventions does the nurse anticipate? *Select all that apply.*
    a. Immediately stop the infusion.
    b. Discontinue the PCA pump.
    c. Administer naloxone per standing orders.
    d. Administer supplementary oxygen.
    e. File an incident report.

98. A client is hospitalized in a long-term care facility because of Alzheimer disease. The client is incontinent of urine and feces. The nurse has delegated incontinent care to unlicensed assistive personnel (UAP). How frequently should the nurse advise that the UAP check the client for dryness?
    a. Every 2 hours
    b. Every hour
    c. When the client appears restless.
    d. Before meals and at bedtime

99. A client with epilepsy is taking phenytoin. What long-term effects should the nurse advise the client can occur with prolonged administration of phenytoin? *Select all that apply.*
    a. Gingival hypertrophy
    b. Hirsutism
    c. Hypertrophy of facial subcutaneous tissue
    d. Dementia
    e. Anemia

100. A 60-year-old client has undergone a nerve-sparing prostatectomy and has been advised by his physician that he may not recover normal sexual functioning. The client is very concerned about this and asks the nurse for more information. Which of the following information should the nurse include? *Select all that apply.*
    a. Retrograde ejaculation may occur.
    b. Recovery rates vary but can take up to a year or more.
    c. If sexual functioning is going to return, it will do so within a month.
    d. Attempts at sexual intercourse are usually avoided for 1 month after surgery.
    e. Anxiety can interfere with sexual functioning.
    f. Other forms of sexual intimacy are more important than sexual intercourse.

101. A client is receiving end-of-life care and tells the nurse that he has not always lived the way he should have or treated his children well. Which of the following responses is the **most** appropriate?
    a. "What kinds of things have you done?"
    b. "There are things that you regret."
    c. "I'm sure those things don't matter anymore."
    d. "It's not too late to ask for forgiveness."

102. A client who was prescribed increasing dosages of baclofen to relieve muscle spasms should have taken 80 mg daily in 4 divided doses but misunderstood and took 80 mg four times a day, resulting in an overdose and pronounced CNS depression. Which of the following treatments does the nurse anticipate?

    a. Administration of naloxone.

    b. Administration of atropine.

    c. Supportive care only.

    d. Administration of flumazenil.

103. A client has been diagnosed with Parkinson disease and has been prescribed levodopa. Which of the following are contraindications to levodopa? *Select all that apply.*

    a. Narrow-angle glaucoma

    b. Macular degeneration

    c. Pregnancy

    d. Melanoma

    e. Cataracts

104. A 78-year-old client with a history of diabetes mellitus type 2, GERD, and hypertension is hospitalized with pneumonia and rings the call bell at 11 PM, complaining of being unable to sleep and having "indigestion" and "heartburn." Which of the following initial interventions is **most** indicated?

    a. Administer antacid per prn order.

    b. Administer acetaminophen per prn order.

    c. Administer hypnotic per prn order.

    d. Assess cardiac and respiratory status.

105. A client is upset that the physician has refused to order a stronger pain medication for the client and berates the nurse, calling the nurse "worthless and stupid" when the nurse brings the prescribed medication. Which of the following ego defense mechanisms is the client exhibiting?

    a. Compensation

    b. Reaction formation

    c. Displacement

    d. Regression

106. When determining whether or not a client is a candidate for restraints, which of the following would be considered an appropriate reason for a restraint?

    a. Current dangerous behavior

    b. History of falls

    c. Recent violent attack on a staff member

    d. Refusal to cooperate with treatment

107. A 52-year-old client is undergoing menopause. Which of the following physical sign or symptom is often attributed to decreased estrogen production associated with menopause?

    a. Weight loss

    b. Excessive sleeping

    c. Increased fat deposits on hips and abdomen

    d. Increased metabolic rate

108. An older client has been sleeping poorly at night, and her daughter states that the client has always loved music and suggests that listening to music might relax the client. Which type of music is most likely to help the client relax?
   a. Classical music
   b. Jazz
   c. Single instrument music (guitar, piano)
   d. Client's favorite music

109. If a client's waist measurement is 38 inches and the hip measurement is 45 inches, what is the client's waist-to-hip ratio. *Record your answer rounded to two decimal places.*
   _____waist-to-hip ratio

110. If a client is to have a nasogastric (NG) tube inserted for intermittent feedings, which of the following is an appropriate task to delegate to unlicensed assistive personnel?
   a. Inserting the NG tube
   b. Verifying tube position
   c. Administer tube feedings
   d. Reposition a displaced NG tube

111. A client received a unit of packed red blood cells; 2 hours after the transfusion had been initiated, the client developed severe chills and a 2°C elevation of temperature. The client had no dyspnea, swelling, or urticaria. Which of the following is the **most** likely cause of the client's symptoms?
   a. Circulatory overload
   b. Acute hemolytic reaction
   c. Febrile nonhemolytic reaction
   d. Allergic reaction

112. A client with prostate cancer has been given the option of various treatments and asks the nurse for advice. Which of the following is the **most** appropriate response?
   a. "Let's discuss the different options and how you feel about them."
   b. "I can't help you to make a decision about your treatment."
   c. "You need to discuss this decision with your physician."
   d. "I would choose surgery if I were in your position."

113. If a client with psoriasis is to begin NB-UVB phototherapy, how long should the initial treatment be?
   a. 30 seconds to 1 minute
   b. 1 to 2 minutes
   c. 5 to 10 minutes
   d. 15 to 20 minutes

114. A neonate has severe congenital abnormalities that make death imminent, and the NICU team believes that further attempts at treatment or feeding are not warranted and that palliative care only should be provided. When speaking with the parents about this, which of the following is the **best** approach?

a. Tell the parents that the team suggests that all food and treatment will be withheld.
b. Tell the parents that the team suggests a change in care plan to focus on comfort measures.
c. Tell the parents that any further efforts at treatment are futile as the infant is dying.
d. Tell the parents that the best thing is to let nature take its course.

115. A client has an open draining wound infected with MRSA and is on contact precautions. If the nurse is entering the room to care for the client, when are gloving and gowning necessary?

a. When the nurse has direct contact with the wound or drainage.
b. When the nurse has direct contact with the client's body, wound, or drainage.
c. When the nurse enters the room for any type of patient or environmental contact.
d. When drainage is not contained by a dressing.

116. Clients taking anticholinergic drugs, such as benztropine mesylate (Cogentin), to relieve muscle tremors and muscle rigidity associated with Parkinson disease should be advised to avoid which of the following?

a. Overheating
b. Overeating
c. Excessive fluid intake
d. Skipping meals

117. Following procurement of organs from a standard criteria donor (donor younger than 50 years who suffered brain death), within what time period should the heart and lungs be transplanted?

a. 4-6 hours
b. 8-12 hours
c. 24 hours
d. 36 hours

118. A nurse who is a friend on a social media site with a coworker finds that the coworker has written on the media site confidential information about a well-known client's health history (information obtained from the client's her). What is the **most** appropriate response?

a. Tell the coworker that the information must be deleted from the site.
b. Advise the client that the security of the EHR has been breached.
c. Do nothing as this is not a serious problem.
d. Report the incident to an appropriate supervisor/administrator.

119. In order to ensure adequate protein intake during pregnancy, how many additional grams of protein should the woman ingest daily during the second half of the pregnancy? *Report your answer using a whole number.*

_____grams

120. Following application of a right BK prosthesis for an amputated limb, the client returns for evaluation, and the nurse notes that the client has an unstable gait and the right hip and knee are showing signs of slight flexion contractures. The client admits to infrequent use of the prosthesis. Which of the following interventions are **most** indicated? *Select all that apply*.

    a. Providing sympathetic encouragement
    b. Arranging for retraining
    c. Chastising the client for failure to use the prosthesis
    d. Suggesting the client meet with a counselor

Answers and Explanations

1. 75 drops per minute:
Calculation:
Volume (mL) × drop factor/total minutes = flow rate.
3 hours and 20 minutes = 200 minutes.
1,000 × 15/200 = 75 drops/min.

2. A, C, and E: Mastitis is a bacterial infection of the breast, most often caused by *Staphylococcus aureus* from the infant, so the mother can continue to breastfeed. The usual treatment includes antibiotics (such as penicillin G or erythromycin). Pain control is achieved with ibuprofen or acetaminophen and alternating hot and cold compresses. The mother should be encouraged to massage her breasts in a hot shower and to pump or express milk on the infected side to prevent an abscess from forming.

3. A, B, and E: Parents should be advised to follow the manufacturer's directions for securing a car seat. Infants should be placed in rear-facing car seats with no padding underneath the infant. The shoulder straps should be fed through slots at or below the infant's shoulders and the harness positioned with the clasp at midchest. The car seat should be positioned so that the infant's head does not fall forward. For neonates, bolsters (such as a rolled infant blanket or diaper) should be placed beside the infant's head to maintain it in a neutral position.

4. B, C, and D: Clients with a Holter monitor (usually in place for 24 to 48 hours) should avoid using wireless electronic devices, such as remote controls, iPads, and laptops, because these may interfere with the monitor. They may use desktop computers but should stay at least 10 feet away from routers. Although microwaves and other equipment may be used in the home, the client should avoid direct or close contact. The client may not shower or bathe until the monitor is removed. Clients may be asked to exercise and drink caffeinated beverages so the effects can be monitored.

5. A: For insertion of a nasogastric tube, the client should be placed in the high Fowler's position with the head tilted forward because this position helps to close the trachea and open the esophagus, facilitating correct insertion. The nurse should examine the nasal passages by occluding one naris and then the other while the client is breathing through the nose and should use the side with the best airflow. The length of the tube should be estimated, the end of the tube is lubricated, and then the tube is inserted slowly. The client may suck on ice cubes or swallow small sips of water during the procedure.

6. B: Because the liver is located on the right side, the client should be positioned in the right side-lying position with a folded towel or small pillow under the biopsy site to apply pressure for at least three hours after the procedure is completed. The client should avoid straining or coughing. If this procedure is done on an outpatient basis, upon discharge the client should be advised to avoid any heavy lifting, strenuous exercise, or straining for one week.

7. D: Gastric secretions are usually acidic, ranging from 1 to 4 pH, although medications may alter the acidity, so depending on the pH alone is not adequate. Additionally, tube feedings usually have a pH of about 6.6, so aspirating with continuous feedings to check the pH is not effective. Intestinal fluid is less acidic than gastric secretions, usually 6 or higher. A pH of greater than 7 often indicates that the end of the tube is located in the respiratory system rather than the gastrointestinal system. Note that some nasogastric tubes contain built-in pH sensors.

8. A: The client is exhibiting signs of obstruction. Because the secretions are very thick, the best action is to increase the humidification to help loosen the secretions and suction the tracheostomy tube. Suction should not be used during insertion of the suction catheter because this removes oxygen and may traumatize the tracheal tissue, but suction should be used for 5 to 10 seconds while the catheter is removed. Suctioning for longer periods should be avoided because it may result in hypoxia.

9. C: Continuous bubbling in the water seal chamber indicates a system air leak. Intermittent bubbling occurs with pneumothorax as the air flows from the chest cavity into the chamber. The water level in the water seal chamber should fluctuate. If the fluctuation stops, this is generally an indication of a problem, such as obstruction of the chest tube or inadequate suction. However, it may also indicate reexpansion of the lung. The collection chamber is monitored for drainage. The suction control chamber should exhibit gentle bubbling.

10. B: The client is exhibiting signs of caregiver neglect: her dirty, disheveled appearance and her loss of weight, which may indicate that she is not receiving sufficient food or sufficient assistance with eating. A client with moderate Alzheimer's disease is not usually able to manage self-care without assistance. For example, clients may forget where their clothing is or believe they have already bathed, changed clothes, and eaten when they haven't done so.

11. C: Medications with antithrombotic properties, such as aspirin or nonsteroidal anti-inflammatory drugs (NSAIDs), are usually avoided the morning of a surgery, although other routine medications may generally be taken with a sip of water a few hours before scheduled surgery. Some medications, such as warfarin, may be discontinued for a few days prior to surgery because of the increased risk of bleeding. All medications (prescription and over the counter [OTC]) should be reviewed with the client, and instructions about use of the medication in relation to the surgery should be provided.

12. 112 micrograms: One milligram contains 1,000 micrograms, and 1 gram contains one million micrograms. Although the symbol μg is used to represent micrograms, the Food and Drug Administration (FDA) and the Institute for Safe Medication Practices (ISMP) recommend against using this symbol because it may easily be confused with the abbreviation for milligrams (mg). The abbreviation mcg is sometimes used. Calculation: 0.112 mg × 1,000 = 112 micrograms.

13. C: Clients with rubella (German measles) must be maintained on droplet precautions. Standard precautions apply to all clients regardless of other precautions.

Contact	Use personal protective equipment (PPE), including gown and gloves, for all contact with the client or the client's immediate environment. Clients should be in private rooms or >3 feet from other clients.
Droplet	Use a mask while caring for the client. Clients should be in a private room or >3 feet away from other clients with a curtain separating them. The patient must be masked for transport.
Airborne	Place the client in an airborne infection isolation room, and use ≥N95 respirators (or masks) for client care.

14. A: All of the laboratory results are within the normal range except for the platelet count. The normal range for platelets is 150,000 to 450,000, so 119,000 is low, indicating thrombocytopenia, which may increase the risk of bleeding and bruising. A decrease in platelets may indicate aplastic anemia, alcohol toxicity, prolonged hypoxia, iron-deficiency anemia, megaloblastic anemia, or viral infection. Severe infection may also suppress platelets. The risk of bleeding with invasive procedures is usually minimal until the count drops below 50,000, and the risk is most severe with counts below 20,000.

15. B, C, D, and F: Diabetic ketoacidosis (DKA) occurs when the amount of insulin is insufficient, resulting in hyperglycemia. Indications include polyuria and polydipsia, hyperventilation (Kussmaul respirations), blurred vision, weakness, headache, abdominal pain, orthostatic hypotension, and mental status changes. Clinically, the primary indications are hyperglycemia, dehydration, electrolyte imbalance, and acidosis. The primary causes of DKA are missing a dose of insulin, illness/infection, and untreated diabetes mellitus. Illness and infection can increase the need for insulin even if food intake is decreased.

16. B: A minor cannot sign a surgical consent unless she is emancipated. Although a surgeon may, in an emergency, perform surgery on a minor without parental or legal guardian consent, every effort should be made to locate a parent or guardian. If reached by telephone, the parent or guardian can give consent verbally, but two witnesses should listen to the conversation and document that consent was given for the procedure, noting the name of the person granting consent.

17. C: For intermittent tube feedings, the client should be positioned with the head of the bed elevated to 30° to prevent aspiration. The client should remain in this position for at least an hour after each feeding, and the head of the bed should stay elevated to at least 30° at all times if he is receiving continuous feedings. Placement of the tube should be verified through aspiration and assessing the pH of aspirant prior to every intermittent feeding and at least every 12 hours for continuous feeding.

18. C: Although 60% of the adult's body is composed of water, 67% of this amount is intracellular fluid (ICF), 25% is interstitial fluid (ISF) (found in the spaces between cells, tissues, and organs), and 8% is plasma volume (PV). ISF and PV are classified as extracellular fluids. Fluid balance is extremely important for life because death usually occurs when 20% to 25% of the total body water is lost, such as through dehydration.

19. A: Whole blood is rarely administered nowadays, although it may be given for extreme loss of blood volume when the red blood cells and the plasma need replacement. The most

commonly used blood products are packed red blood cells and fresh frozen plasma, so whole blood is usually separated into these components. Red blood cells are preferred for most indications because the extra plasma found in whole blood may result in transfusion-associated circulatory overload.

20. D: These symptoms are consistent with hypoparathyroidism and hypocalcemia, so the physician is likely to monitor the calcium level. One complication of thyroidectomy is trauma to or inadvertent removal of the parathyroid glands, resulting in hyperphosphatemia and hypocalcemia because of decreased intestinal absorption of dietary calcium as well as decreased resorption from bone related to inadequate parathormone. Hypocalcemia causes tetany, which may manifest as numbness, tingling, and stiffness in the hands, feet, and face and muscle spasms and contractions. Clients may experience anxiety, depression, and hypotension.

21. A: Constipation and fecal impaction are common with chemotherapy and opioids. Chemotherapeutic agents may cause dysfunction of the autonomic nerves, resulting in abdominal discomfort, and rectal emptying may be slowed. Opioids slow the intestinal motility, so the combination increases the risk of obstruction. The client should have an abdominal examination and abdominal x-ray to evaluate for obstruction before further treatments because the client has not been passing flatus and has increasing pain and nausea.

22. C: Although difficulty with urination, frequency, and urgency are the usual signs of urinary tract infection (UTI), these may be absent in elderly clients, who frequently exhibit nonspecific symptoms, such as anorexia, hyperventilation, low-grade fever, and new onset of urinary incontinence. General fatigue/malaise is the most common presenting symptom in older adults. Cognitive function may also be impaired, and those with dementia may show a sudden cognitive decline. The most common causative agent for UTI in elderly clients is *Escherichia coli.*

23. A: Although protocols for dealing with medication errors may vary from one institution to another, in most cases, the correct response is to notify the physician, notify the supervisor, and complete an incident report. The nurse should not attempt to cover the mistake by obtaining a physician's order after the fact. Usually, documenting an error on the client's record consists only of documenting the actual treatment given—in this case the acetaminophen—but omitting further information about the error and documenting that only in the incident report.

24. A, B, and C: Although African-Americans have a lower risk than Caucasians for skin cancer and osteoporosis; they have a higher risk for a number of other diseases:
- Hypertension: Forty-one percent have hypertension compared to 27% of Caucasians.
- Diabetes mellitus: The incidence is 60% higher than for Caucasians with about two-and-a-half times as many amputations and more than five times as much kidney disease.
- Asthma: The rate of death is three times that of Caucasians.
- Lung cancer: African-American males have twice the incidence of lung cancer than do Caucasian males.
- Heart disease.

- Stroke: The risk is twice that of Caucasians, and resulting deaths are four times higher.

25. Correct order:
A: (First) VI. Cleanse the prosthetic eye according to the manufacturer's directions.
B: (Second) IV. Identify landmarks on the prosthetic eye for the inner and outer areas and superior and inferior aspects.
C :(Third) I. Raise the upper eyelid.
D: (Fourth) III. Slide the prosthesis under and behind the upper eyelid.
E: (Fifth) II. Pull the lower eyelid down.
F: (Sixth) V. Check the positioning.

26. C: These are indications that the client may be experiencing hearing loss. Hearing loss may be insidious, with the client not being fully aware that his hearing is impaired. Because hearing loss may impair the person's ability to hear his own voice as well as others' voices, he may begin slurring his words or dropping word endings. Clients may react to hearing loss by becoming depressed, withdrawn, and irritable, and they may believe that people are whispering or talking behind their backs because they cannot hear what people are saying.

27. B, C, and E: Although unlicensed assistive personnel (UAP) can check routine temperatures and vital signs, they should not be responsible for assessing the condition of a client who is acutely ill. UAP may empty catheter bags and measure urinary output as long as they have been trained in the proper techniques, and they may assist ambulatory clients to walk to the bathroom or help clients with a bedpan. The nurse who delegates the task is always responsible for supervising the UAP and ensuring that the task is completed appropriately.

28. A: Engorgement often occurs in the first two to three days after delivery as the mother begins to produce milk and nurse the infant. Because the infant's intake the first few days is usually very small, the production of milk may exceed demand, resulting in breasts that are swollen, taut, and painful. The mother should be encouraged to continue to nurse and gently massage the breast toward the nipple. Application of cold compresses may relieve discomfort. The mother may take acetaminophen for pain. Engorgement usually lasts only 24 to 48 hours.

29. 21 drops per minute:
Calculation:
Volume (mL) × drop factor/total minutes = flow rate.
250 × 10 = 2,500.
2 hours = 120 minutes.
2,500/120 = 20.83 = 21 drops per minute.

30. Correct order:

Milliliter	Centiliter	Deciliter	Liter	Dekaliter	Hectoliter	Kiloliter

A: II. Milliliter
B: I. Deciliter.
C: III. Dekaliter.
D: V. Hectoliter.
E: IV. Kiloliter.

31. A, B, C, and E: Organ meats, such as liver, and some seafood, such as sardines, mackerels, and scallops, are high in purines and should be avoided. All meats contain purines, so their intake should be limited to 4 to 6 ounces per day. Broth made from meats should be avoided. Because alcohol impairs the elimination of uric acid, wine intake should not exceed 10 ounces daily. Foods high in fat also impair elimination, so high-fat foods, such as avocados and ice cream, should be limited.

32. A: Although all of these are important, histamine is released in response to the antigen, causing erythema and edema, which can result in airway obstruction, so the primary concern is to ensure patency of the airway. This may require intubation. Epinephrine should be administered as soon as possible, and oxygen is provided at 100% high flow. Intravenous fluids are provided to combat hypotension. Albuterol may be given to relieve bronchospasm. If shock continues, diphenhydramine and methylprednisolone may be required.

33. 50 drops/minute:
Calculation:
Volume (mL) × drop factor/total minutes = flow rate.
250 × 60/5 × 60 = 15,000/300.
15,000/300 = 50 drops per minute.

34. C: One grain is equal to 60 to 65 mg (the calculation depends on the manufacturer), so 325 mg is approximately equivalent to five grains of aspirin. Grains are used in the apothecary method of measurement, but only a few medications are still provided using this measurement because most are now provided using metric measurements, such as milligrams. Household measurements, such as ounces and teaspoons, are also used for medications, so nurses should be familiar with conversions among the different measurement systems.

35. 120 mL.:
Calculation:
40 (kg) × 15 (mg per kg) = 600 mg per day.
600 (mg per day) × 10 (total days) = 6,000 mg total.
250/5 = 6,000/x.
250 × x = 250x.
5 × 6,000 = 30,000.
250x = 30,000.
30,000/250 = 120 mL.

36. Two teaspoons: Milliliters are metric measurements, and teaspoons are household measurements. Five milliliters is approximately equivalent to one teaspoon, so the child will require two teaspoons for 10 mL of oral suspension. Oral suspensions are often prescribed in household measurements to reduce the chance of medication errors for those unfamiliar with the metric system.

37. C: In the event of a fire, the client must be evacuated as quickly as possible. Because the client has not yet ambulated and the repaired hip must remain abducted, transferring the client to a wheelchair or attempting to carry the client is precluded. Transferring the client to a gurney is too time-consuming. The best solution to moving a client to a safe area as quickly as possible is to move the client in the bed.

38. A: Restraints cannot be applied as the first intervention, so the nurse must attempt other interventions first, such as trying to camouflage the IV with clothing or dressings. Tying a length of IV tubing to the bedrail and allowing the client to pull on it may distract the client. Restraints may result in injuries and should be avoided whenever possible. Vest restraints have resulted in a number of deaths, so many facilities no longer allow their use.

39. B, C, D, and F: Although advanced age may be a barrier to learning, age should not be a concern for a 55-year-old unless she has cognitive impairment. However, fear and lack of literacy may impact the client's ability to learn. Clients who are weak and frail may not be able to concentrate fully, and those who are hard of hearing may miss important points, especially if the nurse is unaware of the hearing deficit. Asking questions is usually a good sign that the client is alert and attentive.

40. 0.25 mL:
Calculation:
1 (mg)/1 (mL) = 0.25 (mg)/x (mL).
$1 \times x = 1x$.
$1 \times 0.25 = 0.25$.
$1x = 0.25$.
$x = 0.25$ mL.

41. D: The nurse should assess the client's level of pain. Deep breathing, coughing, and turning may be very painful in the first 24 to 48 hours after major surgery, but they are necessary to prevent atelectasis and other complications. Clients who are in pain are often very reluctant to cooperate, so the nurse should ensure that the client has received adequate analgesia prior to the first time she is asked to deep breathe, cough, and turn.

42. B and E: The elbow comprises the simplest type of joint: the hinge. The only movements a hinge joint can perform are flexion and extension. Flexion involves the biceps brachii, brachialis, and brachioradialis muscles, and extension uses the triceps brachii. Three bones (the humerus, ulna, and radius) come together at the elbow but in two different joints—the hinged elbow joint and the pivot proximal radioulnar joint, which allows the forearm to supinate and pronate.

43. C: After a cast is removed, the skin is covered with fatty deposits and dead skin. The nurse should apply a cold-water enzyme wash to the skin, leave it in place for about 20 minutes, and then rinse or soak the leg in warm water to remove the enzyme wash. The skin can then be gently washed with warm water and mild soap, but it should not be rubbed vigorously or scrubbed. The skin should be gently patted dry, and an emollient is applied.

44. A: The correct method of indicating that information has been documented on the wrong record is to draw a straight line (one only) through the incorrect documentation, write "error" above it, and initial the correction. No attempt should be made to obliterate the entry with correction fluid, erasure, or drawing multiple lines through it because the entry must remain readable for legal reasons so that it does not appear that the client's record has been altered.

45. A: Numbness of the thumb and index finger, inability move the thumb to touch the tips of the other fingers, and capillary refill time greater than three seconds are all indications

that the radial nerve is compressed. While the arm is supported, the elastic bandage on the forearm should be removed and reapplied more loosely, and then the circulation is reevaluated to determine if this alleviates the problem. If the numbness, impaired movement, and slow capillary refill persist, then further evaluation is indicated.

46. B: The Braden Scale is used to determine if the client is at risk for developing pressure sores. The scale assesses six different areas with scores of 1 to 4 or 1 to 3. The lower the total score, the higher the risk. The six areas are sensory perception, moisture, activity, mobility, usual nutrition pattern, and friction and sheer. The Braden Scale is used to help identify the need for a support surface and the type of support surface appropriate for the client's needs.

47. D: Healthcare providers should have priority for protection from injury because if they are injured, then no one will be available to provide care to the others who are injured. Police officers and firefighters are usually the first responders in a disaster, and they must determine when it is safe for healthcare providers to enter the area and provide care. In some cases, this may mean that care for the injured is delayed because of unsafe conditions.

48. B: The statement that indicates the client has not made informed consent is "I told the doctor I didn't want to know anything about the surgery, and she agreed." The physician has a responsibility to inform the client of the risks and benefits of the treatment and any alternative treatment options even if the client does not want this information. A client who refuses to receive the information may be in denial or may not yet be emotionally prepared to deal with the reality of the treatment.

49. C: Although these are all important considerations, the installed height, the ratio of computers to staff, and the brand of computer are focused on the needs of the staff. However, the positioning of the computer screens away from the line of sight of clients and visitors is essential for maintaining client confidentiality. The screens must be positioned so that others cannot read what is being documented about a client. Computers must be kept in a secure area. In some cases, privacy screens or filters may be used.

50. D: The trough time is when the blood level is at its lowest (in the trough), so the serum trough level should be drawn immediately before a scheduled dose of the medication is due. Blood levels of a drug may also be measured at the peak time, and this will vary from drug to drug and should always be checked and the time prescribed. When drawing blood for trough and peak levels, it's important that the medication doses be administered on time.

51. 1,140 calories:
Calculation:
75 (g protein) × 4 = 300 (calories).
120 (g carbohydrate) × 4 = 480 (calories).
40 (g fat) × 9 = 360 (calories).
300 + 480 + 360 = 1,140.

52. B: The nurse should contact the admissions department and ask that the client be reassigned to a different room. Although superstitions may seem irrational at times, fear and anxiety can negatively impact recovery. Anxiety before surgery is common, and severe anxiety can result in increased time necessary for induction and an increased need for analgesia in the postoperative period. Superstitions can compound the fear because the

client may feel that the negative outcomes he fears (pain, disability) are more likely to occur.

53. A, C, and D: Because this client is transient and homeless, he probably does not have easy access to a computer or friends and family who can help, so he will most likely have to rely on public agencies and services, such as self-help programs, community agencies (including mental health outreach services), and government agencies (such as Medicaid or Social Security). Although the nurse can provide homeless clients with information, follow-up can be poor among homeless and transient populations.

54. C: At 3 L/min per nasal cannula, the client should receive about 32% FiO_2. Nasal cannulas deliver low concentrations of oxygen, but they are relatively safe and easily tolerated, although they may cause drying and irritation of nasal passages. The FiO_2 measurement may be affected by nasal obstruction and breathing patterns. FiO_2 per L/min:
1 L/min: 24%.
2 L/min: 28%.
3 L/min: 32%.
4 L/min: 36%.
5 L/min: 40%.
6 L/min: 44%.

55. A: The statement "I need my husband to take care of financial matters" suggests that the client's wife has not accepted that her husband's condition will continue to deteriorate and, because of behavioral and language difficulties, he will not be able to manage their financial affairs. She will need to assume responsibilities that were previously handled by her husband, who will become increasingly dependent. This change in roles can be very difficult for a spouse, especially as the behaviors worsen and profound personality changes occur.

56. C: Alcohol, benzodiazepines, and barbiturates pose the greatest risk to life if clients attempt to undergo "cold-turkey" withdrawal. Patients may experience seizures, heart attacks, or strokes. Withdrawal from alcohol may result in delirium tremens (DTs). Clients undergoing withdrawal from opiates, such as heroin, may experience severe physical symptoms (nausea, vomiting, pain, muscle cramping, dyspnea, tremors, palpitations, and sweating) but they are rarely life threatening. Those withdrawing from cocaine and marijuana have milder withdrawal symptoms (anxiety, insomnia, headaches, and depression).

57. D: In a crisis situation, such as a client shouting at the nurse and refusing to stop smoking marijuana, the best initial response is to remain calm and simply repeat the request. Challenges and threats often cause the client who is angry and belligerent to escalate her behavior. The nurse should not intrude on the client's personal space and should be aware of body language and nonverbal communication so as not to appear to be challenging. If possible, the nurse should try to identify the cause of the client's behavior and to state that, "You're feeling nervous about the tests," to determine if the nurse is understanding correctly.

58. A, B, C, and E: Criteria for PTSD include (1) experiencing or witnessing a traumatic event and reliving the experience (flashbacks, dissociative episodes, hallucinations, illusions, and nightmares), (2) exhibiting avoidance behavior (detachment, decreased emotional responsiveness and affect, impaired memory related to the trauma, and phobic/avoidant

behavior related to things that remind the client of the trauma), and (3) a state of chronic hyperarousal (insomnia, poor concentration, blackouts, poor memory, and hypervigilance). Symptoms usually present within three months of a traumatic event, although the reaction may be delayed for many months or years in some individuals.

59. A: Clients should never flush needles or sharps down the toilet but should instead store and dispose of them in accordance with state or local regulations. In some places, needles and sharps must be placed in special sharps containers, but in other places, they may be placed in any secure, puncture-proof container with a lid. People who must dispose of needles and sharps in the community should contact their local refuse disposal service for information about disposal.

60. 0.4 mL:
Calculation:
$10 \text{ (mg)}/1 \text{ (mL)} = 4 \text{ (mg)}/x \text{ (mL)}$.
$10 \times x = 10x$.
$4 \times 1 = 4$.
$10x = 4$.
$4/10 = 0.4 \text{ mL}$.

61. A, D, and F: Peripheral arterial insufficiency is characterized by throbbing, cramping pain that increases with exercise; shiny skin with decreased hair; pale color on elevation; and redness on dependency. The skin is cool to the touch because of impaired circulation. Clients may complain of numbness and tingling and reduced sensation. Capillary refill is greater than two seconds. Ulcerations tend to occur on the tips of the toes or at the sites of trauma and are deep and well delineated.

62. Order of actions:
A: (First) V. Hang the irrigation solution bag with the bottom being 20 inches above the stoma.
B: (Second) IV. Apply the irrigation sleeve over the stoma.
C: (Third) III. Apply gloves, lubricate the cone tip, and insert it into the stoma, holding it securely.
D: (Fourth) II. Allow the solution to flow in for 5 to 10 minutes and then clamp the tubing and close the top of the irrigation sleeve.
E: (Fifth). I. Allow 15 to 20 minutes for evacuation and then fold the sleeve, secure it, and leave it in place for 30 to 45 minutes before removing it.

63. C: Because these signs and symptoms are indicative of obstructive sleep apnea, the client will likely be scheduled for a nocturnal polysomnogram. For the test, which is generally conducted in a sleep center, electrodes are placed on the head, face, and body as well as sensors to evaluate respiratory effort, snore, airflow, and oxygen saturation. The client spends the night in the sleep center so the different stages of sleep can be observed.

64. D: The fetal heart rate (FHR) and nonstress test measure the fetus's heart rate and accelerations during a 20- to 40-minute period. It is done during the daytime with the mother in the semi-Fowler's position with support placed beneath the right hip so the uterus is displaced to the left. An ultrasound transducer is placed on the abdomen to measure the FHR, and a tocodynamometer is used to measure fetal movement. A normal

(reactive) result is ≥2 accelerations of the FHR of 15 bpm above baseline for ≥15 seconds. An abnormal (nonreactive) result is 0 to 1 acceleration of the FHR in a 40-minute period.

65. A, B, C, and E: An aphasia assessment includes observations of spontaneous speech (fluent, nonfluent, grammatical errors, and slow or hesitant speech), comprehension of spoken language (ability to follow simple and then more complex commands), comprehension of written language (ability to read and follow written commands), ability to name items (but not describe), ability to recall four named items (immediately, not after five minutes), and the ability to write. The nurse should observe the client carefully during the assessment for signs of frustration or fatigue.

66. C: The nurse should take the child to a separate treatment area for unpleasant or painful procedures so the child can consider her own room as a safe place. Because the nurse must obtain two specimens (aerobic and anaerobic) from the leg wound, the best position for the child is in the mother's arms (facing the mother in a comfort hold), and a nurse assists to keep the leg from moving because the child will likely react by kicking.

67. B: The area of contact for the automated external defibrillator (AED) pads must be dry, so the nurse should wipe the chest dry with an available dry cloth or ask someone else to do it while she continues cardiopulmonary resuscitation (CPR). The chest should not be wiped with alcohol because this could cause a spark and a fire when the AED shocks the heart. The pads should also not be placed over medicine patches, pacemakers, or implanted defibrillators. Different models of AEDs have slightly different directions, but most have audible directions and pictures that are easy to follow.

68. C: Dressings over intravenous (IV) insertion sites are usually left undisturbed if they are transparent and allow clear visibility and if there is no tenderness until the rotation time for the IV. However, gauze dressings must be changed every 48 hours. If a gauze dressing is under a transparent dressing, then the dressing change schedule remains at 48 hours. In any case, the dressing should be changed if it loosens or is compromised or if signs of infection are evident.

69. D: All neonates should be screened for hearing loss, according to the U.S. Preventive Services Task Force. Although those with identifiable risk factors, such as family history, admission to a neonatal intensive care, and craniofacial abnormalities, have up to 20 times the risk of other infants of having hearing loss, about half of infants with hearing loss have no identifiable risk factors. Testing is recommended for all neonates within one month of birth. Those who fail the hearing test should undergo a complete evaluation by three months.

70. 9 mL:
Calculation:
20 (kg) × 45 (mg) = 900 mg in 24 hours.
900/2 = 450 mg each dose (every 12 hours).
250 (mg)/5 (mL) = 450 (mg)/x (mL).
250 × x = 250x.
5 × 450 = 2,250.
250x = 2,250.
25x = 225.
225/25 = 9 mL.

71. D: Rate response: The pacing rate increases when the sensors note increased activity. Rate smoothing: A pacemaker function prevents excessive changes in the pacing rate. Rate drop response: The pacing rate increases above the normal pacing rate with sudden bradycardia. Mode switching: The pacemaker switches from atrial tracking mode to nontracking mode with atrial fibrillation. Pacemakers may be permanent or temporary and may include single-chamber, dual-chamber, and biventricular pacing. Pacemakers are classified with a five-letter pacemaker code indicating the chamber paced, chamber sensed, response to sensing, programmability, and pacing functions.

72. B: The "5 A's" of the smoking cessation intervention include the following:
Step 1: Ask all clients about tobacco use at every visit. Questions about smoking should be included in all history and physical assessments.
Step 2: Advise all clients who smoke to stop smoking, advising them that smoking is harming their health.
Step 3: Assess clients' willingness to stop smoking. If they are unwilling, ask questions about why.
Step 4: Assist the client to stop smoking. Establish a quit plan with a quit date and a plan for intervention.
Step 5: Arrange for follow-up.

73. B, C, D, and F: Those with hypertension should engage in regular aerobic exercise, such as walking, for 30 minutes most days and should switch to the dietary approaches to stop hypertension (DASH) diet, which is high in fruits and vegetables and low in saturated fat and should limit alcohol to no more than one drink per day for females and two for males, but they need not completely eliminate alcohol. Smoking cessation is essential as is losing weight for those who are overweight.

74. A: Muslims use the left hand, which is considered unclean, for toileting, so the nurse should use the left hand to cleanse the client's rectal area. For the same reason, the nurse should be careful to always pass food, medications, and other items to the client using the right hand and not the left. Wearing gloves to provide rectal cleansing is required by standard precautions and is unrelated to the woman's cultural and religious beliefs.

75. A, C, D and E: Energy-conservation techniques include sitting down to perform activities instead of standing and keeping frequently used items close at hand but at arm level, so the person does not have to reach up or bend down because these activities require increased energy. The client should plan ahead to avoid extra movements; ask for help when needed; and use correct body mechanics, including pushing items instead of pulling them. The client should be advised to watch for stress signals, such as dyspnea or fatigue.

76. A: 24 months: Although children develop at different rates, generally, by age 24 months a child is able to understand about 300 words and is beginning to use two- and three-word sentences ("want candy"). 16 to 18 months: Says and understands 7 to 20 words and can point to body parts. 13 to 15 months: Says and understand 4 to 6 words but understands more and can point to items he wants. 12 months: Says and understands a few words, such as "Mama" and "Dada," and can imitate animal sounds, such as "moo" and "woof."

77. A, C, E, and F: Anoxic brain injuries result from insufficient blood flow and oxygen to the brain, resulting from trauma, near-drowning, choking, cardiac arrest, trauma, drug

overdose, and operative complications. Mild anoxic brain injury: Decreased ability to concentrate, memory impairment, decreased balance, and restlessness. Severe anoxic brain injury: Same as mild anoxic brain injury as well as unclear mumbled speech, dysphasia, seizures, and spasticity. Critical anoxic brain injury: Impaired ability to communicate, semicomatose state but able to open eyes; however, she has inconsistent response to environmental stimuli.

78. D: The primary focus of treatment for osteomyelitis is intravenous (IV) antibiotic therapy, based on the results of a wound culture. IV antibiotics are administered continuously for three to six weeks, and then oral antibiotics are administered for up to three months. If the wound does not respond adequately to antibiotic therapy, then surgical debridement is indicated, during which time antibiotic-impregnated beads may be inserted into the wound. The infected area is immobilized to reduce pain and to reduce the risk of pathological fractures. Warm, wet soaks may be used to increase circulation, and analgesia may be used to reduce pain.

79. C: Although brain damage can occur during labor and delivery, it is more often caused by a lack of oxygen than from compression. In most cases, compression results in cranial molding, which is a relatively benign condition that resolves within a few days of birth. Compression occurs during the second stage of labor, with molding being more pronounced if there is a disparity between the size of the fetal head and the maternal bony pelvis. The bones of the baby's skull are soft and flexible with sutures that allow the plates of the skull to overlap if necessary.

80. A: Because this client faces many challenges in the home environment, the most appropriate referral is to an occupational therapist. The occupational therapist can meet with the client to determine her goals and may observe her carrying out activities of daily living (ADLs) to evaluate her abilities and deficits and can then advise her about modifications needed in the home environment and assistive devices so she can remain independent for as long as possible.

81. A, B, C, and E: If the nurse is teaching a group of clients about risk factors for diabetes mellitus, type 2, the nurse should include the following:
- Obesity
- Hypertension and/or heart disease
- 45 years and older (risk increases with age)
- Non-Caucasian race: African American, Asian, Hispanic, Pacific Islander
- History of diabetes mellitus in family
- High level of LDL cholesterol or low level of HDL cholesterol and high level of triglycerides
- History of polycystic ovarian syndrome

82. A: Clients who are hearing impaired often are reluctant to say so but may try to compensate by reading lips. Because their hearing of their own voice may also be impaired, they may speak more loudly than usual. Even clients who are quite adept at lip reading may misunderstand some words, resulting in answering incorrectly. If a client appears to have hearing impairment, the nurse should ask the client directly if he or she is having trouble hearing the nurse and ask how to best communicate.

83. A, B, C, and E: When a client is discharged 48 hours after delivery of an infant, the client should be apprised of danger signs that could indicate infection or other complications. Constant fatigue, although debilitating, is usually normal so soon after delivery. Danger signs include:
- Temperature higher than 38°C/100.4°F
- Difficulty urinating
- Swelling, redness, or pain in one or both legs
- Increased vaginal bleeding or foul vaginal discharge
- Swelling, masses, or red streaks in the breasts or bleeding nipples
- Blurred vision, persistent headache
- Depression, overwhelming feeling of sadness

84. C: If the nurse notes a scattered red rash on a client's trunk, and the individual lesions are about 0.5 cm in diameter and are flat, nonpalpable, and circumscribed, this type of lesion would be classified as a macule. Macular lesions include those associated with petechiae, measles, and scarlet fever. Freckles are benign macules. A patch is similar to a macule but larger than 1 cm. Papules are solid, elevated, and less than 1 cm in diameter. Nodules are similar to papules but larger than 1 cm.

85. B: If the client has stress incontinence while playing golf, she should certainly be encouraged to urinate immediately before playing golf and to wear incontinence pads for security, but the most effect technique is likely the "knack," which is the use of precisely timed muscle contractions (Kegel exercises). The client should contract the pelvic muscles immediately before stressful events, such as the golf swing, and maintain the contraction until the event is over. This maneuver provides support to the proximal urethra, preventing incontinence.

86. C: If a client has had a recent BK amputation of the right leg and the nurse notes an unusual pattern of swelling after removing the elastic wrap, which the client had applied, the most likely reason for this observation is incorrect wrap technique in which the pressure from the wrap is uneven. The nurse should point out the swelling and discuss the reasons, demonstrating the correct wrap procedure and then observing the client rewrap the stump.

87. A, B, C, and F: If a client has recurrent episodes of constipation and fecal impaction, interventions that should be part of bowel training include scheduled toileting, such as attempting to defecate at the same time each day. The client should be advised to increase fluid intake and eat high-fiber foods. Stool softeners may be taken but not daily laxatives, which may in time make constipation worse. Stimulants, such as a suppository or a hot cup of coffee, may help to promote defecation. Routine exercise may help to stimulate intestinal contractions.

88. D: Gait disturbances:
- Parkinsonian gait: slight flexion of hips and knees, short shuffling steps, trunk leaning forward, and no arm swing
- Ataxic gait: uncoordinated and unsteady, wide-based, staggering, high stepping, flat-footed step
- Geriatric gait: decreased speed and balance, slight flexion of hips and knees, stooped posture, and short or shuffling steps

- Scissors gait: short, slow, stiff steps with thighs crossing while moving forward

89. B: If a client has bilateral pain, enlarged and swollen metacarpophalangeal and proximal interphalangeal joints, swan-neck deformity, and ulnar deviation, these signs and symptoms are consistent with rheumatoid arthritis (RA), an autoimmune disorder that results in inflammation and damage to the joints. RA may also affect other organs of the body. Clients typically experience periods when the disease exacerbates and symptoms worsen. Treatment includes NSAIDs, analgesics, disease-modifying antirheumatic drugs (DMARDs), and biologics.

90. A, B, and C: A client with pelvic skin traction for low back pain (as well as any client on bedrest with decreased mobility) is at risk of the development of the following:
- Orthostatic hypotension: Vessels in the lower extremities lose tone and then dilate when the person stands, resulting in decreased blood flow to the brain and other parts of the body.
- Muscle weakness: Lack of movement results in weakness of muscles.
- Venous stasis: Blood flow slows when vessels lose their tone, resulting in increased risk of thrombus formation.

91. 1680 calories: In order to calculate a client's necessary caloric intake to maintain body weight, the first step is to convert the client's weight in pounds in kilograms:
- $132/2.2 = 60$

Then, the caloric requirement (usually between 25 and 30 calories per kg) is multiplied by the number of kilograms:
- $60 \times 28 = 1680$ calories

Clients who are exceptionally active, such as athletes, may need to have a higher number of calories, so caloric requirements must be individualized.

92. A and C: If a client has had repair of a right fractured hip and has an overhead trapeze on the bed to assist with movement, the client should receive instructions on the proper use of the assistive device:
- The client should always grasp the bar with both hands before moving in order to move smoothly and prevent straining the muscles.
- After grasping the bar, the client should flex the unaffected (in this case left) knee and hip and place the foot flat on the bed.
- In one movement, the client should pull on the trapeze while pushing down on the left foot and moving the body.

93. A and D: If a 6-year-old child has influenza with a fever and cough, the statements by the child's caregiver that suggest a need for information include:
- "If his fever gets too high, I'll give him a bath in cold water": This could lower the child's fever too quickly. If the child's fever is high (> 102°F/39°C), then the child may be bathed with lukewarm water.
- "I've been giving him baby aspirin to lower his fever": Children should not be administered any salicylate for viral infections because this places the child at risk for developing Reye syndrome, which can cause progressive encephalopathy, liver failure, and death.

94. D: The snack with the lowest number of calories per serving is the apple; however, it has very little protein. When calculating calories, each gram of fat is equal to 9 calories and each gram of carbohydrate and protein is equal to 4 calories. Insoluble fiber grams are not absorbed and can be subtracted from the carbohydrate total:

- Lunch meat: $(6 \times 9) + (1 \times 4) + (7 \times 4) = 86$ calories
- Peanuts: $(14 \times 9) + (5 \times 4) - (1 \times 4) + (7 \times 4) = 170$ calories
- Cheese: $(9 \times 9) + (1 \times 4) + (7 \times 4) = 113$ calories
- Apple: $(0.3 \times 9) + (25 \times 4) - (5 \times 4) + (0.5 \times 4) = 84.7$ calories

95. The steps to combining doses of two different insulins from two vials in one syringe include:

Step	Procedure
1	(A) I. Cleanse top of vials.
2	(B) II. Inject air into vial 1.
3	(C) VI. Inject air into vial 2.
4	(D) V. Withdraw medication from vial 2.
5	(E) IV. Change needles.
6	(F) III. Withdraw medication from vial 1.

96. C: If teaching a client to use a metered-dose inhaler without a spacer, the inhaler should be positioned 1 to 2 inches away from the client's lips for administration of a dose of inhaled medication. The client should be advised to exhale and then to deliver a dose while breathing in slowly for about 5 seconds, followed by holding the breath for 10 seconds before exhaling. If an adult has difficulty with coordinating breathing and delivering of a dosage or holding the inhaler at the correct distance, then a spacer should be used. Children should also use a spacer.

97. A, C, D, and E: If a client has received an overdose of opioid per PCA pump because the limit for maximum dosage was set far too high, resulting in the client's being pale, hypotensive, somnolent, and barely responsive with a respiratory rate of 6 breaths per minute, the nurse should immediately stop the infusion. The nurse should also administer naloxone per standing order (or immediately consult the physician to obtain the order). Because the respirations are so slow, supplementary oxygen will generally be administered. Because an error occurred in setting the parameters of dosage on the PCA, an incident report must be filed.

98. A: If a client with Alzheimer disease is incontinent of urine and feces and incontinent care has been delegated to UAP, then the UAP should be advised to check the client for dryness on a regular schedule of every 2 hours. Eating and drinking often trigger urination and/or bowel movements, so scheduling checks after meals is advisable. However, if the client appears restless or pulls at clothing at other times, the UAP should check for dryness then as well.

99. A, B, and C: The long-term effects of prolonged use of phenytoin include a condition referred to as "Dilantin facies," which is characterized by gingival hypertrophy, hirsutism, and hypertrophy of facial subcutaneous tissue. Clients must be advised to maintain good

dental care. Additionally, clients may develop osteoporosis, so supplementary vitamin D is usually advised. Clients with low levels of albumin (usually associated with renal disease or malnutrition) may have more severe effects.

100. A, B, D, and E: If a 60-year-old client has undergone a nerve-sparing prostatectomy and has been advised that he may not recover normal sexual functioning and the client is concerned and asks the nurse for more information, the nurse should include the following:
- Retrograde ejaculation may occur.
- Recovery rates vary but can take up to a year or more.
- Attempts at sexual intercourse are usually avoided for 1 month.
- Anxiety can interfere with sexual functioning.
- The client may want to explore other forms of sexual intimacy even though these are not likely as important to the client as sexual intercourse at this time.

101. B: If a client receiving end-of-life care tells the nurse that he has not always lived the way he should have or treated his children well, the most appropriate response is: "There are things that you regret," which is stating the point that the client is making without being judgmental or questioning. At the end of life, clients often think back over their lives and consider both positive and negative aspects. They often are not seeking advice but rather an opportunity to verbalize feelings.

102. C: There is no antidote for an overdose of muscle relaxants, such as baclofen. Therefore, treatment consists of supportive care. The client should receive large volumes of intravenous fluids to prevent the development of crystalluria, and may require mechanical ventilation if respirations are severely depressed. The client should be placed on cardiac monitoring. If other CNS depressant drugs are taken along with the overdose of muscle relaxant, the client is more at risk.

103. A, C, and D: Contraindications to levodopa include narrow-angle glaucoma, pregnancy, and melanoma (or suspicious skin lesions that may be melanoma). Additionally, levodopa should not be given to clients with psychoses and must be monitored carefully if administered to clients with a history of cardiac problems. Levodopa interacts with numerous drugs, so the client's list of medications should be reviewed by a pharmacist.

104. D: If a 78-year-old client with a history of diabetes mellitus, type 2, GERD, and hypertension is hospitalized with pneumonia and rings the call bell at 11 PM, complaining of being unable to sleep and having "indigestion" and "heartburn," the initial intervention should be to assess the client's cardiac and respiratory status before deciding how to proceed. The nurse should never assume to know the reason for a client's symptoms without conducting an assessment.

105. C: If a client is upset that the physician has refused to order a stronger pain medication for the client and berates the nurse, calling the nurse "worthless and stupid" when the nurse brings the prescribed medication, the ego defense mechanisms that the client is exhibiting is displacement, which is the transference of feelings from one target to another. Compensation is compensating for a perceived weakness by emphasizing a strength. Reaction formation is covering up unacceptable thoughts/behaviors by emphasizing the opposite. Regression is reverting to an earlier level of development.

106. A: When determining whether or not a client is a candidate for restraints, only current behavior should be considered. If the client currently poses a danger to others or to self and no other reasonable alternative exists, then restraints may be considered. Restraints cannot be applied as a preventive measure for such things as history of violent attack against a staff member or a history of falls. There must be evidence of current risk.

107. C: Physical signs and symptoms often attributed to decreased estrogen production associated with menopause include increased fat deposits on hips and abdomen, often associated with weight gain and decreased metabolic rate. Clients may have difficulty sleeping and develop restless leg syndrome and heart palpitations. Hot flashes are common. Clients lose subcutaneous fat in the labia and are more at risk for problems with the lower urinary tract, such as stress incontinence and bladder and vaginal infections.

108. D: If an older client has been sleeping poorly at night, and the daughter states that the mother has always loved music and suggests listening to music might relax the client, the nurse should ask about the client's favorite music. Tastes in music are very individual. For example, while classical music may seem relaxing to some, others may find it boring or irritating. If the client is not in a private room, then the client should use earphones.

109. 0.84: If a client's waist measurement is 38 inches and the hip measurement is 45 inches, then the calculations are:
- Waist measurement/Hip measurement = waist-to-hip (WTH) ratio.
- $38/45 = 0.8444 = 0.84$.

According to the National Institute of Diabetes and Digestive and Kidney Diseases (NIDDK), a female is considered obese if the WTH ratio is greater than 0.8, and a male is considered obese if the WTH ratio is greater than 1.

110. C: If a client is to have a nasogastric tube inserted for intermittent feedings, an appropriate task to delegate to unlicensed assistive personnel (UAP) is to administer the tube feedings if the person has been trained in doing so. However, an RN or LVN/LPN must verify the tube position first because this cannot be delegated to UAP. UAP cannot insert or reposition a displaced NG tube. UAP can be advised to monitor the client's condition and to report any changes in condition, such as dyspnea or nausea.

111. C: If a client who received a unit of packed red blood cells developed severe chills and a 2°C elevation of temperature 2 hours after initiation of the transfusion and the client had no dyspnea, swelling, or urticaria, the most likely cause of the client's symptoms is febrile nonhemolytic reaction. This reaction results from antibodies against the leukocytes that remain in the PRBCs. This is the most common transfusion reaction and is generally treated with nonaspirin antipyretics, such as acetaminophen and ibuprofen. The transfusion is usually resumed after acute hemolytic reaction is excluded.

112. A: If a client with prostate cancer has been given the option of various treatments and asks the nurse for advice, the most appropriate response is: "Let's discuss the different options and how you feel about them." The nurse must avoid trying to directly influence the client's choice; however, since the client asked for advice, this is a good opportunity for the client to express feelings and concerns about the diagnosis and treatment. Additionally, talking through the options may help the client reach an independent decision.

113. B: If a client with psoriasis is to begin NB-UVB phototherapy, the initial treatment is 1 to 2 minutes long with the time increased gradually by 10% to 15% until the optimal duration is reached. Treatments are usually done 3 times weekly to a maximum of 20 to 30 treatments. The phototherapy dosage is adjusted so that only slight erythema occurs during treatment. If the dose is too high, the client may experience marked erythema or burns.

114. B: If a neonate has severe congenital abnormalities, death is imminent, and the NICU team feels that no further attempts at treatment or feeding are warranted, the best approach is to tell the parents that the team suggests a change in care plan to focus on comfort measures. The nurse should avoid such phrases as "stopping" or "withdrawing" treatment of feeding because these terms may make the parents feel as though they are starving or killing their infant, although the exact plan for care should be explained.

115. C: If a client is on contact precautions because of a MRSA infection and has an open, draining wound, the nurse should glove and gown whenever entering the room for any type of patient or environmental contact. MRSA can be spread from the client to surfaces, such as the bedrails or bedside table, on the hands. The gloves and gown should be removed and placed into a receptacle near the door and inside of the client's room.

116. A: Clients taking anticholinergic drugs to relieve muscle tremors and muscle rigidity associated with Parkinson disease should be advised to avoid overheating. Clients taking anticholinergics should be advised to avoid high environmental temperatures or activities, which may increase internal temperature, such as excessive exercise during warm weather. Because anticholinergics interfere with the body's ability to perspire, the body cannot adequately cool if overheated. Anticholinergics are often used as adjuncts to primary Parkinson drugs.

117. A: Following procurement of organs from a standard criteria donor (donor younger than 50 years who suffered brain death), the heart and lungs should be transplanted within 4 to 6 hours, liver and pancreas within 12 hours, and the kidney within 24 hours. Organ and tissue recovery is carried out in the operating room with members of the recovery team present and transportation to the recipient available. The corneas and skin can be harvested for up to 2 hours after death and bone up to 36 hours. Heart valves can be harvested up to 72 hours after death.

118. D: If a nurse who is a friend on a social media site with a coworker finds that the coworker has written on the media site confidential information about a well-known client's health history (information obtained from the client's her), the most appropriate response is to report the incident to an appropriate supervisor/administrator as soon as possible because breaching the security of the EHR is illegal and unethical. In most cases, this type of breach will result in the guilty person being fired.

119. 25 grams: While the average woman should have approximately 46 grams of protein daily, pregnancy increases the demand for protein in order to expand the blood volume and support fetal growth and maternal nutrition. By halfway through the pregnancy, the average woman should have increased the intake of protein by 25 grams. If mothers are vegetarian or vegan, they should especially seek guidance about their diet from a dietitian to ensure that their protein intake is adequate.

120. A and B: Flexion contractures and impaired gait can occur if the client fails to routinely use the prosthesis, but clients may find it easier at times to use a wheelchair, and then this can become a habit. The interventions that are most indicated are to provide sympathetic encouragement without chastising the client, but pointing out the problems that are arising and arranging for a period of retraining, as retraining may be essential to ensuring the client understands and follows instructions for use of the prosthesis.

Practice Test #2

1. A client has received 10 mg of morphine sulfate subcutaneously. When does the nurse anticipate the maximal period of respiratory depression will occur?
   a. 7 minutes
   b. 30 minutes
   c. 60 minutes
   d. 90 minutes

2. How many hours of activity per day are necessary to prevent disuse syndrome with muscle atrophy and joint contracture?
   a. 6 hours
   b. 4 hours
   c. 2 hours
   d. 1 hour

3. The nurse is one of the first on the scene of a bus accident and is triaging injured riders. Place the following injured clients (Roman numerals) into the correct triage classification.
   I.   40-year-old woman with arterial bleed
   II.   20-year-old male with sprained wrist, small cuts, and bruises
   III. 14-year-old female with severe crush injuries to the head and chest and dilated, non-responsive pupils
   IV.   56-year-old male with fractured femur

Minor injury (Ambulatory injured)	Immediate care	Delayed care	Unsalvageable
a.	b.	c.	d.

4. A client nearing death has an Advance Directive in his records indicating that he does not want intravenous fluids or other invasive procedures, but the client's physician has ordered IV fluids. Which of the following initial actions by the nurse is **most** appropriate?
   a. Notify the bioethics committee.
   b. Inform the physician of the Advance Directive regarding intravenous fluids.
   c. Administer intravenous fluids.
   d. Contact a supervisor to resolve the issue.

5. A client has been instructed in the application and use of anti-embolic compression stockings. Which of the following statements by the client indicates a need for more teaching? *Select all that apply.*
   a. "After I apply the stocking, I roll the top back down about 2 inches to hold the stockings in place."
   b. "I remove the stocking and reapply about every day or two."
   c. "To apply, I turn the stocking inside out while holding onto the toe."
   d. "I apply a small amount of baby powder to my legs before applying the stockings."
   e. "These stockings help prevent blood clots."

6. A client with a demand pacemaker complains that he has developed persistent chronic hiccupping and is experiencing mild discomfort in the chest. Which of the following causes does the nurse suspect?

    a. Pacemaker syndrome
    b. Dislocation of a lead
    c. Esophageal reflux
    d. Myocardial infarction

7. Which of the following are common neurological changes associated with aging? *Select all that apply.*

    a. Dementia occurs.
    b. Threshold for sensory input increases.
    c. Perspiration is reduced.
    d. Short-term memory is impaired.
    e. Muscles atrophy.

8. When examining an 80-year-old client with chronic COPD receiving home health care, the nurse notes that over the previous 48 hours the client has developed scattered painful pustular lesions on the right arm near the elbow (see photo), on the back of the neck, the face, and on both legs.

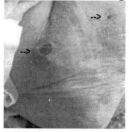

Which of the following does the nurse suspect is the **most** likely cause of the lesions?

    a. Psoriasis
    b. Herpes zoster
    c. MRSA
    d. Contact dermatitis

9. A Turkish-speaking client is scheduled for a colonoscopy, and the nurse must provide printed directions to the client, but directions are not available in Turkish. Which of the following is **most** appropriate?

    a. The nurse contacts a medical translator to translate.
    b. The client's 10-year-old daughter translates the directions.
    c. The nurse draws pictures and pantomimes directions.
    d. Client's daughter is advised to tell her parent to seek a translator.

10. While a dosage of oral morphine has approximately 25% bioavailability, what percentage is the bioavailability of an intravenous dose of morphine? *Record your answer using a whole number.*

11. The nurse is teaching the mother of a newborn to care for the umbilical cord. What should the nurse advise the mother to do if the cord becomes soiled with urine or feces?
    a. Swab with alcohol.
    b. Wipe with a dry cloth.
    c. Wash with mild soap and water, rinse and dry.
    d. Swab with povidone-iodine.

12. A client is in acute postoperative pain, and the physician orders 85 mg of meperidine (Demerol®) stat. The vial contains 100 mg in 2 mL. How many milliliters should the nurse administer? *Record your answer using a decimal number.*

13. The physician has ordered that a client recovering from back surgery be logrolled. The client has a draw sheet in place, and the nurse and an assistant are positioned with one on each side of the bed. Place the steps to logrolling (Roman numerals) in the correct sequence from first to last.
    I.   Grasping draw sheet at shoulder and lower hips, roll patient on count of three.
    II.   Place a small pillow between client's knees.
    III.   Place pillows along length of client's back.
    IV.   Cross client's arms across chest.
        a. (First)
        b. (Second)
        c. (Third)
        d. (Fourth)

14. The physician has ordered that a 132-pound client with increased intracranial pressure receive 0.5 g of mannitol per kg in an IV solution. How many grams should be in the total mannitol dose? *Record your answer using a whole number.*

15. When applying the leads for a 12-lead electrocardiogram, the nurse places V1 and V2 at the fourth intercostal space to the right and left of the sternum. Which of the remaining leads is placed at the fifth intercostal space on the left midclavicular line?
    a. Lead V3
    b. Lead V4
    c. Lead V5
    d. Lead V6

16. A client is recovering from a stroke and the nurse is doing range-of-motion exercises. Which movements should be included for ROM of the elbow on the weak side? *Select all that apply.*
    a. Abduction and adduction
    b. Hyperextension
    c. Supination and pronation
    d. Flexion and extension
    e. Rotation

17. The nurse is assisting a client to adjust crutches to the proper measurement. With the client in standing position, where should the tips of the crutches be placed?
    a. 2 to 3 inches directly to the side of the client's legs
    b. 4 to 6 inches to the side of the client's legs and 4 to 6 inches in front of feet
    c. 2 to 3 inches to the side of the client's legs and 4 to 6 inches in front of feet
    d. 4 to 6 inches directly to the side of the client's legs

18. A client who is very confused removed a diamond ring and threw it on the floor. Which of the following is the **most** appropriate action?
    a. Give the ring to a visiting granddaughter for safekeeping.
    b. Place the ring in the client's bedside stand in an envelope clearly marked "Valuables."
    c. Replace the ring on the client's finger.
    d. Place the ring in a secured container, according to organizational policy.

19. If the first day of a pregnant woman's last menstrual period fell on May 1, 2013, what is the expected delivery month and year? *Record your answer using the month (word) and year (whole number).*

20. Twenty micrograms (µg) are equal to how many milligrams? *Record your answer using a decimal number.*

21. A physician orders chest physiotherapy for a 4-year-old child with cystic fibrosis, but the respiratory therapists are off duty, so the physician tells the nurse to do the therapy. The nurse, however, rarely works in pediatrics, has never done chest physiotherapy, and does not know the procedure. Which of the following is the **most** appropriate response by the nurse?
    a. Ask the child's mother to explain the procedure.
    b. Check the procedure manual and attempt to do the therapy.
    c. Refuse to do the procedure.
    d. Advise the physician that the nurse will try to locate another staff person knowledgeable about chest physiotherapy.

22. A pregnant woman has experienced repeated vaginal monilial infections. When educating the client about the infection, which information should the nurse include? *Select all that apply.*
    a. Advise client to bathe daily.
    b. Explain the effects of increased estrogen production.
    c. Advise client to wear cotton panties and avoid nylon or pantyhose.
    d. Suggest client use panty liners to protect clothing.
    e. Advise the client to avoid wearing any panties.

23. When drawing up a dosage of subcutaneous heparin, how much air should be drawn into the syringe after the correct dosage is obtained?
    a. 1 mL
    b. 0.6 mL
    c. 0.2 to 0.3 mL
    d. 0.01 mL

24. Lochia serosa usually is evident on days 4 to 10 postpartum. When teaching the client about postpartum care, how should the nurse describe lochia serosa?
    a. Dark red discharge with small clots
    b. Yellowish discharge
    c. Pinkish to brownish discharge
    d. Clear watery discharge

25. The Z-track injection technique should be used with which of the following? *Select all that apply.*
    a. Iron
    b. Haloperidol
    c. Heparin
    d. Hydroxyzine (Vistaril®)
    e. Insulin

26. A Mexican-American client states that she and her family live next door to her brother and his family and that they share goods, services, and childcare. How is this type of family classified?
    a. Nuclear
    b. Dual career/dual earner
    c. Extended
    d. Extended kin network

27. The physician has ordered sublingual nitroglycerin for a client. Which of the following are contraindications for administration of sublingual or buccal medications? *Select all that apply.*
    a. Client is edentulous.
    b. Client has mild dementia.
    c. Mucous membranes are red and irritated.
    d. Client is dehydrated.
    e. Client has productive aphasia.

28. The nurse is teaching a new breastfeeding mother about breast care, but the mother has engorgement and asks if she should quit breastfeeding. Which information should the nurse include? *Select all that apply.*
    a. "Continue to nurse every 2 to 3 hours."
    b. "Gently massage the breast toward the nipple while breastfeeding."
    c. "Apply hot compresses to the breast."
    d. "Acetaminophen or ibuprofen is safe to use to relieve pain."
    e. "Engorgement usually recedes in 24 to 48 hours."

29. When administering a capsule that is individually wrapped to a client, when should the wrapping be removed?
    a. When initially obtained from the medicine cart
    b. When placed in the medicine cup
    c. Prior to entering the client's room
    d. At bedside in the client's presence

30. Which of the following are important factors in facilitating attachment between a newborn and mother?
    a. Rooming in
    b. Swaddling and holding the infant
    c. Knowledge of childcare
    d. Beginning breastfeeding within 24 hours of birth

31. Which of the following are controlled substances (Schedules I through V) regulated by the Drug Enforcement Agency (DEA)? *Select all that apply.*
    a. Codeine
    b. Ibuprofen
    c. Diphenhydramine (Benadryl®)
    d. Hydrocodone

32. Which of the following ethnic groups has the highest risk of developing diabetes mellitus type 2 and should be routinely screened for diabetes?
    a. Hispanics
    b. Asians
    c. Caucasians
    d. African-Americans

33. A hospice client is receiving high doses of opioid analgesia and is exhibiting nocturnal myoclonus with restless leg movement and involuntary jerking. Which of the following responses would the nurse expect?
    a. Discontinue opioids.
    b. Reduce dosage by half and administer a benzodiazepine.
    c. Administer naloxone.
    d. Administer flumazenil.

34. A 16-year-old female has been sexually active for two years but was recently treated for a gonorrhea infection. The nurse is teaching the adolescent about safe sex practices. Which of the following statements by the adolescent indicate a need for more information? *Select all that apply.*
    a. "I'm never going to have sex again until I'm married, so I don't need to know about safe sex!"
    b. "I should never have any kind of sex unless my partner wears a condom."
    c. "We don't need to use a condom for oral sex."
    d. "I'm confused about different birth control methods."
    e. "Birth control pills are more effective than diaphragms."

35. A client receiving high doses of hydromorphone (Dilaudid®) develops acute respiratory depression with a drop in blood pressure. Which of the following treatments is most indicated?
    a. Naloxone
    b. Naproxen
    c. Flumazenil
    d. Nortriptyline

36. A 20-year-old client has taken forty 500-mg tablets of acetaminophen with 4 ounces of alcohol in a suicide attempt. The client is **most** at risk for which of the following?
   a. Gastrointestinal hemorrhage
   b. Respiratory depression
   c. Liver failure
   d. Brain damage

37. A client with bipolar disorder is taking lithium to control symptoms. Which of the following statements indicates the need for further education?
   a. "I need to have regular tests for thyroid function."
   b. "Once I'm stabilized, I won't need further testing."
   c. "I should avoid taking ibuprofen."
   d. "It's important for me to avoid dehydration."

38. Which of the following antibiotics is contraindicated in children younger than 8 years?
   a. Tetracycline
   b. Augmentin
   c. Azithromycin
   d. Amoxicillin

39. A nurse notes that clients of one surgeon have developed at least twice as many infections as clients of other surgeons on the unit. Which of the following is the **most** appropriate action?
   a. Report the physician to the hospital administration.
   b. Ask the physician why his rate of infections is so high.
   c. Report the observations to the infection control nurse.
   d. Say nothing as infection rates vary from time to time.

40. Which type of laxative agent is usually the safest for most people?
   a. Bulk laxatives
   b. Stool softeners
   c. Stimulants
   d. Osmotics/saline

41. Prior to drawing blood for blood gas analysis, the nurse conducts the modified Allen test to ensure there is adequate collateral circulation. The nurse asks the client to extend the wrist over a rolled towel and make a fist. Place the following steps (Roman numerals) in order from first to last.
   I.   Ask the client to open and close the hand until the skin blanches.
   II.   Palpate the ulnar and radial pulses and apply pressure to both arteries.
   III.   Observe the hand for color.
   IV.   Release the ulnar artery while maintaining pressure on the radial artery.
   a. (Step 1)
   b. (Step 2)
   c. (Step 3)
   d. (Step 4)

42. What is the critical point for PO2 (the "ICU" point), the percentage point at which there is marked decrease in oxygen saturation? *Record your answer using a whole number.*

43. A client with heart failure has been prescribed the DASH diet (dietary approaches to stop hypertension) and must limit sodium intake to 2300 mg per day. Which of the following statements by the client indicates a need for further education?
    a. "All I really have to do for this diet is stop adding salt to foods."
    b. "I can have 2 or 3 servings of nonfat or low-fat dairy products each day."
    c. "I should have 4 or 5 servings of both vegetables and fruits daily."
    d. "I should limit lean meat, poultry, and fish to 6 ounces per day."

44. A client has immune thrombocytopenic purpura. The client's platelet count is 19,000. Which initial treatment does the nurse expect?
    a. Splenectomy
    b. Immunosuppressive therapy
    c. Observation only
    d. Platelet administration

45. A client is being assessed for neutropenia. The client's total white blood cell count is 5200 with 45% neutrophils and 5% bands. What is the absolute neutrophil count (ANC)? *Record your answer using a whole number.*

46. Each staff person has an individual password that allows access to electronic health records. Under which of the following circumstances should a nurse allow another staff person to use his/her password?
    a. A physician asks to use the password to access records of a former client.
    b. Another nurse asks to use the password because he has forgotten his own.
    c. The nurse's supervisor asks to use the password to access client records.
    d. The nurse should not allow anyone else to use the password, regardless of circumstances.

47. The nurse is part of an interdisciplinary team in a rehabilitation unit. Which of the following statements by a client is **most** important to be communicated to the social worker on the team?
    a. "I can't afford to hire anyone to help me when I am discharged."
    b. "I'm worried about falling when I go home."
    c. "I need to learn how to get in and out of the shower."
    d. "I'm not sure what kinds of adaptive equipment I will need."

48. An 84-year-old female with COPD in an extended-care facility is alert and responsive and has been maintained on low-flow oxygen and nebulizer treatments, but the client, who is bedridden, has removed the oxygen and refused nebulizer treatments, telling the nurse that she is ready to die and only wants comfort measures. Which of the following actions by the nurse is **most** appropriate?
    a. Insist the client take treatments as ordered by the physician.
    b. Notify the physician of the client's refusal.
    c. Ask family members to intervene.
    d. Remind the client that committing suicide is contrary to her religious beliefs.

49. If a client's LDL cholesterol is 100, HDL cholesterol is 50, and triglycerides are 150, what is the client's total cholesterol? *Record your answer using a whole number.*

50. The nurse is conducting a physical examination of a client's abdomen. Place the examination techniques listed below (Roman numerals) in the correct sequence, from first to last.

    I.   Percussion
    II.   Palpation
    III.   Inspection
    IV.   Auscultation
      a. (First)
      b. (Second)
      c. (Third)
      d. (Fourth)

51. The nurse is conducting an examination of the abdomen and auscultating for bruits. Label the lettered points on the diagram with Roman numerals identifying the position of the arteries.

    I.   Femoral
    II.   Aorta
    III.   Iliac
    IV.   Renal

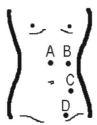

      a.
      b.
      c.
      d.

52. A female client is scheduled for a routine pelvic exam. Which of the following should the nurse ask the client to do prior to the exam?

      a. Refrain from drinking.
      b. Urinate.
      c. Wash perineal area.
      d. Perform relaxation exercises.

53. The nurse is inserting an intravenous line into the right arm and has identified a potential insertion site. Place the steps (indicated in Roman numerals) of venipuncture in the proper sequential order.

    I.   Palpate vein.
    II.   Cleanse skin.
    III.   Apply tourniquet.
    IV.   Perform venipuncture.
      a. (First)
      b. (Second)
      c. (Third)
      d. (Fourth)

54. A client is receiving oxygen per nasal cannula at 3L/minute. Which of the following is the approximate inspired oxygen concentration (FiO2)?

      a. 60%
      b. 50%
      c. 40–42%
      d. 28–32%

55. A client is taking nebulizer treatments for asthma, and the nurse is instructing the client in the correct method for measuring peak expiratory flow rates (PEFR) after treatment. The nurse prepares the meter with the indicator at the base of the scale. Place the following steps (Roman numerals) in the correct order from first to last.
   I.   Client sits upright or stands.
   II.   Client places the meter in the mouth and seals lips.
   III. Client expels air through the meter as forcefully as possible.
   IV.   Client takes a deep breath.
      a. (First)
      b. (Second)
      c. (Third)
      d. (Fourth)

56. Following a lumbar puncture, a client develops a severe headache that persists 24 hours and is unrelieved by bedrest or oral fluids. Which of the following interventions does the nurse anticipate?
      a. Bedrest for 3 days
      b. Opioid analgesia
      c. Epidural blood patch
      d. Intravenous fluids

57. The nurse is assisting a client who is to undergo a thoracentesis. Which of the following is the optimal position for the procedure?
      a. Lying prone with arms above head
      b. Side lying on the unaffected side
      c. Side lying on the affected side
      d. Upright position, leaning forward over an over-bed tray table

58. A client has experienced 48 hours of severe repeated bouts of vomiting. Which acid-base imbalance is of most concern?
      a. Respiratory acidosis
      b. Respiratory alkalosis
      c. Metabolic acidosis
      d. Metabolic alkalosis

59. A client is scheduled for hemodialysis twice weekly through an arteriovenous fistula in the left arm. Following each hemodialysis treatment, the nurse should evaluate the client for which of the following because of risks associated with hemodialysis? *Select all that apply.*
      a. Fluid volume deficit
      b. Fluid volume excess
      c. Bleeding
      d. Metabolic acidosis
      e. Pulmonary edema

60. A client with liver failure and ascites is having a paracentesis to relieve severe dyspnea resulting from abdominal fluid accumulation. Prior to the procedure, the nurse assists the client to urinate. Which of the following is the **most** important reason to have the patient urinate?
    a. Patient comfort
    b. Prevention of incontinence
    c. Prevention of bladder puncture
    d. Fluid displacement

61. A client is to be discharged with a tracheostomy. Which of the following should the nurse **most** stress when educating the client about home management? *Select all that apply.*
    a. Bowel care
    b. Pulmonary hygiene
    c. Dietary supplements
    d. Tracheostomy care
    e. Exercise program

62. A 72-year-old client with Parkinson disease is recovering from pneumonia and is to be discharged, but he remains weak and has poor control of his hands because of tremors. A home health aide will visit three times weekly to assist the client to bathe, and his daughter will visit every evening after work to help with laundry and housework. Which of the following referrals is **most** indicated to allow the client to remain independent in his home?
    a. Home meal delivery program (Meals on Wheels)
    b. Friendly Visitors program
    c. Hospice
    d. Occupational therapist

63. A client is receiving hospice and palliative care, including analgesia and other comfort measures. Which of the following indicates the client is undergoing life review? *Select all that apply.*
    a. The client looks through old photo albums.
    b. The client states that her analgesia is not adequate.
    c. The client reminisces about her children when they were young and her parenting skills.
    d. The client states that she is ready to die.
    e. The client states she does not want her children to have a funeral for her.

64. A mother brings her child to the clinic because of repeated bouts of head lice. Which of the following statements by the mother suggests a need for education? *Select all that apply.*
    a. "I've repeatedly used mayonnaise and olive oil treatments."
    b. "I spent hours combing nits from my child's hair."
    c. "I washed her clothing and bedding in hot water and dried in a hot dryer for 20 minutes."
    d. "I warned my child not to use anyone else's comb or brush."
    e. "I treated the dogs for lice as well."

65. A client comes to the emergency department with scalding burns covering his entire left arm, anterior and posterior surfaces. Using the rule of nines, how much total body surface area (TBSA) has been burned? *Record your answer using a whole number.*

66. A client has been on prolonged bedrest following surgery. The nurse notes that the patient has pain in the right calf on palpation with dorsiflexion of the ankle. Which of the following causes does the nurse suspect?
    a. Arthritis
    b. Muscle strain
    c. Compartment syndrome
    d. Deep vein thrombosis

67. A client had a craniotomy for a basal meningioma and is being monitored postoperatively. The client's baseline blood pressure and pulse were BP 138/72 and P 82. Temperature was 97.5°F/36.4°C. The client is awake and responding. Which of the following findings **most** indicates possible increasing intracranial pressure?
    a. Patient restless, BP 146/80 and P 90. Temperature 98.2°F/36.7°C.
    b. Patient restless and complaining of headache. BP 160/64 and P 70. Temperature 99.4°F/37.4°C.
    c. Patient sleeping. BP 142/76 and P 86. Temperature 97.8°F/36.6°C.
    d. Patient complaining of headache, BP 160/110, P 92. Temperature 98°F/36.7°C.

68. A client is being discharged with an implantable cardioverter-defibrillator (ICD), and the nurse is educating the client about home management. The client asks what he should do if the ICD fires one time but he has no other symptoms. Which of the following is the best advice?
    a. "Call 9-1-1."
    b. "Go to the emergency department when recovered from the firing."
    c. "Resume normal activities."
    d. "Lie down and rest and report the event to the physician by telephone."

69. The nurse is monitoring a client's cardiac rhythm when an abnormal rhythm occurs. Which of the following cardiac rhythms does the ECG strip (see image) indicate?

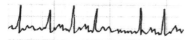

    a. Ventricular fibrillation
    b. Ventricular tachycardia
    c. Atrial fibrillation
    d. Atrial flutter

70. A client is to be discharged on warfarin (Coumadin®) therapy, and the nurse is teaching the client about the medication. Which of the following statements by the client indicates that the client's education has been effective? *Select all that apply.*
    a. "I should use a soft toothbrush."
    b. "My stools will routinely be black."
    c. "Swimming is a good choice for exercise."
    d. "I should wear a Medical Alert bracelet."
    e. "I should avoid all green, leafy vegetables."

71. A client has had a central catheter inserted for administration of parenteral nutrition. An X-ray was taken to ensure correct positioning prior to commencing infusions. The X-ray report indicates that the catheter tip is in the right atrium. Which of the following actions by the nurse is correct?
    a. Hold the infusion and notify the MD.
    b. Gently withdraw the catheter 2 to 3 inches.
    c. Begin the infusion as the catheter is placed correctly.
    d. Gently insert the catheter 2 to 3 inches further.

72. A client was to receive 1 g of vancomycin intravenously in 200 mL of iso-osmotic solution over 60 minutes per infusion pump. However, the IV administration was discontinued after 45 minutes because the client developed nausea and chills. How many milligrams of vancomycin did the client receive? *Record your answer using a whole number.*

73. A client is receiving enteral feedings through a nasogastric tube, and the nurse is administering the client's medications. Which of the following can be administered through the NG tube? *Select all that apply.*
    a. Hard extended-release capsules (opened, crushed, and dissolved)
    b. Pills (crushed and dissolved)
    c. Enteric-coated tablets (crushed and dissolved)
    d. Liquid suspension
    e. Soft-gel capsules (dissolved)
    f. Sublingual wafer (dissolved)

74. The nurse is monitoring a client following postoperative cardiac catheterization and is checking the client's oxygen saturation (SPO2) per pulse oximetry. The nurse recognizes that the SPO2 should be maintained above what percentage in most clients to ensure adequate oxygenation? *Record your answer using a whole number.*

75. An older adult has become very confused after surgery for repair of a hip fracture. The client has repeatedly tried to climb over the bedrails and the nurse is considering placing the client in a Posey vest that is secured to the bed. Which of the following must the nurse consider when applying restraints to a client? *Select all that apply.*
    a. An alternate method should be tried prior to applying a restraint.
    b. Confused clients are almost always safer in restraints.
    c. Restraints must be removed and the client reassessed at least every 2 hours.
    d. A written policy for application of restraints must be in place.
    e. The most restrictive restraint should be applied.
    f. The nurse does not need an order for a restraint if the client is in danger.

76. The nurse is working with mothers and newborns. When educating a new mother about security measures to protect her infant, which of the following should the nurse include?
    a. "Never leave your infant unattended for more than 5 minutes."
    b. "Only allow people in hospital attire to remove the infant from the mother's room."
    c. "Notify your assigned nurse if anyone attempts to carry the child from the room in his/her arms."
    d. "Anyone with a hospital ID can be considered safe."

77. The nurse must administer 120 mg of amoxicillin oral suspension to a child. However, the only dosage available in the pharmacy is 200 mg per 5 mL. How many milliliters of suspension should the nurse administer? *Record your answer using a whole number only.*

78. Based on clinical findings, the physician suspects that a 65-year-old client has kidney disease and has ordered a blood-urea-nitrogen (BUN) test. Which of the following results is within normal limits?
    a. 5 mg/dL
    b. 15 mg/dL
    c. 40 mg/dL
    d. 100 mg/dL

79. A physician has ordered the HbA1c test for a client who complains of increased thirst and urination. Which of the following results (on two separate testings) is the lowest value considered diagnostic for diabetes mellitus?
    a. 3.5 to 4.5%
    b. 4.5 to 6%
    c. 5.7 to 6.4%
    d. ≥6.5%

80. A client with an artificial eye is too ill to remove the eye, but the lids are crusted and irritated, so the nurse must remove the prosthesis for cleaning and to inspect the eye socket. The nurse has washed hands and applied disposable gloves. Place the remaining steps to removing the prosthesis (Roman numerals) in the correct order.
    I.   Gently retract the upper lid.
    II.   Exert slight pressure below the eyelid and slip index finger under prosthesis.
    III.   Break suction and slide prosthesis out of eye.
    IV.   Gently retract the lower eyelid against the orbital ridge with the thumb.
    a. (First)
    b. (Second)
    c. (Third)
    d. (Fourth)

81. If a nurse accidentally punctures a finger with a needle after withdrawing blood from a client, which of the following actions should be carried out first?
    a. Notify a supervisor.
    b. Wash the puncture area with soap and water.
    c. Apply pressure to the wound.
    d. File an incident/injury report.

82. When withdrawing blood from a peripheral vein in the arm and using a tourniquet, what is the maximum duration of time in minutes that the tourniquet should be left in place? *Record your answer using a whole number.*
        _____minute(s)

83. Which of the following factors increase the risk of developing deep vein thrombosis (DVT)? *Select all that apply.*
    a. Being underweight
    b. Smoking
    c. Having surgery
    d. Taking oral contraceptives
    e. High-protein diet
    f. Immobility

84. A client with COPD must have the arterial blood gas (ABG) test and asks the nurse to explain the purpose of the test. Which of the following information should the nurse include? *Select all that apply.*
    a. ABGs measure the levels of carbon dioxide, oxygen, and acidity in the blood.
    b. ABGs help to evaluate the effectiveness of treatment.
    c. ABGs measure the degree of anemia that has developed.
    d. ABGs can help to determine the need for supplemental oxygen.

85. The nurse is doing a digital removal of stool for a client with a large fecal impaction resulting from opioid use when the client feels faint, and assessment of vital signs shows a marked decrease in pulse. Which of the following is the **most** likely reason for the change in pulse rate?
    a. Stimulation of the vagus nerve
    b. Onset of shock
    c. Internal bleeding
    d. Anxiety

86. A 15-year-old client took a full bottle of extra-strength acetaminophen in a suicide attempt 5 hours prior to admission to the emergency department for treatment, and the serum level of the drug is 180 mcg/mL. Which of the following interventions does the nurse anticipate? *Select all that apply.*
    a. Antidote: 72-hour N-acetylcysteine (NAC) protocol
    b. Supportive care
    c. GI decontamination with activated charcoal
    d. Monitoring of hepatic function
    e. Psychiatric consultation

87. The nurse has inserted a nasogastric tube and aspirated gastric contents to check the pH with color-coded pH paper. The aspirate is dark brown, and pH measures slightly less than 5 according to the color chart. What does this pH usually indicate?
    a. Gastric aspirate
    b. Intestinal aspirate
    c. Respiratory aspirate
    d. Inconclusive results

88. A client who is to undergo electroconvulsive therapy for severe depression is quite anxious about the treatment and asks the nurse what to expect after treatment. Which of the following information should the nurse include? *Select all that apply.*
   a. The client will experience confusion for a short time.
   b. Headache and muscle soreness are common.
   c. Some degree of memory loss, usually transient, may occur.
   d. Possible urinary incontinence may occur for 12 hours.
   e. The client may experience hallucinations for 2 to 3 weeks.

89. A 40-year-old male client has been diagnosed with Huntington disease and his spouse asks the nurse if their 3-year-old son should be tested to determine if the son inherited the genetic disorder. Which of the following is the **most** appropriate response?
   a. "It's best to go ahead and have testing completed so that you don't have to worry about it."
   b. "You should discuss the pros and cons about this with a genetic counselor."
   c. "That's a bad idea. Your son may not want to know if he has the disease."
   d. "Most authorities recommended letting your child decide when he is older and can make an informed decision about testing."

90. Following femoral catheterization for percutaneous coronary intervention (PCI), the client has increasing pain in the catheterization site, and the nurse notes visible edema and induration surrounding the site. The nurse suspects a hematoma and notifies the physician. Which of the following interventions does the nurse anticipate? *Select all that apply.*
   a. Apply pressure to the site.
   b. Mark margins of edematous, indurated area.
   c. Monitor hemoglobin and hematocrit.
   d. Maintain bedrest.
   e. Administration of clotting factors.

91. If both parents are carriers of the defective gene for a disease with an autosomal recessive inheritance, what percentage chance does each child have of inheriting the gene from both parents and developing the disorder? *Report your answer using a whole number.*
   _____%

92. A client has been diagnosed with immune thrombocytic purpura (ITP). Which of the following signs and symptoms indicate increased thrombocytopenia? *Select all that apply.*
   a. Frequent nosebleeds
   b. Petechiae and increased bruising
   c. Temporary changes in vision
   d. Numbness and tingling in distal limbs
   e. Confusion

93. A client seen in the emergency department for influenza asks for an antibiotic prescription. Which of the following guidelines are important in helping the client decrease the risk of developing an antibiotic-resistant infection? *Select all that apply.*
   a. Stop taking antibiotics as soon as symptoms subside.
   b. Do not take antibiotics for viral infections, as they do no good.
   c. Do not take preventive antibiotics to avoid infection.
   d. Follow prescription directions when taking antibiotics.
   e. Take the same antibiotic for every infection.

94. A client who received an IV antibiotic mistakenly believed she was receiving opioid analgesia and reported a few minutes later that the medication had relieved her pain. Which of the following is the **most** likely reason for the client's response?

    a. The client was lying about having pain.
    b. The antibiotic actually relieved the pain.
    c. The client experienced a placebo effect.
    d. The client's pain subsided coincidentally.

95. A client has suffered a severe traumatic brain injury and is being treated in the ICU. Which of the following interventions does the nurse anticipate to control intracranial pressure? *Select all that apply.*

    a. Elevate the head of the bed.
    b. Administer oxygen to maintain a PaO_2 >85 mm Hg.
    c. Maintain neutral alignment of the head.
    d. Administer sedation to prevent or reduce agitation.
    e. Maintain body temperature below normal limits.

96. A pregnant client is keeping a "kick count" log during the last trimester. Which of the following may indicate fetal distress?

    a. Fewer than 5 movements within 2 hours
    b. Fewer than 5 movements within 1 hour
    c. Fewer than 10 movements within 2 hours
    d. Fewer than 10 movements within 1 hour

97. Which of the following are intrinsic factors that increase risk of falls in older adults? *Select all that apply.*

    a. Sensory impairment
    b. Steep and unlit stairs
    c. Throw rugs and loose carpet
    d. Chronic illness
    e. Medications

98. During which stage of injury repair does the wound show evidence of erythema and edema, and phagocytosis begins?

    a. Proliferation
    b. Inflammation
    c. Hemostasis
    d. Maturation

99. A client with heart failure has a left ventricular ejection fraction of 38%. When educating the client about managing the condition, which of the follow advice should the nurse include? *Select all that apply.*

    a. The client should take frequent rest periods.
    b. The client should avoid strenuous activities.
    c. The client should stop all exercises.
    d. The client should stop smoking.
    e. The client should limit alcohol intake to 2 to 3 drinks daily.

100. Which type of behavior modification is **most** likely to benefit a client who has a severe phobia regarding spiders?
    a. Positive reinforcement
    b. Negative reinforcement
    c. Desensitization
    d. Aversion therapy

101. A pregnant client at 36 weeks' gestation has partial placenta previa and has been on bedrest at home for the previous 4 weeks. The client has started to have occasional contractions and is beginning to experience increasing vaginal bleeding. What intervention does the nurse anticipate?
    a. Tocolytic, observation, and supportive care
    b. Immediate induction and vaginal birth
    c. Transfusions and eventual vaginal birth
    d. Cesarean delivery

102. If the nurse is providing education to a male client who is HIV positive, which of the following information should the nurse include? *Select all that apply.*
    a. Need to use condoms for every sexual encounter.
    b. Need to tell sexual or needle-sharing partners about HIV status.
    c. Signs and symptoms indicating increased viral load and infections.
    d. Importance of maintaining a healthy lifestyle.
    e. Availability of support groups.

103. If a group includes only members selected on a specific basis, such as women with a history of domestic or partner abuse, how is this type of group classified?
    a. Homogeneous
    b. Closed
    c. Heterogeneous
    d. Task

104. Which of the following is the primary focus of cognitive behavioral therapy (CBT)?
    a. Gaining reward by repeating good behavior
    b. Understanding the underlying causes of behavior
    c. Acknowledging the effect behavior has on others
    d. Identifying automatic thoughts and correcting errors in thinking

105. A nurse reviewed a client's progress in smoking cessation, praising the client for being successful but suggesting the client might stop having coffee in the morning since that caused an urge to smoke. Following this session, the client appeared upset and complained that the nurse believed she was doing poorly because she wanted a cigarette with her morning coffee. Which type of cognitive distortion is the client exhibiting?
    a. Overgeneralization
    b. Mental filter
    c. All-or-nothing thinking
    d. Magnification

106. A client has accidentally splashed a toxic (although not caustic) substance in his right eye and the nurse must flush the eye. Which of the following steps are correct? *Select all that apply.*

    a. Position client head down and on the left side.

    b. Irrigate with bulb syringe tip about one-half inch above eye.

    c. Flush for about 5 minutes.

    d. Hold eyelid open with thumb and index finger while flushing.

    e. Hold an emesis basin against left face to contain irrigant.

107. A postoperative client whose oxygen saturation has been stable at 96% to 98% suddenly shows a drop to 80%. What initial response is **most** indicated?

    a. Notify physician.

    b. Administer oxygen.

    c. Assess client and reposition pulse oximeter.

    d. Collect an arterial specimen for ABGs.

108. A client has had 4 pregnancies. She experienced one miscarriage at 12 weeks, had one stillborn birth at 34 weeks, a healthy son at 38 weeks, and a healthy daughter at 40 weeks. How would the client's obstetric history be classified?

    a. Gravida 3, Para 2

    b. Gravida 4, Para 4

    c. Gravida 4, Para 3

    d. Gravida 4, Para 2

109. Which of the following immunizations is usually administered to neonates within hours of birth?

    a. Rotavirus

    b. Polio

    c. Hepatitis A

    d. Hepatitis B

110. Using Naegele's rule for estimating the due date for a pregnancy, if a client's last menstrual cycle started on September 6 and ended September 10, when is the client's approximate due date?

    a. June 6

    b. June 13

    c. June 10

    d. June 17

111. In many cultures, pregnancy is viewed as a natural rather than a medical condition. How does this affect prenatal care?

    a. Pregnant women often seek prenatal care later and less frequently.

    b. These views have little effect on prenatal care.

    c. Pregnant women believe prenatal care is harmful to the fetus.

    d. These views often result in increased rates of fetal mortality.

112. A fundamentalist Muslim woman and her spouse come to the emergency department when the pregnant woman develops premature contractions and slight vaginal bleeding; however, the only physician available is a male. Which of the following initial responses is **most** appropriate?

    a. Ask the woman's permission for treatment by a male physician.

    b. Ask the woman's husband's permission for treatment by a male physician.

    c. Delay examination by a physician until a female physician can be located.

    d. Proceed with examination by the male physician.

113. Which cephalic presentation is most common during delivery of a neonate?

    a. Vertex

    b. Face

    c. Military

    d. Brow

114. Two Mexican immigrant families live closely together and share goods, services, and childcare. To which of the following family structures does this model correspond?

    a. Kinship network

    b. Binuclear

    c. Nuclear

    d. Extended

115. A 65-year-old client who recently retired from many years of working full-time for a company has become increasingly unmotivated and states he feels as though he has no purpose. Which of the following recommendations are **most** appropriate? *Select all that apply.*

    a. Volunteer or get a part-time job.

    b. Participate in community activities.

    c. Join a senior citizen's group.

    d. Be thankful he can afford to retire.

    e. Ask to have retirement reversed.

116. The first-time mother of a 6-month old infant is concerned that the child's physical development is delayed because the child cannot crawl. Which of the following is the **most** appropriate response?

    a. "Most infants can crawl by 9 months."

    b. "Most infants can crawl by 6 months."

    c. "Don't worry, infants vary widely in abilities."

    d. "Look at all your child can do!"

117. A 14-year-old client has been diagnosed with celiac disease after a long history of diarrhea, anemia, and weight loss. What type of diet does the nurse anticipate the client will require?

    a. High protein

    b. Dairy free

    c. Low carbohydrate

    d. Gluten free

118. A 68-year-old client states he decided not to take the herpes zoster (shingles) immunization because his friend had the immunization and still developed shingles. Which of the following information should the nurse include when discussing this issue with the client? *Select all that apply.*

   a. Shingles rarely occurs after immunization.
   b. The immunization decreases the severity of infection.
   c. The immunization decreases the likelihood of postherpetic syndrome.
   d. The immunization cuts the chance of developing shingles in half.
   e. The client should never take advice from friends.

119. A nulliparous client has been admitted after 12 hours of mild contractions at home. On examination, the client is found to be fully effaced and dilated to 3 cm. Contractions are every 5 minutes and last approximately 60 seconds. The client asks the nurse approximately how long it should take to get to 10 cm dilation. Which of the following is the **most** appropriate response?

   a. Approximately 3 hours
   b. Approximately 4 hours
   c. Approximately 5 hours
   d. Approximately 7 hours

120. The nurse is serving on the performance improvement committee, which has agreed to some changes in procedures on the basis of evidence-based research. If the committee wants to convince staff members to comply with the changes, which of the following actions should the committee carry out first?

   a. Identify and gain support of key staff.
   b. Explain the consequences of failure to comply.
   c. Determine a reward system for compliance.
   d. Clearly outline expectations in written format.

Answers and Explanations

1. D: The period of maximal respiratory depression after subcutaneous injection of morphine sulfate is approximately 90 minutes while it is 30 minutes for intramuscular and 7 minutes for intravenous. The respiratory center sensitivity should return to normal within 3 hours, but minute volume may remain impaired for up to 5 hours, so clients should be monitored carefully for indications of respiratory depression. IV morphine peaks at approximately 20 minutes while IM peaks at 30 to 60 minutes and SQ at 50 to 90 minutes.

2. C: Two hours of activity are necessary in each 24-hour period to prevent disuse syndrome with muscle atrophy and joint contractures, but periods of exercise should be spaced and not done all at one time. Exercises may include ambulation, active and passive range-of-motion exercises, isometric exercises, and resistive isometric exercises. Clients should be encouraged to do as much independently as possible, and children may engage in active play activities.

3.

Minor injury	Immediate care	Delayed care	Unsalvageable
A. II Sprain, cuts	B. I Arterial bleed	C. IV Fx femur	D. III Crush injuries

A-II: Minor injuries can safely be attended to later. The injured are generally alert and responsive and ambulatory ("walking wounded"). B-I: People with life-threatening injuries must be tended to immediately, so they have first priority. C-IV: People with moderate to serious injuries that are not immediately life threatening can receive delayed care and are second priority. D-III: Those who are unsalvageable, meaning their injuries are incompatible with life, have the lowest priority.

4. B: As an advocate for the client, the nurse has a responsibility to inform the physician that the client's Advance Directive specifically states he is not to receive intravenous fluids. Many times, physicians order treatments without referring to the Advance Directive, so the nurse should always be aware of client's preferences and should communicate them. If the physician insists on the treatment, then the nurse should contact a supervisor to determine if there is an organizational policy regarding the issue.

5. A and B: Anti-embolic compression stockings must be applied properly, or they can have a constrictive effect. The stocking must be without wrinkles and the top must not be turned down as this makes a constrictive band that can impair venous circulation. The stockings should be removed and reapplied at least every 8 hours so that the skin can be examined and wrinkles removed. The client correctly holds onto the toe and turns the stocking inside out before applying, and putting a small amount of baby powder or talcum powder on the skin may make application easier.

6. B: Chest discomfort and hiccupping are often indications that the atrial lead of a pacemaker has become dislodged and is stimulating the phrenic nerve, resulting in persistent hiccupping. If phrenic nerve stimulation is caused by output, then reprogramming may alleviate the problem, but if leads are displaced, then they must be replaced, and this is a medical emergency. In some cases, a lead may be too close to the diaphragm, resulting in repeated stimulation, especially if the patient is very thin.

7. B, C, D, and E: Neurological changes associated with aging include short-term memory loss, but dementia does not normally occur unless there is an underlying disorder. Peripheral nerve cells may begin to degenerate, causing muscles of the arms and legs to atrophy. The threshold for sensory input may increase and vibratory sensation may decrease. Autonomic changes cause reduced perspiration so that core temperature is higher before sweating is induced. Post-operative delirium is more likely to occur in older adults than younger.

8. C: *Staphylococcus aureus* is a common skin bacterium, and some strains, such as methicillin-resistant *Staphylococcus aureus* (MRSA), are especially virulent. Skin infections with pustular lesions may develop and spread quickly. Common manifestations of MRSA infections include impetigo, cellulitis, boils, abscesses, and rashes. Because the infection may spread systemically to internal organs, the infection must be aggressively treated with antibiotics.

9. A: While ideally printed materials should be available in a number of languages, if none are available in the language needed, then the nurse should contact a medical translator. Telephone translation services are available if speakers cannot be found locally. Children should not be asked to translate for adults as they may not completely understand and may not translate correctly. The nurse should not depend on diagrams and pantomime if medications or specific treatments are involved, and non-English speakers may not have personal access to people who can adequately translate.

10. 100%: Bioavailability refers to the amount of a drug that is absorbed unchanged into the systemic circulation. Morphine is poorly absorbed through the oral route because of the way it is metabolized in the intestines and liver, but medications that are administered intravenously immediately enter the systemic circulation and the bioavailability is 100%. Intramuscular and transdermal administration of medications also have high bioavailability, so when switching a client from oral medications to another form, the dosage may need to be adjusted.

11. C: If the umbilical cord becomes soiled with urine or feces, it should be washed with mild soap and water, rinsed, and dried. Wiping with alcohol is no longer recommended as it may increase irritation of the surrounding skin. The cord should not be covered with clothing and should be protected by folding the top of the diaper under the cord instead of covering the cord with the diaper. The baby should not be immersed in water until the cord falls off in 10 to 14 days.

12. 1.7 mL: The calculation is as follows:
Required dose X amount of solution/mg of medication.
85 X 2/100
85 X 0.02 = 1.7 mL.
Using an algebraic formula
100/2 = 85/x
100 x = 170
100x/100 = 170/100
x = 1.7 mL

13. A-II: Place a small pillow between client's knees. B-IV: Cross client's arms across chest in preparation for turn. C-I: Grasping draw sheet at shoulder and lower hips, roll patient on count of three. D-III: (Opposite nurse) Place pillows along length of client's back to provide support and maintain the person in the side-lying position. After the client is positioned, the nurse should check body alignment and client's comfort level to determine if more pillows or rolled bath blankets are needed for support.

14. 30 g: To convert pounds to kilograms, divide pounds by 2.2 (132/2.2 = 60). Then, multiply the kilograms of weight by the per-kilogram dose (60 X 0.5 = 30 g). When converting kilograms to pounds, multiply kilograms by 2.2. Mannitol is an osmotic diuretic that is used to increase excretion of sodium and water in order to reduce ICP and brain mass, especially after traumatic brain injury. Mannitol may also be used to shrink the cells of the blood-brain barrier to facilitate other medications breaching this barrier.

15. B: Lead V4. The 12-lead ECG gives a picture of electrical activity from 12 perspectives through placement of 10 body leads:
4 limb leads for both arms and both legs
Precordial leads:
V1: right sternal border at 4th intercostal space
V2: left sternal border at 4th intercostal space
V3: midway between V2 and V4
V4: left midclavicular line at 5th intercostal space
V5: horizontal to V4 at left anterior axillary line
V6: horizontal to V5 at left midaxillary line

16. B and D: The elbow range of motion should include the following:
Flexion: Bend elbow until the hand is level with the shoulder.
Extension: Straighten elbow until arm is almost vertical (150 degrees) without forcing.
Hyperextension: Bend elbow and extend lower arm as far back as possible (10 to 20 degrees) beyond vertical.
Range-of-motion exercises for the elbow can be incorporated into activities of daily living. Eating, bathing, shaving, combing the hair, and brushing the teeth all involve both flexion and extension of the elbow.

17. B: When conducting measurements for crutches with a client in standing position, the tips of the crutches should be placed approximately 4 to 6 inches to the side and 4 to 6 inches in front of the client's feet. The crutch pads should be 1.5 to 2 inches below the axilla and the client cautioned not to bear weight under the axilla but to hold the crutches against the lateral chest wall to prevent nerve damage. The client's elbows should be slightly flexed (15 to 30 degrees) when grasping the handgrip.

18. D: Because the client is confused, the nurse should place the ring in a secured container, according to organizational policy, which may vary widely. The ring should not be given to a friend or family member without consent and should not be replaced on the client's finger as the client may remove it again. The nurse should document when the ring was found, where it was found, and where it was placed for safekeeping. If witnesses are required, their names should be documented as well.

19. February 2014: Depending on the formula one uses, the exact date may vary. Starting with the first day of the last menstrual period on May 1, 2013, and using Naegele's formula, subtract 3 months and add 6 days. This would place the delivery date at February 7, 2014. Another formula adds 9 months and 7 days, placing the delivery date at February 8. Still other formulas place the date at February 5. Generally, gestation is considered to be 280 days in duration.

20. 0.02: A microgram (µg) is one-millionth of a gram (g). There are 1000 milligrams in a gram and 1000 micrograms in a milligram. In order to convert micrograms to milligrams, divide the micrograms by 1000 (20/1000 = 0.02 mg). To convert milligrams to micrograms, multiply the milligrams by 1000 (0.02mg X 1000 = 20 micrograms). Other conversions:
mg to cg = mg/10; cg to mg = cg X 10
g to cg = g X 100; cg to g = cg/100
mg to g = mg/1000; g to mg = g X 1000

21. D: The nurse should not attempt a procedure for which the nurse has not been trained and is not familiar. Chest physiotherapy may result in injury to a child if done incorrectly. The nurse should tell the physician that he has not been trained to do chest physiotherapy on children but will attempt to locate another staff person knowledgeable about the procedure. Nurses should not rely on parents or other family members to explain procedures.

22. A, B, and C: Increased estrogen production during pregnancy promotes hyperplasia of vaginal mucosa and increased production of mucus. This can create a warm, moist environment that promotes *Candida* monilial infection. The client should be advised to bathe daily and wear cotton panties but to avoid wearing nylon panties or pantyhose, panty liners, and tight clothing as these can increase the temperature and prevent airflow. The client should also be advised not to douche. Topical treatments that can be used include miconazole, butoconazole, clotrimazole, tioconazole, nystatin, or terconazole.

23. C: After withdrawing the correct dosage of heparin into a syringe, approximately 0.2 to 0.3 mL of air should be drawn into the syringe. This air helps to clear the remaining drug from the syringe and to "lock" the medication into the tissue. After the air is drawn into the syringe, the cap should be replaced carefully and the syringe pointed needle down so that the air bubble rises to the top of the syringe. Heparin injection sites should be rotated with usual sites in the upper and lower abdomen and anterior thighs.

24. C: **Lochia rubra** (days 1 to 3 or 4): Dark red discharge with small clots (smaller than nickel size). Larger clots may indicate hemorrhage or bleeding from vaginal lacerations. **Lochia serosa** (days 4 to 10): Pinkish to brownish discharge, gradually lightening as the number of red blood cells decreases. **Lochia alba** (persists an additional 2 to 85 days with average of 24 days): Yellowish discharge. Lochia alba ceases when the cervix closes. This decreases the chance of uterine infection.

25. A, B, and D: The Z-track injection technique is especially indicated for IM drugs that are irritating to the tissues, such as iron, haloperidol, hydroxyzine, and interferon. Procedure:
Fill syringe, including approximately 0.3 mL of air to provide an air lock.
Choose site (avoid deltoid). Don gloves and cleanse skin in a circular pattern.
Place 3 fingers or ulnar surface of nondominant hand on skin and pull skin laterally.
Inject at 90 degrees over 3 to 5 seconds in the spot that fingers or hand was initially placed.

Hold needle in place for 10 seconds.
Withdraw needle and release tissue.

26. D: **Extended kin network:** Two nuclear families live closely together and share goods, services, and childcare. This model is common in Hispanic families. **Nuclear:** Husband-wife-children model in which the mother usually stays home and cares for the children while the husband is the wage earner (7% of American families). **Dual career/dual earner:** Both parents work (66% of two-parent families) although one may work more than the other. **Extended:** Multigenerational or shared households with friends or family who share childcare responsibilities.

27. C and D: Sublingual and buccal medications should not be administered if the mucous membranes in the mouth are red and irritated or if the client is dehydrated, because these conditions may interfere with absorption of the medication. While severe confusion may pose a problem, as long as the client is cognizant enough to cooperate with administration, dementia alone is not a contraindication. Being edentulous is not a contraindication because sublingual wafers absorb readily and do not have to be held in place for extended periods.

28. A, B, D, and E: Production of milk sometimes outstrips demand in the first 2–3 days because the baby ingests small amounts, so the breasts often become engorged. Nursing frequently (every 2–3 hours) and gently massaging the breast toward the nipple while nursing can help reduce engorgement. If the areola is hard, some milk should be manually expressed to soften the areola before the infant latches on. Breast pumps and heat (except in a shower) may increase engorgement. Cold compresses, acetaminophen, or ibuprofen may provide relief. Engorgement usually recedes within 24 to 48 hours.

29. D: While all solid medications, such as pills, tablets, and capsules, should be delivered to the client in a disposable paper medicine cup, all individually wrapped doses should be opened in the presence of the client after verifying the client's identification with two identifiers. Prior to administration, the client should be assessed for level of consciousness, nausea and vomiting, and difficulty swallowing. Calibrated medicine cups are used for liquid preparations of 5 mL or more, but smaller amounts should be measured in a syringe for accuracy.

30. A: While knowledge of childcare is helpful to a new mother, it does not necessarily promote attachment between a newborn and mother. Important factors include frequent contact, starting as soon after birth as possible; breastfeeding, ideally starting within 60 minutes of birth; and utilizing rooming-in so that the baby stays with the mother rather than in a nursery, allowing the mother to respond readily to the infant's needs. New mothers should be reassured that bonding may take time and that it is normal if the mother does not feel an immediate attachment.

31. A and D: Schedule I drugs, such as cocaine and LSD, have high potential for abuse and no accepted medical use. Schedule II drugs pose potential for abuse and addiction and include most commonly used narcotics (codeine, hydrocodone). Schedule III drugs, such as anabolic steroids and intermediate-acting barbiturates, have lesser potential for abuse. Schedule IV drugs, including benzodiazepines, may lead to limited physical or psychological dependence. Schedule V drugs, including cough suppressants, have low potential for abuse. Schedule VI drugs include those with low potential for abuse and addiction, such as OTC drugs like ibuprofen and diphenhydramine (Benadryl®).

32. D: African-Americans have the greatest risk of developing diabetes mellitus type 2, although risks are also high for Mexican Americans, Native Americans and Hawaiians, and some Asian Americans, all of whom also have high rates of hypertension and obesity. Risk is also increased if a family member has the disease. Diabetes mellitus type 2 is the most prevalent type, accounting for 90% to 95% of cases of diabetes, and is closely associated with obesity.

33. B: Nocturnal myoclonus is a toxic effect of opioid analgesics. Toxicity may occur because they have metabolites that are neuroexcitatory. The medication dosage should be reduced by at least half and a benzodiazepine administered. The drug may also be changed to an equianalgesic, but opioids should not be discontinued as the client may experience withdrawal and inadequate pain control. Naloxone is not an effective solution for toxicity, and flumazenil is a benzodiazepine antagonist.

34. A, C, and D: Most people who are sexually active remain so, so even though the adolescent may be adamant that she is not going to have sex again until she is married, the nurse should advise her that ALL people need to know about safe sex and that she can share what she has learned with her friends. Many people believe that a condom is not necessary for oral sex, but they are mistaken. "I'm confused about different birth control methods" is a clear indication that information is needed.

35. A: Naloxone (Narcan®) is an opioid antagonist and should be administered if clients exhibit signs of acute respiratory and/or circulatory depression, although it must be used cautiously with opioid addiction as clients may experience withdrawal symptoms. For an opioid overdose in an adult client, the usual initial dose is 0.4 to 2 mg intravenously, repeated at 2- to 3-minute intervals. If the client does not have adequate response after administration of 10 mg, then other causes for the symptoms should be explored.

36. C: The maximum adult dosage of acetaminophen in 24 hours is 4 g. A single dose of 20 to 25 g can result in hepatic necrosis and liver failure with 25 g often resulting in death. The toxic reaction of acetaminophen is potentiated by alcohol. Clients often exhibit mild symptoms of nausea, vomiting, and abdominal pain in the first two days after overdose but by the second or third day, signs of liver injury become evident with elevations of transaminase, lactic hydrogenase, and bilirubin and prolonged prothrombin time. Oral N-acetylcysteine is administered to prevent or reduce liver damage.

37. B: A complete initial assessment, ongoing assessments, frequent evaluations of lithium levels, and client education are all essential. Plasma levels of lithium must be frequently monitored for lithium toxicity, which can lead to death. The normal therapeutic range of lithium is 0.6 to 1.4 mEq/L for adults. About 1 client in 25 develops goiter from lithium-induced hypothyroidism, so clients must be evaluated for thyroid disease prior to beginning therapy and on a regular basis afterward. Clients should avoid NSAIDs and dehydration.

38. A: Children younger than 8 years should not receive tetracycline because it can result in discoloration and inadequate calcification of permanent teeth if taken during the process of tooth calcification. Because this process is usually completed by the time the child is 8, the medication may be used in older children. The pediatric dose is 20 to 50 mg/kg orally in 4 equal doses over 24 hours. Discoloration and inadequate calcification of permanent teeth may also result from fetal exposure to tetracycline.

39. C: The nurse should report the observations to the infection control nurse. The nurse should avoid making assumptions about cause and effect until an investigation is concluded. While increased rates of infection may indicate surgeon negligence, they can also indicate that the physician simply has more clients on the unit than other physicians, that an operating room is contaminated, that surgical procedures are not followed by all surgical staff, or that the physician has clients who are immunocompromised or more susceptible to infection because of condition.

40. A: Bulk laxatives, such as Metamucil® and Citrucel®, are usually the safest for most people because their action most closely mimics human physiology. The polysaccharides or cellulose derivatives contained in the laxatives combine with fluids in the intestine to form gels, which stimulate peristalsis and evacuation. Clients must be advised to drink adequate liquids because bulk laxatives may induce constipation if clients are dehydrated. Clients should be encouraged to increase bulk naturally in the diet through eating bran, fruits, and vegetables.

41. A-II, B-I, C-IV, D-III: The modified Allen test is conducted to ensure that the ulnar artery provides adequate circulation, including collateral circulation, so that the radial artery can be used to obtain an arterial blood sample. The patient extends the wrist over a rolled towel and makes a fist. Steps:
A. (Step 1) II. Palpate the ulnar and radial pulses and apply pressure to both arteries.
B. (Step 2) I. Ask the client to open and close the hand until the skin blanches.
C. (Step 3) IV. Release the ulnar artery while maintaining pressure on the radial artery.
D. (Step 4) III. Observe the hand for color. The hand should regain natural color within 5 seconds if circulation is adequate.

42. 60 percent: Each hemoglobin molecule has four iron-containing heme sites to which oxygen can bind. As oxygen binds to the heme, the hemoglobin becomes saturated. The SO2 level is the percentage of total heme sites in the blood saturated with oxygen. At 80 to 90 PO2, hemoglobin is fully saturated so increased PO2 can't increase saturation. The critical point for PO2 is 60% because below this point there is a marked decrease in saturation. PO2 of 60 usually corresponds to SO2 of 91%, which is referred to as the "ICU" point.

43. A: Simply not adding extra salt to food is insufficient because many foods, especially processed foods, are very high in sodium. Clients need to follow dietary guidelines and learn to read labels. DASH nutrient goals (based on a 2100 calorie diet) limit Na to 1500 to 2300 mg, total fat 27%, protein 18%, and carbohydrates 55%.
Grains (whole grains preferred): 6 to 8 daily
Vegetables and fruits: 4 to 5 each daily
Milk products (non- or low-fat): 2 to 3 daily
Lean meat, poultry, fish: ≤6 ounces daily
Nuts, seeds, legumes: 4 to 5 weekly
Fats and oils: 2 to 3 daily
Sweet/added sugar: ≤5 weekly

44. D: Once the platelet count drops below 50,000, the blood's ability to clot is impaired. If a client is scheduled for an invasive procedure, the risk of bleeding increases at this level; otherwise, risk is not generally significant until the platelet count drops to below 20,000. At this level, clients usually begin to develop signs of bleeding, such as petechial, nosebleeds,

bleeding gums, and increased menstrual flow and require administration of platelets. For milder thrombocytopenia, observation and steroids are indicated with immunosuppressive therapy and splenectomy used for more severe disease.

45. 2600: The absolute neutrophil count (ANC) is calculated indirectly based on the total white blood cell count and percentages of neutrophils and bands:
ANC = Total WBC X (% neutrophils + % bands/100)
ANC = 5200 X (45 + 5/100) = 5200 X 0.50 = 2600 mm³
A normal ANC for adults is 1800 to 7700, so this is within normal range. The risk of infection increases markedly when the ANC falls to 1000, and risk is severe at 500.

46. D: Passwords are used to protect client's records from unauthorized access, so anyone who is authorized should be able to access the records with his/her own password. Therefore, the nurse should not allow anyone else to use his/her password. Passwords can also be used to track an individual nurse's activity in the electronic health record, so the nurse may be putting his/her own career in jeopardy by allowing someone else to use the password.

47. A: The nurse should communicate the client's financial concerns to the social worker: "I can't afford to hire anyone to help me when I am discharged." The social worker will have knowledge about resources and qualifications for applying for assistance, such as Medicaid. The social worker can assess the client's income and support system to help determine the best plan for the client. Concerns about necessary equipment and managing self-care, such as showering safely, should be communicated to physical and occupational therapists.

48. B: Clients who are alert and responsive have the right to refuse any treatment, so the most appropriate action is for the nurse to notify the physician and ensure that orders are in place for comfort measures, such as adequate analgesia. The nurse should not insist that the client accept treatments against her wishes, as this may be construed as coercion, and should not ask family members to intervene. Most religions view refusing life-prolonging treatments as different from active suicide, but it is inappropriate to use religious beliefs to make clients feel guilty.

49. 180: The formula for calculating total cholesterol is LDL + HDL + (triglycerides/5).
100 + 50 + (150/5) = 100 + 50 +30 = 180
An alternate formula is LDL + HDL + (Triglycerides X 0.20).
100 + 50 + (150 X 0.20) = 100 + 50 +30 = 180
The optimal total cholesterol level is below 200. Optimal LDL is below 100. Optimal HDL is ≥60. Normal triglyceride level is below 150.

50. A: (First) III Inspection, B (Second) IV Auscultation, C (Third) I Percussion, D (Fourth) II Palpation. While the usual order of examination techniques is to begin with examination and then progress to palpation, percussion, and finally auscultation, because stimulating the abdomen may increase bowel sounds and contractions, the nurse should examine the abdomen differently from least invasive to most, beginning with inspection. This is followed by auscultation to assess normal bowel sounds, then percussion to assess for gas, fluid, and consolidated masses, and finally to palpation.

51. A-II Aorta, B-IV Renal, C-III Iliac, D-I Femoral:

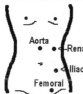 Auscultation should be done gently to avoid stimulating bowel contractions over the sites indicated on the diagram. For hypertensive patients, the renal arteries should be assessed bilaterally as bruits may be heard, suggesting arterial occlusion. Systolic bruits are fairly common and often benign, but bruits that have both systolic and diastolic components indicate turbulent blood flow. Aortic, iliac, and femoral bruits may be heard with peripheral arterial insufficiency.

52. B: The client should always urinate prior to a pelvic exam. When positioning the client for the exam, the client's head should be elevated slightly as this helps relax abdominal muscles. The client should be advised to keep her arms at her side or folded across her chest and not over her head as this position may cause the abdominal muscles to tense. The nurse should explain the steps to the procedure and ensure that the speculum is warmed prior to the examination.

53. A-III Apply tourniquet, B-I Palpate vein, C-II Cleanse skin, and D-IV Perform venipuncture: The nurse should carefully examine the veins for potential puncture sites prior to performing the venipuncture. The nurse may apply a tourniquet or heat and hold the arm in dependent position. Once a vein has been selected, the tourniquet can be released while the nurse prepares materials. Then the tourniquet is applied, the vein palpated, and the skin cleansed, with venipuncture last. The nurse should avoid palpating the vein after the skin is cleansed unless wearing sterile gloves.

54 D: A nasal cannula at 3L/min delivers an FiO2 of approximately 28–32%. The flow rate for nasal cannulas ranges from 0.5 L/min (21–24% FiO2) to 6 L/min (40–44% FiO2), but should not be administered at a higher flow rate because the FiO2 will not increase, and it can result in drying of the mucous membranes. Face masks, non-rebreathing masks, partial re-breathing masks, and Venturi masks can be used if a higher FiO2 is needed.

55. A-I Client sits upright or stands. B-IV Client takes a deep breath. C-II Client places the meter in the mouth and seals lips. D-III Client expels air through the meter as forcefully as possible. The client should repeat this procedure 2 to 5 times, noting the highest number achieved. Following treatment, the client's PEFR should be within 20% of personal best, and if results are <80% of personal best, treatment may be inadequate for client's condition.

56. C: Headaches occur in about one-fifth of clients following lumbar puncture, but the headaches are usually relieved by the client's lying flat and drinking ample fluids. If headaches are severe and persistent, then this usually indicates a hole in the dura mater, and an epidural blood patch may be applied with an autologous blood specimen. The blood is injected in a small amount at the site of the lumbar puncture to create a blood clot that serves as a "patch."

57. D: The optimal position for a thoracentesis is an upright position with the client sitting and leaning over an over-bed tray table with the shoulders and upper arms supported by a pillow as this position expands the intercostal space, making insertion easier. If the client is unable to tolerate a sitting position, then the client should be positioned in the side-lying position on the unaffected side so that the thoracentesis insertion site is easily accessed.

58. D: Severe vomiting can result in metabolic alkalosis because of loss of chloride in the emesis. In a compensating measure for chloride loss, bicarbonate increases. Metabolic alkalosis may also result from gastric suctioning, diuresis, hypokalemia, and excessive mineralocorticoid or sodium bicarbonate intake. Other laboratory findings include increased pH, normal PCO2 if compensated but increased if noncompensated. Symptoms include dizziness, confusion, anxiety, muscle cramping, tingling, seizures, tetany, tachycardia, arrhythmias, nausea, vomiting, anorexia, and compensatory hypoventilation.

59. A and C: Excess fluid is removed quickly from the body during hemodialysis. This can sometimes result in fluid deficit, especially if the client has run a fever or had inadequate fluid intake. Because heparin is administered during the treatment to prevent clots from forming, the client is at increased risk of bleeding. The presence of fluid volume excess, metabolic acidosis, and pulmonary edema should be evaluated prior to hemodialysis since clients are unable to excrete adequate fluids or waste products because of impaired kidney function.

60. C: The large accumulation of fluid that can occur with ascites makes palpating the bladder difficult, so the bladder must be emptied prior to a paracentesis in order to prevent inadvertent puncture of the bladder when the needle or trocar is inserted. Clients should be positioned in upright or high Fowler's position because this helps to keep the intestines toward the back of the peritoneal cavity, preventing intestinal laceration. Usually only 4 to 5 L of fluid are removed at one time. If larger volumes are removed, the client is at risk of hypotension.

61. A, B, and D: Clients with a tracheostomy are at increased risk of fecal impaction because they cannot perform the Valsalva maneuver to bear down, so they need to be educated about bowel care and advised to use stool softeners routinely and laxatives and suppositories as needed. Additionally, they need to understand the importance of pulmonary hygiene to prevent atelectasis and infection and should be confident in all aspects of tracheostomy care, including information about what to do if the tracheostomy tube falls out.

62. A: Because of his weakness and tremors, the client will probably have difficulty preparing meals, so referral to a home meal delivery program (such as Meals on Wheels) is probably the best referral since arrangements have already been made for personal care and housekeeping. Home meal delivery programs usually provide meals 5 to 7 days a week at low cost ($2 to $4 is common). The meals are often delivered midday with a hot entrée, and many programs also provide a sandwich or other light meal for evening as well as breakfast foods (such as cereal) for the next day.

63. A and C: During a life review, clients reflect on their lives, their successes and failures, and their relationships. Some clients may begin to organize old photographs or look through photo albums. Others may want to reminisce and talk about their lives and families. Some talk about their children and parenting skills. They may talk about things they regret or choices they have made. People often try to validate that their lives had purpose through their life reviews.

64. A and E: The mother is using nonstandard treatments with mayonnaise and olive oil. While some anecdotal reports suggest this is helpful, according to the CDC there is no evidence to support these treatments. The mother should use OTC or prescription

shampoos intended to treat lice. While linens and clothes used by the child should be washed and dried in a hot air cycle for at least 5 minutes to prevent spread, treating pets, such as cats and dogs, does no good as they do not spread head lice.

65. 9%: According to the rule of nines, body surface area (BSA) is sectioned into areas that are primarily multiples of 9:
Head: 9%
Anterior trunk: 18% (9% chest and 9% abdomen)
Posterior trunk: 18% (9% upper back and 9% lower back and buttocks)
Legs: 18% each (9% anterior and 9% posterior)
Arms: 9% each (4.5% anterior and 4.5% posterior)
Genitals: 1%
The percentage of BSA that is burned is important when calculating potential fluid loss and the need for fluid and electrolyte replacement.

66. D: A positive Homan's sign—pain on palpation of the calf with dorsiflexion of the ankle—is indicative of deep vein thrombosis (DVT) although this sign occurs in only about 10%, so the absence does not preclude DVT. DVT is associated with inactivity, such as prolonged bedrest or sitting for long periods while flying, and is a complication of surgery. Clients may have pain and tenderness, erythema, elevated temperature, and unilateral edema although some exhibit no overt symptoms.

67. B: Increasing intracranial pressure is indicated by increasing BP with widening pulse pressure, decreasing pulse, and increasing temperature. The client's initial BP was 138/72 with a pulse pressure of 66 but is now 160/64 with a pulse pressure of 96. The initial pulse was 83 and has decreased to 70. Baseline temperature was 97.5°F/36.4°C and is now increased to 99.4°F/37.4°C. Restlessness and headache are early indications of increasing intracranial pressure. Clients may also have an alteration in consciousness, change in pupillary reactions, and increasing dyspnea.

68. D: If an implantable cardioverter-defibrillator fires one time and is not associated with other cardiac symptoms, this is not a medical emergency, and the patient should be advised to lie down to rest until he feels recovered from the stress of the firing and to telephone the physician to report the event. Multiple firings are a medical emergency, and the client or family member should call 9-1-1 as the firings may indicate recurrent ventricular fibrillation/ventricular tachycardia or a fractured lead. A single firing associated with symptoms (chest pain, dizziness, syncope, and shortness of breath) is also a medical emergency.

69. C: The irregular rhythm is an atrial fibrillation, which is characterized by a rapid, very irregular pulse with an atrial rate of 300 to 600 and ventricular rate of 120 to 200. Because the beats are rapid and ineffectual, the atria do not empty adequately, so blood begins to pool, increasing risk of thrombus formation and emboli. Because stroke volume decreases, cardiac output decreases, leading to myocardial ischemia and palpitations.

70. A, C, and D: Because clients are at risk for bleeding, they should use soft toothbrushes. Swimming is a good choice for exercise because the water exerts even pressure. Clients should always wear a Medical Alert bracelet or necklace indicating they are taking the anticoagulant. Stools should not be black as this is a sign of bleeding. While green leafy

vegetables are high in vitamin K, they can be eaten in normal amounts and do not need to be restricted.

71. A: The nurse should hold the infusion and notify the MD that the catheter tip is incorrectly placed, as it should be in the superior vena cava rather than the right atrium. Infusing the solutions directly into the right atrium may result in tissue damage. While the catheter needs to be withdrawn a few inches and another X-ray taken to ensure correct placement, this procedure should only be done by a physician or a specially trained nurse.

72. 750 mg: The simplest solution to the problem is to convert 1 g to 1000 mg and then, since the infusion was set for 60 minutes and three-fourths of the time elapsed, simply multiply 1000 X 0.75 = 750 mg. If using an algebraic formula:
$1000/60 = x/45$
$60x = 45,000$
$6 x = 4500$
$6x/6 = 4500/6$
$x = 750$ mg

73. B, D, and E: Pills may be crushed and diluted in 10 to 15 mL of water to be added to the NG tube feeding. Liquid forms of medications are easiest to add. Soft-gel capsules can be opened at one end and drained, but some dosage is usually lost, so dissolving the capsule in warm water first (and removing the remains of the gel capsule) is a better solution. Extended-release capsules should be opened but NOT crushed before adding to the tube. Enteric-coated tablets should not be crushed or administered per NG tube, and sublingual wafers are not absorbed through the GI tract.

74. 95%: The oximeter uses light waves to determine oxygen saturation (SPO2) and utilizes an external oximeter attached to a finger or earlobe. If a client has marked vasoconstriction, the earlobe may provide more accurate readings than the finger. Oxygen saturation should be maintained >95% although some patients with chronic respiratory disorders, such as COPD, may have lower SPO2. Oximetry is often used postoperatively to assess peripheral circulation and when patients are on mechanical ventilation.

75. A, C, and D: Restraints are used to restrict movement, activity, and access. Guidelines for restraints not part of routine care (surgical restraints, arm boards) include:
A written policy must be in place.
An assessment must be completed prior to application of restraints.
An alternative method should be tried before applying a restraint.
Restraints cannot be applied without a written order.
The least restrictive effective restraint should be used.
The nurse must remove the restraint, assess, and document findings at least every 2 hours.

76. C: While security measures may vary somewhat, generally infants should only be removed from the mother's room in a crib and never carried in someone's arms. Mothers should be informed to never leave their infants unattended, even for a few minutes to use the bathroom. If no family member is present, the mother should call her nurse. The mother should not assume hospital attire or ID alone are sufficient identification and should remain wary of any strangers asking questions about the infant.

77. 3 mL: A simple algebraic formula provides the answer:
Mg in suspension/mL = Desired dose/x (mL needed)
200/5 = 120/x
200x = 600
200x/200 = 600/200
x = 3 mL dose

78. B: Fifteen mg/dL is within normal limits (range is 8–21 for ages 14 to adult; 5–17 for newborns; 7–17 for children to 13 years; 10–31 for adults >90 years. Urea (nonprotein nitrogen compound) is an end product of protein metabolism. BUN is usually evaluated with creatinine. The normal ratio of BUN/creatinine is 15:1 to 24:1. A BUN >100 mg/dL is a critical value. Signs of an elevated BUN include restlessness, confusion, acidemia, nausea and vomiting, and coma.

79. D: While there is not total agreement about the results of HbA1c tests, generally levels of ≥6.5% are considered diagnostic of diabetes mellitus. Values of 5.7 to 6.4% are considered pre-diabetic by most authorities. Lower values are within normal limits. Because hemoglobin retains excess blood glucose and red blood cells live about 120 days, the HbA1c test shows the average blood glucose levels over a 3-month period. HbA1c is used to diagnose diabetes and monitor long-term diabetic therapy.

80. A-IV Gently retract the lower eyelid against the orbital ridge with the thumb. B-I Gently retract the upper lid. C-II Exert slight pressure below the eyelid and slip the index finger under the prosthesis. D-III Break suction and slide the prosthesis out of the eye. Once the prosthesis is removed, clean the prosthesis with soap and water and rinse well with running water to remove all soap and residue. Dry and polish the prosthesis. Retract eyelids, wash socket with clean washcloth or gauze pad moistened with warm water or NS. Wash eyelid margins with mild soap and water and dry.

81. B: If a nurse accidentally punctures a finger with a needle after withdrawing blood from a client, the nurse should immediately wash the puncture area with soap and water, being careful not to apply pressure but to allow the injury to bleed freely to facilitate washing out any virus or bacteria that may have been injected into the wound. Then, the incident should be reported to a supervisor, an incident/injury report filed, and follow-up assessment carried out.

82. 1 minute: Leaving a tourniquet in place for longer than a minute may cause the blood to concentrate below the tourniquet, and this can increase values for some tests, such as packed cell volume. The tourniquet should be applied to locate an appropriate vein and then released while the nurse puts on gloves, cleanses the site, and assembles equipment. The tourniquet is then reapplied immediately before the draw.

83. B, C, D, and F: The following factors increase the risk of developing deep vein thrombosis (DVT):
- Being overweight
- Smoking
- Having surgery
- Taking oral contraceptives

- Undergoing prolonged sitting or bedrest during which the calf muscles do not contract to help circulate the blood
- Older than 60 years
- Having some medical conditions, such as blood-clotting disorder, cancer, heart failure, pregnancy, or inflammatory bowel disease
- Immobility

84. A, B, and D: If a client with COPD asks the nurse why the client is having the arterial blood gas (ABG) test, the nurse should explain to the client that ABGs measure the levels of carbon dioxide, oxygen, and acidity (pH level) in the blood, help to evaluate the effectiveness of treatment, and help to determine the need for supplemental oxygen. ABGs are also carried out to help diagnose and monitor certain disorders, such as metabolic disorders and kidney disease.

85. A: If the nurse is doing a digital removal of stool for a client with a large fecal impaction resulting from opioid use, the client feels faint, and assessment of vital signs shows a marked decrease in pulse, the bradycardia has likely resulted from stimulation of the vagus nerve. Oil retention enemas should be given prior to attempting digital removal of stool, as the procedure can be very painful for the client and cause rectal bleeding.

86. A, B, D, and E: If a 15-year-old client is admitted to the emergency department 5 hours after taking a large overdose of acetaminophen and the serum level of the drug is still 180 mcg/mL, then the client should receive the 72-hour N-acetylcysteine (NAC) protocol and supportive care in an attempt to minimize hepatic damage. Hepatic function must be monitored carefully. It is too late for GI contamination with activated charcoal. The Rumack-Matthew nomogram is used to determine the need for treatment. The client should also receive a psychiatric consultation.

87. B: If the nurse has inserted a nasogastric tube and aspirated gastric contents to check the pH with color-coded pH paper and the aspirate is dark brown with a pH of slightly less than 5 according to the color chart, this pH usually indicates intestinal aspirate rather than gastric aspirate. Gastric aspirate may vary in color from cloudy to green to tan to brown with pH less than 4, while intestinal aspirate may be yellow or brown but the pH is usually greater than 4. Respiratory secretions may look like saliva and have a pH greater than 5.5.

88. A, B, and C: Because the dosage of ECT used now is less than in the earlier days of treatment, the memory loss associated with ECT is less severe, but still may occur. Confusion for a short time after the treatment as well as headache and muscle soreness are common. Clients receive medication prior to the treatment to reduce the severity of seizures induced by ECT. ECT should not result in urinary incontinence or hallucinations.

89. D: If a male client has been diagnosed with Huntington disease and his spouse asks the nurse if their 3-year-old son should be tested to determine if he inherited the genetic disorder, the most appropriate response is: "Most authorities recommend letting your child decide when he is older and can make an informed decision about testing." Since there is no treatment that can alter the course of the disease, there are ethical concerns regarding testing children.

90. A, B, C, and D:. If following femoral catheterization for PCI the client has increasing pain in the catheterization site and the nurse notes visible edema and induration, indications of a

hematoma, the nurse should anticipate applying pressure to the site to control the bleeding, marking the margins of the edematous, indurated area to determine if bleeding continues, monitoring hemoglobin and hematocrit to determine if blood transfusions are needed, and maintaining bedrest.

91. 25%: If both parents are carriers of the defective gene for a disease with an autosomal recessive inheritance, each child has a 25% chance of inheriting the gene from both parents and developing the disorder. Each child has a 50% chance of inheriting the gene from only one parent and becoming a carrier:

	N	R
N	N N	N R Carrier
R	N R Carrier	RR Disease

N = normal gene; R = recessive mutated gene

92. A and B: If a client has been diagnosed with immune thrombocytic purpura, signs and symptoms that indicate increased thrombocytopenia are frequent nosebleeds, petechiae, and increased bruising. Clients may also experience very heavy menstruation and may have blood in the stool or urine. Because platelets are essential for clotting of the blood, the platelet count must be monitored for those with ITP, although excessive bleeding is not usually a major concern until the platelet count drops below 50,000 per microliter of blood. Vision changes, numbness, and tingling are associated with thrombocytosis.

93. B, C, and D: If a client seen in the emergency department for influenza asks for an antibiotic prescription, the nurse should provide the following guidelines to help the client decrease the risk of developing an antibiotic-resistant infection:
- Do not stop taking antibiotics until the entire prescription is gone.
- Do not take antibiotics for viral infections (such as influenza and the common cold) because they do no good.
- Do not take preventive antibiotics to avoid infections.
- Follow prescription directions when taking antibiotics.

94. C: If a client who received an IV antibiotic mistakenly believed she was receiving opioid analgesia and reported a few minutes later that the medication had relieved her pain, the most likely reason for the client's response is the placebo effect. The belief that a medication is for pain control can trigger the release of endorphins that, in turn, result in a reduced perception of pain. This does not mean that the pain the client was feeling was imaginary or exaggerated.

95. A, C, and D: If a client has suffered a traumatic brain injury and is being treated in the ICU, the nurse should expect to elevate the head of the bed and keep the client's head in neutral alignment. The nurse will likely administer oxygen to maintain the PaO_2 at > 90 mm Hg (85 mm Hg is hypoxic) and will administer sedation to prevent or reduce agitation. Additionally, cerebral perfusion pressure should be maintained at > 70 mm Hg and body temperature maintained within normal limits.

96. C: While there are different methods of doing a "kick count," which actually counts movements rather than kicks, the usual standard is that the fetus should have at least 10 movements within a 2-hour period. However, clients may perceive movement differently, and a fetus in a rest cycle may be less active, so one finding of decreased activity is usually not a concern. Fetal activity may be depressed if the mother takes certain drugs, such as methadone or heroin, or uses alcohol or tobacco.

97. A, D, and E: Intrinsic factors that increase risk of falls in older adults include sensory impairment (decrease vision and hearing) and chronic illness that interferes with strength and/or mobility. Other intrinsic factors include medications that may cause weakness or dizziness. Extrinsic factors include environmental concerns, such as steep and unlit stairs, throw rugs, and loose carpets. While falling is not a normal experience of aging, falls are most common in people older than 65 years. Falls occurring in hospitals often occur with transfers or ineffective equipment.

98. B: The wound shows evidence of erythema and edema and phagocytosis begins during the inflammation stage of injury repair. Stages:
   I. Hemostasis: During first few minutes. Platelets seal off the vessels and secrete substances that cause vasoconstriction. Thrombin stimulates the clotting mechanism, forming a fibrin mesh.
   II. Inflammation: Over days 1-4. Inflammatory response and phagocytosis occurs.
   III. Proliferation: Over days 5-20. Fibroblasts produce collagen to and granulation tissue starts to form. Epithelization contracts wound.
   IV. Maturation: After day 21 to 2 years. Collagen tightens to reduce scarring. The tissue gains tensile strength.

99. A, B, and D: If a client with heart failure has a left ventricular fraction of 38%, this is classified as heart failure (< 40% EF). Normal EF is 50 to 70%. Risk of dysrhythmias occurs if the EF falls to below 35%. While the client should avoid strenuous exercise and should take frequent rest periods, maintaining a routine of regular exercise, such as walking, is important to maintain adequate cardiac output. The client should stop smoking and limit alcohol intake to 1 to 2 drinks daily.

100. C: The type of behavior modification that is most likely to benefit a client who has a severe phobia regarding spiders is desensitization. With desensitization, the client is increasingly exposed to the thing the person fears. Clients usually begin by constructing an anxiety hierarchy that indicates the least disturbing and most disturbing aspects of the phobic item and then practicing relaxation techniques before beginning desensitization, which may begin with briefly talking about the feared item and looking at a photo of it.
101. D: If a pregnant client at 36 weeks' gestation has partial placenta previa and has been on bedrest at home for the previous 4 weeks starts to have contractions and increasing vaginal bleeding, the nurse should anticipate a cesarean delivery because of the danger of hemorrhage from partial or complete placenta previa. Fetal lungs are usually mature after 34 weeks. With partial placenta previa, part of the placenta is implanted over the internal cervical os.

102. A, B, C, D, and E: If the nurse is providing education to a male client who is HIV positive, the nurse should include information about the need to use condoms for every sexual encounter and the need to tell sexual or needle-sharing partners about the client's HIV status. The client should understand the signs and symptoms that may indicate an increased

viral load or infection and should also understand the importance of maintaining a healthy lifestyle (eat well, avoid smoking and drinking, exercise routinely). The client should be apprised of the availability of support groups

103. A: If a group includes only members selected on a specific basis, such as women with a history of domestic or partner abuse, this group is classified as homogeneous. A heterogenous group comprises individuals with different diagnoses, ages, and genders. A closed group is one that does not admit new members once the group has formed. A task group is one that meets in order to achieve a particular goal or complete an assignment.

104. D: The primary focus of cognitive behavioral therapy (CBT) is identifying automatic thoughts and correcting errors in thinking. Basically, Beck theorized that clients have cognitive biases that affect their perceptions of the world, so clients need to alter the way they think about people, things, and events because cognitive distortions can lead to false assumptions. Clients are helped to identify negative thinking and to substitute these thoughts for more rational ones.

105. B: If the nurse reviewed a client's progress in smoking cessation and praised her but suggested she stop having coffee in the morning because that caused an urge to smoke and the client became upset and complained the nurse believed she was doing poorly because she wanted a cigarette with her morning coffee, this type of cognitive distortion is a mental filter. With a mental filter, the person tends to focus only on a negative detail and overlook anything positive that has been said.

106. B and D: If a client has accidentally splashed a toxic (although not caustic) substance in the right eye, the steps to flushing the eye include:
- Placing the client with head elevated to 20 degrees and on right side.
- Hold emesis basis against face on right.
- Fill bulb syringe with NS irrigant.
- Hold the right eyelid open with the thumb and index finger.
- Hold tip of syringe about one-half inch above eye and direct flow of irrigant toward the lower conjunctival sac, from inner to outer canthus.
- Flush for about 1 minute.

107. C: If a postoperative client whose oxygen saturation has been stable at 96% to 98% suddenly drops to 80%, the initial response should be to quickly assess the client's condition and reposition the pulse oximeter. In most cases, a sudden change results from incorrect position of the pulse oximeter. Oxygen saturation should be maintained above 95%, although clients with COPD may have a lower oxygen saturation level. Pulse oximeters provide information only about oxygen, not carbon dioxide, and cannot recognize carbon monoxide.

108. C: The obstetric history of a client who has had 4 pregnancies with one miscarriage at 12 weeks, a stillborn birth at 34 weeks, a healthy son at 38 weeks, and a healthy daughter at 40 weeks would be classified as gravida 4, para 3. Gravida refers to the number of pregnancies, regardless of the duration or outcome. Para refers to the number of births after 20 weeks, regardless of whether they are live births or not. This client had 4 total pregnancies (gravida 4) and 3 births after 20 weeks (gravida 3).

109. D: The immunization that is usually administered to neonates within hours of birth is hepatitis B, which is followed by a second dose at 6 to 18 months. A number of other immunizations are recommended during the first year at 2 months, 4 months, and 6 months: rotavirus (to prevent infectious diarrhea), DTaP (diphtheria, tetanus, and pertussis), Hib (*Haemophilus influenzae*), and CV (pneumococcal). IPV (polio) is administered in 2 doses (2 months and 4 months). Additional immunizations begin at about 1 year.

110. B: Naegele's rule for estimating the due date of a pregnancy is:
- Date of onset of last menstrual period (LMP) + 9 months + 7 days = estimated due date
- September 6 + 9 months = June 6 + 7 days = June 13

Naegele's rule does not account for differences in menstrual cycles or number of days in the months (using an average of 28 days), but this method accounts for approximately 280 days, the normal duration of pregnancy. Most physicians use a combination of Naegele's rule and ultrasound during the first trimester to estimate a due date.

111. A: If pregnancy is viewed as a natural rather than a medical condition, then pregnant women often seek prenatal care later and less frequently than typical American women. However, the women from other cultures usually follow cultural traditions related to pregnancy, such as restrictions on types of food or activities. They may also seek the advice of older family members or shamans, so lack of prenatal care does not mean that the pregnancy has not been considered or is necessarily at risk.

112. B: Because Muslim societies are patriarchal and decisions are made by the male in fundamentalist households, the woman's husband should be first asked for permission for the client to be treated by a male physician. If he agrees, then the woman's permission should be sought. If neither agrees, then the examination will need to be delayed until a female physician can be located, but the client and her husband should be advised that this delay may pose a risk to the fetus and/or the mother. If they agree to care by a male physician, then the client's body should be covered as much as possible and a female in attendance.

113. A: The cephalic presentation that is most common during delivery of a neonate is the vertex presentation. With the presentation, the fetal head is fully flexed and the diameter is the smallest, facilitating passage through the birth canal. In most cases, the fetal attitude (relationship of body parts to each other) is flexion and the lie (relationship of fetal long axis to mother's) is longitudinal. Complications may arise if the presentation, lie, and/or attitude are different.

114. A: If two Mexican immigrant families lives closely together and share goods, services, and childcare, this family structure is a kinship network. The families may be related or may be close friends. This family structure is quite common in Mexican-American communities. In an extended family, multiple generations live together as one family. The nuclear family comprises 2 parents and their children. A binuclear family occurs when 2 nuclear families share custody of children, who typically live part of the week with one family and part of the week with the other.

115. A, B, and C: The transition from full-time employment to retirement can be difficult for people, especially those who identify closely with their positions and whose lives have revolved around work. It may take time to become used to a different pace of life, but often taking on a more active role in community activities, taking classes, joining a senior citizen's center, volunteering, or taking part-time employment can help the person repurpose his life. The client should be encouraged to explore various interests. Clients who become depressed may need to seek professional support.

116. A: First-time mothers, especially, often have little experience with children and are unsure of what to expect, so if the mother is concerned that her child cannot crawl at 6 months, then she needs factual information about when to expect the child to crawl: "Most infants can crawl by 9 months." The nurse should also assure the mother that infants may vary in their development. A 6-month old child should be able to sit in tripod position and roll in both directions, but crawling generally follows this, and the child's gross motor skills improve over the next 3 months.

117. D: If a 14-year-old client has been diagnosed with celiac disease after a long history of diarrhea, anemia, and weight loss, the client will require a gluten-free diet. Celiac disease is an autoimmune disorder in which products containing gluten (grains, such as wheat, rye, barley) trigger damage to the intestinal mucosa. Some clients exhibit an itching vesicular rash (dermatitis herpetiformis) on the buttocks, scalp, face, elbows, and knees. Because the damaged intestinal mucosa cannot adequately absorb nutrients, anemia, osteoporosis, muscle wasting, weight loss, and malnutrition are common.

118. B, C, and D: If a 68-year-old client states that he decided not to take the herpes zoster (shingles) immunization because his friend had the immunization and still developed the infection, the nurse should explain that the immunization cuts the chance of developing shingles in half. Additionally, if the person develops shingles after the immunization, the severity of the infection is usually lessened and the likelihood of developing postherpetic syndrome, which can result in severe and long-standing pain, is decreased.

119. D: Because the client is nulliparous, the average rate of dilation is 1 cm per hour, so the approximate time to full dilation of 10 cm is approximately 7 hours. The woman has been progressing at the average rate. The latent phase of stage 1 usually lasts from 10 to 14 hours, and the client was in this phase for 12 hours and has now progressed to the active phase. However, the nurse should stress to the client that there are individual variations with some progressing much more quickly and others more slowly.

120. A: If the performance improvement committee has agreed to some changes in procedures on the basis of evidence-based research and wants to convince staff members to comply with the changes, the best action to carry out first is to identify and gain support of key staff. In all organizations, there are staff members who are influential for various reasons, and they are usually easy to identify. Once these key staff members (key informants) are on board, they can often influence others to comply.

Secret Key #1 - Time is Your Greatest Enemy

Pace Yourself

Wear a watch. At the beginning of the test, check the time (or start a chronometer on your watch to count the minutes), and check the time after every few questions to make sure you are "on schedule."

If you are forced to speed up, do it efficiently. Usually one or more answer choices can be eliminated without too much difficulty. Above all, don't panic. Don't speed up and just begin guessing at random choices. By pacing yourself, and continually monitoring your progress against your watch, you will always know exactly how far ahead or behind you are with your available time. If you find that you are one minute behind on the test, don't skip one question without spending any time on it, just to catch back up. Take 15 fewer seconds on the next four questions, and after four questions you'll have caught back up. Once you catch back up, you can continue working each problem at your normal pace.

Furthermore, don't dwell on the problems that you were rushed on. If a problem was taking up too much time and you made a hurried guess, it must be difficult. The difficult questions are the ones you are most likely to miss anyway, so it isn't a big loss. It is better to end with more time than you need than to run out of time.

Lastly, sometimes it is beneficial to slow down if you are constantly getting ahead of time. You are always more likely to catch a careless mistake by working more slowly than quickly, and among very high-scoring test takers (those who are likely to have lots of time left over), careless errors affect the score more than mastery of material.

Secret Key #2 - Guessing is not Guesswork

You probably know that guessing is a good idea. Unlike other standardized tests, there is no penalty for getting a wrong answer. Even if you have no idea about a question, you still have a 20-25% chance of getting it right.

Most test takers do not understand the impact that proper guessing can have on their score. Unless you score extremely high, guessing will significantly contribute to your final score.

Monkeys Take the Test

What most test takers don't realize is that to insure that 20-25% chance, you have to guess randomly. If you put 20 monkeys in a room to take this test, assuming they answered once per question and behaved themselves, on average they would get 20-25% of the questions correct. Put 20 test takers in the room, and the average will be much lower among guessed questions. Why?

1. The test writers intentionally write deceptive answer choices that "look" right. A test taker has no idea about a question, so he picks the "best looking" answer, which is often wrong. The monkey has no idea what looks good and what doesn't, so it will consistently be right about 20-25% of the time.
2. Test takers will eliminate answer choices from the guessing pool based on a hunch or intuition. Simple but correct answers often get excluded, leaving a 0% chance of being correct. The monkey has no clue, and often gets lucky with the best choice.

This is why the process of elimination endorsed by most test courses is flawed and detrimental to your performance. Test takers don't guess; they make an ignorant stab in the dark that is usually worse than random.

$5 Challenge

Let me introduce one of the most valuable ideas of this course—the $5 challenge:

You only mark your "best guess" if you are willing to bet $5 on it.
You only eliminate choices from guessing if you are willing to bet $5 on it.

Why $5? Five dollars is an amount of money that is small yet not insignificant, and can really add up fast (20 questions could cost you $100). Likewise, each answer choice on one question of the test will have a small impact on your overall score, but it can really add up to a lot of points in the end.

The process of elimination IS valuable. The following shows your chance of guessing it right:

If you eliminate wrong answer choices until only this many remain:	Chance of getting it correct:
1	100%
2	50%
3	33%

However, if you accidentally eliminate the right answer or go on a hunch for an incorrect answer, your chances drop dramatically—to 0%. By guessing among all the answer choices, you are GUARANTEED to have a shot at the right answer.

That's why the $5 test is so valuable. If you give up the advantage and safety of a pure guess, it had better be worth the risk.

What we still haven't covered is how to be sure that whatever guess you make is truly random. Here's the easiest way:

Always pick the first answer choice among those remaining.

Such a technique means that you have decided, **before you see a single test question**, exactly how you are going to guess, and since the order of choices tells you nothing about which one is correct, this guessing technique is perfectly random.

This section is not meant to scare you away from making educated guesses or eliminating choices; you just need to define when a choice is worth eliminating. The $5 test, along with a pre-defined random guessing strategy, is the best way to make sure you reap all of the benefits of guessing.

Secret Key #3 - Practice Smarter, Not Harder

Many test takers delay the test preparation process because they dread the awful amounts of practice time they think necessary to succeed on the test. We have refined an effective method that will take you only a fraction of the time.

There are a number of "obstacles" in the path to success. Among these are answering questions, finishing in time, and mastering test-taking strategies. All must be executed on the day of the test at peak performance, or your score will suffer. The test is a mental marathon that has a large impact on your future.

Just like a marathon runner, it is important to work your way up to the full challenge. So first you just worry about questions, and then time, and finally strategy:

Success Strategy

1. Find a good source for practice tests.
2. If you are willing to make a larger time investment, consider using more than one study guide. Often the different approaches of multiple authors will help you "get" difficult concepts.
3. Take a practice test with no time constraints, with all study helps, "open book." Take your time with questions and focus on applying strategies.
4. Take a practice test with time constraints, with all guides, "open book."
5. Take a final practice test without open material and with time limits.

If you have time to take more practice tests, just repeat step 5. By gradually exposing yourself to the full rigors of the test environment, you will condition your mind to the stress of test day and maximize your success.

Secret Key #4 - Prepare, Don't Procrastinate

Let me state an obvious fact: if you take the test three times, you will probably get three different scores. This is due to the way you feel on test day, the level of preparedness you have, and the version of the test you see. Despite the test writers' claims to the contrary, some versions of the test WILL be easier for you than others.

Since your future depends so much on your score, you should maximize your chances of success. In order to maximize the likelihood of success, you've got to prepare in advance. This means taking practice tests and spending time learning the information and test taking strategies you will need to succeed.

Never go take the actual test as a "practice" test, expecting that you can just take it again if you need to. Take all the practice tests you can on your own, but when you go to take the official test, be prepared, be focused, and do your best the first time!

Secret Key #5 - Test Yourself

Everyone knows that time is money. There is no need to spend too much of your time or too little of your time preparing for the test. You should only spend as much of your precious time preparing as is necessary for you to get the score you need.

Once you have taken a practice test under real conditions of time constraints, then you will know if you are ready for the test or not.

If you have scored extremely high the first time that you take the practice test, then there is not much point in spending countless hours studying. You are already there.

Benchmark your abilities by retaking practice tests and seeing how much you have improved. Once you consistently score high enough to guarantee success, then you are ready.

If you have scored well below where you need, then knuckle down and begin studying in earnest. Check your improvement regularly through the use of practice tests under real conditions. Above all, don't worry, panic, or give up. The key is perseverance!

Then, when you go to take the test, remain confident and remember how well you did on the practice tests. If you can score high enough on a practice test, then you can do the same on the real thing.

General Strategies

The most important thing you can do is to ignore your fears and jump into the test immediately. Do not be overwhelmed by any strange-sounding terms. You have to jump into the test like jumping into a pool—all at once is the easiest way.

Make Predictions

As you read and understand the question, try to guess what the answer will be. Remember that several of the answer choices are wrong, and once you begin reading them, your mind will immediately become cluttered with answer choices designed to throw you off. Your mind is typically the most focused immediately after you have read the question and digested its contents. If you can, try to predict what the correct answer will be. You may be surprised at what you can predict.

Quickly scan the choices and see if your prediction is in the listed answer choices. If it is, then you can be quite confident that you have the right answer. It still won't hurt to check the other answer choices, but most of the time, you've got it!

Answer the Question

It may seem obvious to only pick answer choices that answer the question, but the test writers can create some excellent answer choices that are wrong. Don't pick an answer just because it sounds right, or you believe it to be true. It MUST answer the question. Once you've made your selection, always go back and check it against the question and make sure that you didn't misread the question and that the answer choice does answer the question posed.

Benchmark

After you read the first answer choice, decide if you think it sounds correct or not. If it doesn't, move on to the next answer choice. If it does, mentally mark that answer choice. This doesn't mean that you've definitely selected it as your answer choice, it just means that it's the best you've seen thus far. Go ahead and read the next choice. If the next choice is worse than the one you've already selected, keep going to the next answer choice. If the next choice is better than the choice you've already selected, mentally mark the new answer choice as your best guess.

The first answer choice that you select becomes your standard. Every other answer choice must be benchmarked against that standard. That choice is correct until proven otherwise by another answer choice beating it out. Once you've decided that no other answer choice seems as good, do one final check to ensure that your answer choice answers the question posed.

Valid Information

Don't discount any of the information provided in the question. Every piece of information may be necessary to determine the correct answer. None of the information in the question is there to throw you off (while the answer choices will certainly have information to throw you off). If two seemingly unrelated topics are discussed, don't ignore either. You can be confident there is a relationship, or it wouldn't be included in the question, and you are probably going to have to determine what is that relationship to find the answer.

Avoid "Fact Traps"

Don't get distracted by a choice that is factually true. Your search is for the answer that answers the question. Stay focused and don't fall for an answer that is true but irrelevant. Always go back to the question and make sure you're choosing an answer that actually answers the question and is not just a true statement. An answer can be factually correct, but it MUST answer the question asked. Additionally, two answers can both be seemingly correct, so be sure to read all of the answer choices, and make sure that you get the one that BEST answers the question.

Milk the Question

Some of the questions may throw you completely off. They might deal with a subject you have not been exposed to, or one that you haven't reviewed in years. While your lack of knowledge about the subject will be a hindrance, the question itself can give you many clues that will help you find the correct answer. Read the question carefully and look for clues. Watch particularly for adjectives and nouns describing difficult terms or words that you don't recognize. Regardless of whether you completely understand a word or not, replacing it with a synonym, either provided or one you more familiar with, may help you to understand what the questions are asking. Rather than wracking your mind about specific detailed information concerning a difficult term or word, try to use mental substitutes that are easier to understand.

The Trap of Familiarity

Don't just choose a word because you recognize it. On difficult questions, you may not recognize a number of words in the answer choices. The test writers don't put "make-believe" words on the test, so don't think that just because you only recognize all the words in one answer choice that that answer choice must be correct. If you only recognize words in one answer choice, then focus on that one. Is it correct? Try your best to determine if it is correct. If it is, that's great. If not, eliminate it. Each word and answer choice you eliminate increases your chances of getting the question correct, even if you then have to guess among the unfamiliar choices.

Eliminate Answers

Eliminate choices as soon as you realize they are wrong. But be careful! Make sure you consider all of the possible answer choices. Just because one appears right, doesn't mean that the next one won't be even better! The test writers will usually put more than one good answer choice for every question, so read all of them. Don't worry if you are stuck between two that seem right. By getting down to just two remaining possible choices, your odds are now 50/50. Rather than wasting too much time, play the odds. You are guessing, but guessing wisely because you've been able to knock out some of the answer choices that you know are wrong. If you are eliminating choices and realize that the last answer choice you are left with is also obviously wrong, don't panic. Start over and consider each choice again. There may easily be something that you missed the first time and will realize on the second pass.

Tough Questions

If you are stumped on a problem or it appears too hard or too difficult, don't waste time. Move on! Remember though, if you can quickly check for obviously incorrect answer choices, your chances of guessing correctly are greatly improved. Before you completely give up, at least try to knock out a couple of possible answers. Eliminate what you can and then guess at the remaining answer choices before moving on.

Brainstorm

If you get stuck on a difficult question, spend a few seconds quickly brainstorming. Run through the complete list of possible answer choices. Look at each choice and ask yourself, "Could this answer the question satisfactorily?" Go through each answer choice and consider it independently of the others. By systematically going through all possibilities, you may find something that you would otherwise overlook. Remember though that when you get stuck, it's important to try to keep moving.

Read Carefully

Understand the problem. Read the question and answer choices carefully. Don't miss the question because you misread the terms. You have plenty of time to read each question thoroughly and make sure you understand what is being asked. Yet a happy medium must be attained, so don't waste too much time. You must read carefully, but efficiently.

Face Value

When in doubt, use common sense. Always accept the situation in the problem at face value. Don't read too much into it. These problems will not require you to make huge leaps of logic. The test writers aren't trying to throw you off with a cheap trick. If you have to go beyond creativity and make a leap of logic in order to have an answer choice answer the question, then you should look at the other answer choices. Don't overcomplicate the problem by creating theoretical relationships or explanations that will warp time or space. These are normal problems rooted in reality. It's just that the applicable relationship or explanation may not be readily apparent and you have to figure things out. Use your common sense to interpret anything that isn't clear.

Prefixes

If you're having trouble with a word in the question or answer choices, try dissecting it. Take advantage of every clue that the word might include. Prefixes and suffixes can be a huge help. Usually they allow you to determine a basic meaning. Pre- means before, post- means after, pro - is positive, de- is negative. From these prefixes and suffixes, you can get an idea of the general meaning of the word and try to put it into context. Beware though of any traps. Just because con- is the opposite of pro-, doesn't necessarily mean congress is the opposite of progress!

Hedge Phrases

Watch out for critical hedge phrases, led off with words such as "likely," "may," "can," "sometimes," "often," "almost," "mostly," "usually," "generally," "rarely," and "sometimes." Question writers insert these hedge phrases to cover every possibility. Often an answer choice will be wrong simply because it leaves no room for exception. Unless the situation calls for them, avoid answer choices that have definitive words like "exactly," and "always."

Switchback Words

Stay alert for "switchbacks." These are the words and phrases frequently used to alert you to shifts in thought. The most common switchback word is "but." Others include "although," "however," "nevertheless," "on the other hand," "even though," "while," "in spite of," "despite," and "regardless of."

New Information

Correct answer choices will rarely have completely new information included. Answer choices typically are straightforward reflections of the material asked about and will directly relate to the question. If a new piece of information is included in an answer choice that doesn't even seem to relate to the topic being asked about, then that answer choice is likely incorrect. All of the information needed to answer the question is usually provided for you in the question. You should not have to make guesses that are unsupported or choose answer choices that require unknown information that cannot be reasoned from what is given.

Time Management

On technical questions, don't get lost on the technical terms. Don't spend too much time on any one question. If you don't know what a term means, then odds are you aren't going to get much further since you don't have a dictionary. You should be able to immediately recognize whether or not you know a term. If you don't, work with the other clues that you have—the other answer choices and terms provided—but don't waste too much time trying to figure out a difficult term that you don't know.

Contextual Clues

Look for contextual clues. An answer can be right but not the correct answer. The contextual clues will help you find the answer that is most right and is correct. Understand the context in which a phrase or statement is made. This will help you make important distinctions.

Don't Panic

Panicking will not answer any questions for you; therefore, it isn't helpful. When you first see the question, if your mind goes blank, take a deep breath. Force yourself to mechanically go through the steps of solving the problem using the strategies you've learned.

Pace Yourself

Don't get clock fever. It's easy to be overwhelmed when you're looking at a page full of questions, your mind is full of random thoughts and feeling confused, and the clock is ticking down faster than you would like. Calm down and maintain the pace that you have set for yourself. As long as you are on track by monitoring your pace, you are guaranteed to have enough time for yourself. When you get to the last few minutes of the test, it may seem like you won't have enough time left, but if you only have as many questions as you should have left at that point, then you're right on track!

Answer Selection

The best way to pick an answer choice is to eliminate all of those that are wrong, until only one is left and confirm that is the correct answer. Sometimes though, an answer choice may immediately look right. Be careful! Take a second to make sure that the other choices are not equally obvious. Don't make a hasty mistake. There are only two times that you should stop before checking other answers. First is when you are positive that the answer choice you have selected is correct. Second is when time is almost out and you have to make a quick guess!

Check Your Work

Since you will probably not know every term listed and the answer to every question, it is important that you get credit for the ones that you do know. Don't miss any questions through careless mistakes. If at all possible, try to take a second to look back over your answer selection and make sure you've selected the correct answer choice and haven't made a costly careless mistake (such as marking an answer choice that you didn't mean to mark). The time it takes for this quick double check should more than pay for itself in caught mistakes.

Beware of Directly Quoted Answers

Sometimes an answer choice will repeat word for word a portion of the question or reference section. However, beware of such exact duplication. It may be a trap! More than likely, the correct choice will paraphrase or summarize a point, rather than being exactly the same wording.

Slang

Scientific sounding answers are better than slang ones. An answer choice that begins "To compare the outcomes…" is much more likely to be correct than one that begins "Because some people insisted…"

Extreme Statements

Avoid wild answers that throw out highly controversial ideas that are proclaimed as established fact. An answer choice that states the "process should used in certain situations, if…" is much more likely to be correct than one that states the "process should be discontinued completely." The first is a calm rational statement and doesn't even make a definitive, uncompromising stance, using a hedge word "if" to provide wiggle room, whereas the second choice is a radical idea and far more extreme.

Answer Choice Families

When you have two or more answer choices that are direct opposites or parallels, one of them is usually the correct answer. For instance, if one answer choice states "x increases" and another answer choice states "x decreases" or "y increases," then those two or three answer choices are very similar in construction and fall into the same family of answer choices. A family of answer choices consists of two or three answer choices, very similar in construction, but often with directly opposite meanings. Usually the correct answer choice will be in that family of answer choices. The "odd man out" or answer choice that doesn't seem to fit the parallel construction of the other answer choices is more likely to be incorrect.

Special Report: How to Overcome Test Anxiety

The very nature of tests caters to some level of anxiety, nervousness, or tension, just as we feel for any important event that occurs in our lives. A little bit of anxiety or nervousness can be a good thing. It helps us with motivation, and makes achievement just that much sweeter. However, too much anxiety can be a problem, especially if it hinders our ability to function and perform.

"Test anxiety," is the term that refers to the emotional reactions that some test-takers experience when faced with a test or exam. Having a fear of testing and exams is based upon a rational fear, since the test-taker's performance can shape the course of an academic career. Nevertheless, experiencing excessive fear of examinations will only interfere with the test-taker's ability to perform and chance to be successful.

There are a large variety of causes that can contribute to the development and sensation of test anxiety. These include, but are not limited to, lack of preparation and worrying about issues surrounding the test.

Lack of Preparation

Lack of preparation can be identified by the following behaviors or situations:

Not scheduling enough time to study, and therefore cramming the night before the test or exam
Managing time poorly, to create the sensation that there is not enough time to do everything
Failing to organize the text information in advance, so that the study material consists of the entire text and not simply the pertinent information
Poor overall studying habits

Worrying, on the other hand, can be related to both the test taker, or many other factors around him/her that will be affected by the results of the test. These include worrying about:

Previous performances on similar exams, or exams in general
How friends and other students are achieving
The negative consequences that will result from a poor grade or failure

There are three primary elements to test anxiety. Physical components, which involve the same typical bodily reactions as those to acute anxiety (to be discussed below). Emotional factors have to do with fear or panic. Mental or cognitive issues concerning attention spans and memory abilities.

Physical Signals

There are many different symptoms of test anxiety, and these are not limited to mental and emotional strain. Frequently there are a range of physical signals that will let a test taker know that he/she is suffering from test anxiety. These bodily changes can include the following:

Perspiring
Sweaty palms
Wet, trembling hands
Nausea
Dry mouth
A knot in the stomach
Headache
Faintness
Muscle tension
Aching shoulders, back and neck
Rapid heart beat
Feeling too hot/cold

To recognize the sensation of test anxiety, a test-taker should monitor him/herself for the following sensations:

The physical distress symptoms as listed above
Emotional sensitivity, expressing emotional feelings such as the need to cry or laugh too much, or a sensation of anger or helplessness
A decreased ability to think, causing the test-taker to blank out or have racing thoughts that are hard to organize or control.

Though most students will feel some level of anxiety when faced with a test or exam, the majority can cope with that anxiety and maintain it at a manageable level. However, those who cannot are faced with a very real and very serious condition, which can and should be controlled for the immeasurable benefit of this sufferer.

Naturally, these sensations lead to negative results for the testing experience. The most common effects of test anxiety have to do with nervousness and mental blocking.

Nervousness

Nervousness can appear in several different levels:

The test-taker's difficulty, or even inability to read and understand the questions on the test
The difficulty or inability to organize thoughts to a coherent form
The difficulty or inability to recall key words and concepts relating to the testing questions (especially essays)
The receipt of poor grades on a test, though the test material was well known by the test taker

Conversely, a person may also experience mental blocking, which involves:

Blanking out on test questions
Only remembering the correct answers to the questions when the test has already finished.

Fortunately for test anxiety sufferers, beating these feelings, to a large degree, has to do with proper preparation. When a test taker has a feeling of preparedness, then anxiety will be dramatically lessened.

The first step to resolving anxiety issues is to distinguish which of the two types of anxiety are being suffered. If the anxiety is a direct result of a lack of preparation, this should be considered a normal reaction, and the anxiety level (as opposed to the test results) shouldn't be anything to worry about. However, if, when adequately prepared, the test-taker still panics, blanks out, or seems to overreact, this is not a fully rational reaction. While this can be considered normal too, there are many ways to combat and overcome these effects.

Remember that anxiety cannot be entirely eliminated, however, there are ways to minimize it, to make the anxiety easier to manage. Preparation is one of the best ways to minimize test anxiety. Therefore the following techniques are wise in order to best fight off any anxiety that may want to build.

To begin with, try to avoid cramming before a test, whenever it is possible. By trying to memorize an entire term's worth of information in one day, you'll be shocking your system, and not giving yourself a very good chance to absorb the information. This is an easy path to anxiety, so for those who suffer from test anxiety, cramming should not even be considered an option.

Instead of cramming, work throughout the semester to combine all of the material which is presented throughout the semester, and work on it gradually as the course goes by, making sure to master the main concepts first, leaving minor details for a week or so before the test.

To study for the upcoming exam, be sure to pose questions that may be on the examination, to gauge the ability to answer them by integrating the ideas from your texts, notes and lectures, as well as any supplementary readings.

If it is truly impossible to cover all of the information that was covered in that particular term, concentrate on the most important portions, that can be covered very well. Learn these concepts as best as possible, so that when the test comes, a goal can be made to use these concepts as presentations of your knowledge.

In addition to study habits, changes in attitude are critical to beating a struggle with test anxiety. In fact, an improvement of the perspective over the entire test-taking experience can actually help a test taker to enjoy studying and therefore improve the overall experience. Be certain not to overemphasize the significance of the grade - know that the result of the test is neither a reflection of self worth, nor is it a measure of intelligence; one grade will not predict a person's future success.

To improve an overall testing outlook, the following steps should be tried:

Keeping in mind that the most reasonable expectation for taking a test is to expect to try to demonstrate as much of what you know as you possibly can.
Reminding ourselves that a test is only one test; this is not the only one, and there will be others.
The thought of thinking of oneself in an irrational, all-or-nothing term should be avoided at all costs.
A reward should be designated for after the test, so there's something to look forward to. Whether it be going to a movie, going out to eat, or simply visiting friends, schedule it in advance, and do it no matter what result is expected on the exam.

Test-takers should also keep in mind that the basics are some of the most important things, even beyond anti-anxiety techniques and studying. Never neglect the basic social, emotional and biological needs, in order to try to absorb information. In order to best achieve, these three factors must be held as just as important as the studying itself.

Study Steps

Remember the following important steps for studying:

Maintain healthy nutrition and exercise habits. Continue both your recreational activities and social pass times. These both contribute to your physical and emotional well being.
Be certain to get a good amount of sleep, especially the night before the test, because when you're overtired you are not able to perform to the best of your best ability.
Keep the studying pace to a moderate level by taking breaks when they are needed, and varying the work whenever possible, to keep the mind fresh instead of getting bored. When enough studying has been done that all the material that can be learned has been learned, and the test taker is prepared for the test, stop studying and do something relaxing such as listening to music, watching a movie, or taking a warm bubble bath.

There are also many other techniques to minimize the uneasiness or apprehension that is experienced along with test anxiety before, during, or even after the examination. In fact, there are a great deal of things that can be done to stop anxiety from interfering with lifestyle and performance. Again, remember that anxiety will not be eliminated entirely, and it shouldn't be. Otherwise that "up" feeling for exams would not exist, and most of us depend on that sensation to perform better than usual. However, this anxiety has to be at a level that is manageable.

Of course, as we have just discussed, being prepared for the exam is half the battle right away. Attending all classes, finding out what knowledge will be expected on the exam, and knowing the exam schedules are easy steps to lowering anxiety. Keeping up with work will remove the need to cram, and efficient study habits will eliminate wasted time. Studying should be done in an ideal location for concentration, so that it is simple to become interested in the material and give it complete attention. A method such as SQ3R (Survey, Question, Read, Recite, Review) is a wonderful key to follow to make sure that the study habits are as effective as possible, especially in the case of learning from a textbook. Flashcards are great techniques for memorization. Learning to take good notes will mean that notes will be full of useful information, so that less sifting will need to be done to seek out what is pertinent for studying. Reviewing notes after class and then again on occasion will keep the information fresh in the mind. From notes that have been taken summary sheets and outlines can be made for simpler reviewing.

A study group can also be a very motivational and helpful place to study, as there will be a sharing of ideas, all of the minds can work together, to make sure that everyone understands, and the studying will be made more interesting because it will be a social occasion.

Basically, though, as long as the test-taker remains organized and self confident, with efficient study habits, less time will need to be spent studying, and higher grades will be achieved.

To become self confident, there are many useful steps. The first of these is "self talk." It has been shown through extensive research, that self-talk for students who suffer from test anxiety, should be well monitored, in order to make sure that it contributes to self confidence as opposed to sinking the student. Frequently the self talk of test-anxious students is negative or self-defeating, thinking that everyone else is smarter and faster, that they always mess up, and that if they don't do well, they'll fail the entire course. It is important to decreasing anxiety that awareness is made of self talk. Try writing any negative self thoughts and then disputing them with a positive statement instead. Begin self-encouragement as though it was a friend speaking. Repeat positive statements to help reprogram the mind to believing in successes instead of failures.

Helpful Techniques

Other extremely helpful techniques include:

Self-visualization of doing well and reaching goals
While aiming for an "A" level of understanding, don't try to "overprotect" by setting your expectations lower. This will only convince the mind to stop studying in order to meet the lower expectations.
Don't make comparisons with the results or habits of other students. These are individual factors, and different things work for different people, causing different results.
Strive to become an expert in learning what works well, and what can be done in order to improve. Consider collecting this data in a journal.
Create rewards for after studying instead of doing things before studying that will only turn into avoidance behaviors.
Make a practice of relaxing - by using methods such as progressive relaxation, self-hypnosis, guided imagery, etc - in order to make relaxation an automatic sensation.
Work on creating a state of relaxed concentration so that concentrating will take on the focus of the mind, so that none will be wasted on worrying.
Take good care of the physical self by eating well and getting enough sleep.
Plan in time for exercise and stick to this plan.

Beyond these techniques, there are other methods to be used before, during and after the test that will help the test-taker perform well in addition to overcoming anxiety.

Before the exam comes the academic preparation. This involves establishing a study schedule and beginning at least one week before the actual date of the test. By doing this, the anxiety of not having enough time to study for the test will be automatically eliminated. Moreover, this will make the studying a much more effective experience, ensuring that the learning will be an easier process. This relieves much undue pressure on the test-taker.

Summary sheets, note cards, and flash cards with the main concepts and examples of these main concepts should be prepared in advance of the actual studying time. A topic should never be eliminated from this process. By omitting a topic because it isn't expected to be on the test is only setting up the test-taker for anxiety should it actually appear on the exam. Utilize the course syllabus for laying out the topics that should be studied. Carefully go over the notes that were made in class, paying special attention to any of the issues that the professor took special care to emphasize while lecturing in class. In the textbooks, use the chapter review, or if possible, the chapter tests, to begin your review.

It may even be possible to ask the instructor what information will be covered on the exam, or what the format of the exam will be (for example, multiple choice, essay, free form, true-false). Additionally, see if it is possible to find out how many questions will be on the test. If a review sheet or sample test has been offered by the professor, make good use of it, above anything else, for the preparation for the test. Another great resource for getting to know the examination is reviewing tests from previous semesters. Use these tests to review, and aim to achieve a 100% score on each of the possible topics. With a few exceptions, the goal that you set for yourself is the highest one that you will reach.

Take all of the questions that were assigned as homework, and rework them to any other possible course material. The more problems reworked, the more skill and confidence will form as a result. When forming the solution to a problem, write out each of the steps. Don't simply do head work. By doing as many steps on paper as possible, much clarification and therefore confidence will be formed. Do this with as many homework problems as possible, before checking the answers. By checking the answer after each problem, a reinforcement will exist, that will not be on the exam. Study situations should be as exam-like as possible, to prime the test-taker's system for the experience. By waiting to check the answers at the end, a psychological advantage will be formed, to decrease the stress factor.

Another fantastic reason for not cramming is the avoidance of confusion in concepts, especially when it comes to mathematics. 8-10 hours of study will become one hundred percent more effective if it is spread out over a week or at least several days, instead of doing it all in one sitting. Recognize that the human brain requires time in order to assimilate new material, so frequent breaks and a span of study time over several days will be much more beneficial.

Additionally, don't study right up until the point of the exam. Studying should stop a minimum of one hour before the exam begins. This allows the brain to rest and put things in their proper order. This will also provide the time to become as relaxed as possible when going into the examination room. The test-taker will also have time to eat well and eat sensibly. Know that the brain needs food as much as the rest of the body. With enough food and enough sleep, as well as a relaxed attitude, the body and the mind are primed for success.

Avoid any anxious classmates who are talking about the exam. These students only spread anxiety, and are not worth sharing the anxious sentimentalities.

Before the test also involves creating a positive attitude, so mental preparation should also be a point of concentration. There are many keys to creating a positive attitude. Should fears become rushing in, make a visualization of taking the exam, doing well, and seeing an A written on the paper. Write out a list of affirmations that will bring a feeling of confidence, such as "I am doing well in my English class," "I studied well and know my material," "I enjoy this class." Even if the affirmations aren't believed at first, it sends a positive message to the subconscious which will result in an alteration of the overall belief system, which is the system that creates reality.

If a sensation of panic begins, work with the fear and imagine the very worst! Work through the entire scenario of not passing the test, failing the entire course, and dropping out of school, followed by not getting a job, and pushing a shopping cart through the dark alley where you'll live. This will place things into perspective! Then, practice deep breathing and create a visualization of the opposite situation - achieving an "A" on the exam, passing the entire course, receiving the degree at a graduation ceremony.

On the day of the test, there are many things to be done to ensure the best results, as well as the most calm outlook. The following stages are suggested in order to maximize test-taking potential:

Begin the examination day with a moderate breakfast, and avoid any coffee or beverages with caffeine if the test taker is prone to jitters. Even people who are used to managing caffeine can feel jittery or light-headed when it is taken on a test day. Attempt to do something that is relaxing before the examination begins. As last minute cramming clouds the mastering of overall concepts, it is better to use this time to create a calming outlook.
Be certain to arrive at the test location well in advance, in order to provide time to select a location that is away from doors, windows and other distractions, as well as giving enough time to relax before the test begins.
Keep away from anxiety generating classmates who will upset the sensation of stability and relaxation that is being attempted before the exam.
Should the waiting period before the exam begins cause anxiety, create a self-distraction by reading a light magazine or something else that is relaxing and simple.

During the exam itself, read the entire exam from beginning to end, and find out how much time should be allotted to each individual problem. Once writing the exam, should more time be taken for a problem, it should be abandoned, in order to begin another problem. If there is time at the end, the unfinished problem can always be returned to and completed.

Read the instructions very carefully - twice - so that unpleasant surprises won't follow during or after the exam has ended.

When writing the exam, pretend that the situation is actually simply the completion of homework within a library, or at home. This will assist in forming a relaxed atmosphere, and will allow the brain extra focus for the complex thinking function.

Begin the exam with all of the questions with which the most confidence is felt. This will build the confidence level regarding the entire exam and will begin a quality momentum. This will also create encouragement for trying the problems where uncertainty resides.

Going with the "gut instinct" is always the way to go when solving a problem. Second guessing should be avoided at all costs. Have confidence in the ability to do well.

For essay questions, create an outline in advance that will keep the mind organized and make certain that all of the points are remembered. For multiple choice, read every answer, even if the correct one has been spotted - a better one may exist.

Continue at a pace that is reasonable and not rushed, in order to be able to work carefully. Provide enough time to go over the answers at the end, to check for small errors that can be corrected.

Should a feeling of panic begin, breathe deeply, and think of the feeling of the body releasing sand through its pores. Visualize a calm, peaceful place, and include all of the sights, sounds and sensations of this image. Continue the deep breathing, and take a few minutes to continue this with closed eyes. When all is well again, return to the test.

If a "blanking" occurs for a certain question, skip it and move on to the next question. There will be time to return to the other question later. Get everything done that can be done, first, to guarantee all the grades that can be compiled, and to build all of the confidence possible. Then return to the weaker questions to build the marks from there.

Remember, one's own reality can be created, so as long as the belief is there, success will follow. And remember: anxiety can happen later, right now, there's an exam to be written!

After the examination is complete, whether there is a feeling for a good grade or a bad grade, don't dwell on the exam, and be certain to follow through on the reward that was promised...and enjoy it! Don't dwell on any mistakes that have been made, as there is nothing that can be done at this point anyway.

Additionally, don't begin to study for the next test right away. Do something relaxing for a while, and let the mind relax and prepare itself to begin absorbing information again.

From the results of the exam - both the grade and the entire experience, be certain to learn from what has gone on. Perfect studying habits and work some more on confidence in order to make the next examination experience even better than the last one.

Learn to avoid places where openings occurred for laziness, procrastination and day dreaming.

Use the time between this exam and the next one to better learn to relax, even learning to relax on cue, so that any anxiety can be controlled during the next exam. Learn how to relax the body. Slouch in your chair if that helps. Tighten and then relax all of the different muscle groups, one group at a time, beginning with the feet and then working all the way up to the neck and face. This will ultimately relax the muscles more than they were to begin with. Learn how to breathe deeply and comfortably, and focus on this breathing going in and out as a relaxing thought. With every exhale, repeat the word "relax."

As common as test anxiety is, it is very possible to overcome it. Make yourself one of the test-takers who overcome this frustrating hindrance.

Special Report: Additional Bonus Material

Due to our efforts to try to keep this book to a manageable length, we've created a link that will give you access to all of your additional bonus material.

Please visit http://www.mometrix.com/bonus948/nclexrn to access the information.